# THE DOCTORS
# AND PATIENTS
# HANDBOOK
# OF MEDICINES
# AND DRUGS

*Peter Parish, M.D., is an authority on the ways in which drugs are prescribed and used. He was a member of the British Pharmaceutical Revision Committee from 1968 to 1973. Dr. Parish is a Fellow of the Royal College of General Practitioners, and is currently a professor of clinical pharmacy in Wales. In 1975 and 1976 he was Hill Visiting Professor at the University of Minnesota College of Pharmacy and School of Medicine.*

# PETER PARISH, M.D.

# THE DOCTORS AND PATIENTS HANDBOOK OF MEDICINES AND DRUGS

ALFRED · A · KNOPF · NEW YORK · 1977

THIS IS A BORZOI BOOK
PUBLISHED BY ALFRED A. KNOPF, INC.
Copyright © 1977 by Peter Parish, M.D.
All rights reserved under International
and Pan-American Copyright Conventions.
Published in the United States
by Alfred A. Knopf, Inc., New York.
Distributed by Random House, Inc., New York.

Library of Congress Cataloging in Publication Data
Parish, Peter.
The doctors and patients handbook of medicines
and drugs.
1. Chemotherapy. 2. Drugs—Dictionaries.
I. Title. [DNLM: 1. Drugs—Handbooks. 2. Drug
therapy—Handbooks. QV55 P233d]
RM262.P37       615'.58       76-30658
ISBN 0-394-49407-5
ISBN 0-394-73337-1 pbk.

Manufactured in the United States of America
First Edition

Cover design by Tony Greco

This book is dedicated to

PAT

and to our children

CATHERINE, RICHARD, and CHRISTOPHER.

# CONTENTS

viii / CONTENTS

# ACKNOWLEDGMENTS

In the preparation of this book I have been encouraged by three colleagues and friends: Gail Eaton, Gerry Stimson, and Barbara Webb. They have been a major influence upon my thinking, and I owe them a great debt of gratitude for the added perspectives they have given me on the manifold aspects and problems of health care. I am also grateful to Bill Williams for his support, to Penny Leach for her commonsense advice, to Peter Wells, Tom Rolewicz, and Gary Carlson for their advice, to Sheila Goodall and Lynn Samson for their help in preparing the manuscript, and to Charles Elliott for being such a patient editor. And I wish particularly to thank Millie Owens for her excellent copy-editing.

PETER PARISH

*Cardiff*

# INTRODUCTION

Each year the consumption of drugs increases. Few of us would deny the immense relief from pain and suffering that some drugs provide, but increasing consumption is, inevitably, associated with increasing risks from adverse effects. We ought to ask ourselves whether drug production, sales promotion, and prescription are always in the interests of the individual who seeks relief from symptoms.

Unfortunately, these comments apply to both prescription and over-the-counter drug preparations. The intervention of a doctor may not necessarily offer protection to the consumer. It is a sad fact that a high proportion of adverse drug effects caused by prescription drugs could have been prevented by prescribing doctors. These dangers are increased because poor communication among doctor, pharmacist, and patient often leaves the consumer in almost total ignorance of the benefits and risks of any drug preparation he takes.

It is against such a background that I decided to write this book. My aim is to provide information about drugs to people who have no medical training or knowledge. The information may also interest and benefit doctors, pharmacists, nurses, medical students, and others; I present it, however, principally for the lay person, in the belief that knowledge available to those within the medical profession should be shared by those outside it.

Many may disagree with me—particularly some of my medical colleagues. Some may argue that by providing information about the risks of drugs I will make the reader unnecessarily anxious; that patients given such information will not comply with their doctor's instructions; that they may, in fact, reject a drug treatment altogether out of fear, and that they may lose some of the real benefits that can accrue from the appropriate use of drugs. They may also argue that such knowledge may make some patients more "demanding" about their drug treatments. Finally, they may claim that patients do not really *want* to know—that the element of faith in the doctor and his treatment forms a "magical" core of healing which would be lost if the patient were given knowledge about the drugs being prescribed for him.

Let me give my answers to some of these fears. With regard to patients' anxiety, I would argue that we cannot allow a situation of "ignorance is bliss" to exist in drug treatment. The risks of inappropriate drug use can be serious; further, those risks are often avoidable. All drug treatments involve balancing benefits with risks, and appropriate use of drugs lessens the risks and improves the benefits. That is the message of this book. The appropriate use of drugs, based upon knowledge of their benefits and risks, will not only benefit the consumer but should be in the best interest of doctors, pharmacists, the pharmaceutical industry, and the government.

As for the argument that knowledge may affect the way the patient complies, recent studies have shown that at least two out of five patients do not take prescribed drugs as directed by their doctors. Surveys of unused prescribed drugs found in homes indicate that a large proportion are *never* taken. These observations and other studies suggest that a greater understanding of just what drugs are for, and a greater appreciation of how to obtain maximum benefits for minimum risks, will encourage patients actually to follow the courses of treatment prescribed for them.

Doctors often complain about the "ignorance" of the patient, which hinders his understanding of treatment and the carrying out of instructions on drug use. Yet at the same time doctors are reluctant to "educate" the patient by giving him more information. I see such knowledge as of benefit to both patient and doctor because I see it as enabling them to work together toward the most appropriate treatment. If this results in making the patient more "demanding," fine.

Sharing of knowledge need not alter the patient's respect for his doctor; after all, respect is often described by patients in terms which praise the doctor's manner, sympathetic approach, understanding, and so on. Patients with knowledge about drugs should not be seen as posing any threat to doctors. If an individual feels that knowledge about drugs will weaken his faith in his doctor and his treatment, then, of course, he does not have to read this book. Nor do those who do not wish to know, or those who think it will make them anxious. On the other hand, I believe that it will be useful in improving doctor-patient relationships through a process of mutual education.

I also hope this book will help those who wish to identify over-the-counter drugs which will benefit them most. It should help them to choose, from among the thousands of proprietary drug preparations available, those preparations which contain the drugs most suitable for their needs.

I would like to see a more rational use of self-treatments, including the use of drugs, but without knowledge this is difficult. Therefore, you will find in this book the recommendation that you discuss the selection of a particular drug preparation with a pharmacist, who because of his professional training has a very great knowledge about drugs. Further, adequate and safe self-treatment is unlikely to be practical until the individual has knowledge of the structure and functioning of his body and how it responds to disease, stress, and injury. This depends upon the sharing of knowledge between doctors and lay people. I hope this book is a step in that direction.

# HOW TO USE THIS BOOK

To help you to assess the benefits and risks of any drug which you may take, this book is divided into three parts. Part I should give you sufficient background knowledge to understand how a drug works in the body and how it may produce desired and undesired effects. In Part II, organized according to commonly occurring disorders and the drugs used to treat them, various types of drugs are discussed; each section ends with comments on the drugs of choice. Part III gives the uses, adverse effects, and precautions to be taken for individual drugs, both prescription drugs and those sold over the counter.

Part I is intended to be read by everyone; Part II should be used as a reference on groups of drugs; Part III should be used as a reference on individual drugs. Having read about a drug in Part III, always look back to the appropriate section in Part II covering the drugs to which it belongs.

Although drug treatments of particular disorders are discussed, this book is not about treatments as such, but about drugs. I have included most of the commonly used drug groups. Some I have deliberately excluded because their use is highly technical—for example, general anesthetics and immunosuppressive drugs.

# BASIC PRINCIPLES OF DRUG USE

# THE BASIC PRINCIPLES
# OF DRUG USE

Patients often say to me, "Doctor, those tablets that you prescribed for me—they're not *drugs*, are they?" I have to explain that all medicines are drugs and that coffee, tea, cola, cocoa, tobacco, and alcohol are also drugs. Their anxiety is natural, because the word "drugs" has become associated with the use of mind-active drugs by certain groups of people. This misconception has resulted in a belief that medicines are good and drugs are bad—or as one headmaster said to another, "If I were not on tranquilizers I think I would have finished up on drugs!"

What then is a drug? A drug may be defined as any substance which can alter the structure or function of the living organism. Air pollutants, pesticides, vitamins, and virtually any chemical may be regarded as drugs. Therefore, all medicines are drugs, but not all drugs are medicines. Those drugs used as medicines have been selected because they possess or are thought to possess useful properties. They are used to relieve physical or mental symptoms, to produce an altered state of mind, to treat, prevent, or diagnose disease, and to prevent and end pregnancy.

The term "drug" does not indicate the way that it is used—whether medically or nonmedically, legally or illegally, prescribed by a doctor or not. Similarly, the term "medicine" does not refer specifically to a drug in liquid form; such a preparation is only one of several ways in which a drug may be administered. Medicines can also be given as tablets, capsules, inhalations, injections, and so on.

Until this century most drugs used in treatment were obtained from plants. Now only a few drugs are obtained from their natural source, and most of these are highly purified to remove any unwanted or harmful effects.

The action of a drug is a complex physical and chemical process that may take place locally in certain cells, organs, or special tissues, or more generally upon a variety of cells. Some drugs act outside the cell, some on its surface, and others within the cells. In most cases we still know very little about how drugs actually act within the body, but we know a good deal about the effects of that action.

The effect of most drugs is to stimulate or to depress certain biochemical or physiological functions within the body, although some, such as the antibiotics, deal instead with infecting organisms.

Drugs can be used to attack disease in several different ways. Antibiotics, which destroy invading organisms that are making the patient ill, are known as antimicrobial drugs. At the other end of the spectrum are drugs whose effects can be used to prevent disease, such as the vaccines. Then, between these two extremes, there are drugs whose effects can be used to alter actual body processes, in order to change the course of a disease process. Drugs used in this way are known as pharmacodynamic drugs. They include such drugs as anticoagulants, used to reduce the tendency of blood to clot. There are drugs which can be used to replace elements which the body cannot take in or absorb—such as vitamin $B_{12}$ for the patient with pernicious anemia—and there are drugs which can be used to give the body what it fails to manufacture for itself—for instance, thyroid hormone for the patient with an inactive thyroid gland. Finally, of course, there are all the drugs which are given because their effects relieve symptoms; these include everything from painkillers and tranquilizers to antacids and decongestants.

Any drug produces some undesired effects along with the desired effects. For a drug to be a useful therapeutic agent and a medicine, it must produce more beneficial than harmful effects. If it does not make you better, at least it should not make you worse. Unfortunately, many people do not recognize adverse drug effects (sometimes called "side effects" or "toxic effects"). Drugs are described by their most important useful effect, and it does not occur to the patient that the morphine which he is considering only as a pain reliever, an analgesic, is causing his constipation or his sleepiness or his tight chest. Even doctors are often reluctant to consider the possibility that their treatment has made the patient worse; or they may try to combat the new troubles with further drugs, thus starting up a new chain of adverse effects.

It must always be remembered that a drug's effects are like pellets from a shotgun shell. Some land on target; others do not. We must therefore try to think of a drug in terms of its full spectrum of benefits and risks.

## USE OF DRUGS

### Methods of Administration
Drug effects, both beneficial and harmful, are much affected by the way in which the drug is introduced into the body—the method of administration. There are four routes by which a drug may reach the body. *Topical administration* means applying the drug to the skin (as with ointments) or to the mucous membranes. *Inhalation* means simply that the drug is breathed into the lungs (aerosols for asthma, or general

anesthetics). *Enteral administration* means that the drug is given either by mouth or via the rectum. *Parenteral administration* means that the drug is injected. An injection may be made directly into a nerve for local effect, as when the dentist "deadens" a painful tooth, or it may be made into the spinal cord fluid, as in spinal anesthesia. Otherwise injections are either intravenous (into a vein), intramuscular (into a muscle), or subcutaneous (made under the skin). Some intramuscular injections are now given in prolonged-release forms. These are called "depot" injections; the drug—certain insulins, steroids, and tranquilizers, for instance—is slowly absorbed from the injection site over a period of hours, days, or weeks. These "depot" injections are not without long-term dangers, and the convenience they offer to you or your doctor should not be allowed to mask the hazard. If you are receiving one of these treatments, you should always carry an appropriate warning card.

Intravenous injections ensure that the drug reaches a high concentration in the blood very quickly, and they may produce almost instantaneous effects, as "mainlining" drug abusers know. Intramuscular and other injection routes may produce high or low, prolonged concentrations in the blood, depending upon the drug and the injection technique. But no injection is without risk or difficulty. The drug has to be soluble; dosage must be very exact, and the injection must take place under sterile conditions. Injections are therefore usually reserved for cases in which a rapid effect is essential or the drug is poorly absorbed from the gut or the patient cannot take it by mouth.

Taking drugs by mouth is the most convenient way. Some drugs may be absorbed from the mouth itself (for instance nitroglycerin tablets are allowed to dissolve under the tongue for the treatment of angina). Most are swallowed and absorbed from the stomach and intestine. There can be disadvantages to taking drugs by mouth—some may irritate the stomach and produce vomiting. Others may be destroyed by the acid in the stomach or by digestive juices. These sorts of drugs may need a special coating (called enteric coating) to protect them until they reach the intestine, or they may be taken as a suppository.

## Absorption
The rate and amount of a drug reaching the bloodstream (absorption) determines the time between taking the drug and its onset of action. As we have seen, certain injection methods can ensure quick absorption, but absorption into the bloodstream from the gut is very variable. Rate and extent of absorption can vary from person to person and from time to time in the same person. The best-known example is probably

the absorption of alcohol. Hot food taken with alcohol delays its absorption. The presence of any food in the stomach also delays absorption to some extent, while alcohol taken when the stomach is empty will "go to your head" almost immediately.

Rate and extent of absorption are also dependent upon the solubility of the drug and of the other materials (excipients) used in making it into a tablet or capsule. Drugs given in solution are absorbed more quickly than tablets or capsules swallowed whole. Absorption from these depends upon many factors, including size and solubility of particles, chemical form, and various manufacturing processes, such as the compression force used to make the tablet. These can all affect the rate at which a tablet breaks up and the particles separate in the gut before dissolving. This is the most important step in absorption and determines bioavailability—that is, the amount of drug which becomes available to the body.

## Distribution

Once a drug has been absorbed into the bloodstream, its concentration in the tissue fluids around its target area will determine its effectiveness. This in turn may depend on the concentration of the drug in the blood. As we have seen, different routes of administration can give varying initial blood levels, with intravenous injection giving the highest levels quickly. Whatever the route of administration, different formulations of drugs can give different rates and extents of absorption into the blood. Even so, once a drug is put into the body and absorbed into the bloodstream, different types of drug behave differently. Some pass through the whole body, even across the placenta into an unborn baby. Other drugs are much more limited in their effects. They may be, for example, "filtered" by the placenta, or confined to action in the fluid outside cells.

Some drugs are fairly quickly absorbed and well distributed around the body in the bloodstream, but are as quickly and easily excreted. Aspirin, for example, is normally excreted within a few hours. A one-time dose for a headache has time to be effective, but continuous treatment for arthritis requires regularly repeated doses.

Other drugs are very slowly excreted by the body. They accumulate in various tissues and form long-acting deposits. Digoxin, used to control heart rate, accumulates in this way. At the beginning of treatment it takes several days for the deposit of the drug to accumulate, so high starter doses are normally given. Once the deposit has built up, only maintenance doses are needed to keep the level of the drug at its target site—the heart muscle.

A few drugs actually bind themselves to the proteins of the blood itself, so that, once present in the bloodstream, they remain available for a long period. Suramin, a drug used to treat sleeping sickness, clings so tightly to the blood proteins that a single dose will protect against the illness for three months or more.

Bones and teeth act as reservoirs for certain drugs. Lead, for example, is stored in bones, while the antibiotic tetracycline is stored in both bones and teeth. Many unfortunate children have teeth yellowed by this drug, given to them when they were babies and young children, or to their mothers while the child was in the womb.

Other specialized organs act as reservoirs for some drugs. For example, the antimalarial drug quinacrine, after only a single dose, reaches a concentration in the liver many times greater than the concentration in the blood. Even body fat can act as a storage depot of fat-soluble drugs: an obese person may store much more of such a drug than a thin person.

## Biotransformation

Biotransformation refers to the alteration of a drug from one chemical structure to another. This transformation within the body usually results in the inactivation of a drug so that it can be eliminated from the body. Sometimes a more toxic form of drug may be produced. Biotransformation is often called drug breakdown or drug metabolism. Occasionally, activation of a drug may take place at first, followed by inactivation. Biotransformation involves complex chemical and physical processes which usually take place in the liver. Note how your body reacts to drugs: once a drug has been administered, the body's main concern is to try to get rid of it.

## Elimination

The concentration of a drug in the tissues rises when the rate of absorption exceeds the rate of elimination. Eventually these rates become equal, and thereafter elimination exceeds absorption. The kidneys are the important organs involved in the elimination or excretion of a drug; less important are the bile system, the lungs, sweat, and other body secretions. Drugs excreted in the feces are usually unabsorbed drugs which have been taken by mouth (note how dark your stools are when you take iron tablets) or products excreted in the bile. Drugs may also be excreted in breast milk and affect the baby. Alcohol is eliminated in tears, sweat, bile, gastric juice, saliva, and other secretions, but the small amount of alcohol that is not used up in the body is mainly eliminated in the breath and in the urine (thus breath tests administered to drunken drivers).

## Dosage

There is a direct relationship between dosage of a drug and its effectiveness. Unfortunately the relationship is a very complex one. While any drug will obviously fail to work if the dose given is too small to produce effective levels in the bloodstream, or the formulation is such that the drug cannot be absorbed, or the interval between doses is so great that the drug has been eliminated before the next dose starts to be absorbed, making the drug work is not simply a matter of increasing the dosage—this can also increase whatever adverse effects the drug may have. The person who enjoys the relaxing effects of a glass of whiskey may not make himself more pleasurably relaxed by taking twice the quantity. He may simply become unpleasantly drunk.

The dose of a drug required to produce a specified level of effect in 50 percent of individuals is known as the median effective dose. The dose required to produce toxic effects in 50 percent of individuals is known as the median toxic dose. The ratio of these two, called the therapeutic index, gives an indication of a drug's safety and the relationship between benefits and risks.

Some drugs do not have one single therapeutic index, but many. The antihistamines are an example; they are useful in allergic disorders, but they often cause drowsiness. One therapeutic index for antihistamines might therefore refer to the ratio between their beneficial effects in relieving allergic symptoms and their adverse effect of making the patient sleepy. But that same adverse effect of sleepiness becomes the desired effect of the antihistamine when a manufacturer includes it in a preparation marketed to promote sleep. So another therapeutic index is constructed, this time looking at the ratio between the drug's sleep-inducing properties and other adverse effects.

## Drug Testing and the Placebo Effect

Therapeutic indexes must be based on the performance of drugs in real patients. As we have already seen, innumerable factors having to do with the patient, such as the state of his digestion, his obesity, and his age, may alter a drug's effects. To complicate drug testing further, the placebo effect operates in all sorts of unpredictable ways in different individuals. The word "placebo" (which means "I will please" in Latin) is used to describe any sort of "treatment" without any known specific effect on the condition being treated. Usually the effect of such a "treatment" is good; if you think something will make you feel better it often will. But the placebo effect can operate the other way too: people given dummy tablets in drug trials often complain of side effects such as headaches, nausea, or giddiness.

Most of the medical practice of past centuries was based on placebos; very few therapeutic drugs were known, and treatment therefore rested on the faith the patient had in his doctor and his "medicines." Now many highly effective drugs have been discovered; their very effectiveness has so strengthened the faith which both patients and doctors have in drugs that the placebo effect is still as general as ever. It shows itself most clearly in the testing of painkillers and sedatives, when about four out of ten patients usually report improvement after taking dummy pills. And the effect operates not only when you are given dummy pills; it works when real medicine is given too. The more sure you are that the drug (or operation or other procedure) will do you good, the more likely it is to work well for you. Your faith in the doctor who prescribes for you or the neighbor who suggests a pill or the advertisement which persuades you to buy one over the counter will all have some effect on the way the drug works.

Scientific drug testing has to allow for these faith-healing elements as well as all the other factors that influence a drug's effectiveness. It is also essential to know as much as possible about the disorder which the drug is intended to cure or ameliorate. For example, a cold generally lasts about three or four days if no treatment is given. In testing a cold "cure" we have therefore to be certain that the drug actually shortened the natural course of the illness.

The selection of a proper sample of patients for the drug trial is important too. They must be representative of the population who are to be offered the new treatment. The size of the sample of patients must be statistically representative, and the drug dosage must be carefully and realistically chosen.

Once a sample of patients and a drug regimen have been chosen, the drug testers have to find a way of preventing placebo effects from distorting their results. This is usually done by using what is called a double-blind technique. Identical tablets (or some other preparation) are made, half containing the drug to be tested and the other half containing either an established drug or some inert dummy substance. Half the consenting patients are given the true drug, half are given the dummy, and their responses are compared. Or half the patients may start with the real drug and then change to the dummy tablet after a suitable period, the other half of the sample starting with the dummy tablets and changing to the drug. The point, of course, is that neither the patient nor the prescribing doctor knows at any given point in time whether the "drug" is real or fake, new or old, and thus can have no preconceptions about it.

The results of the trials are subjected to highly complex statistical analyses. They may take several years from start to finish, and cost the drug companies a great deal of money, with no guarantee that at the end they will find they have an effective, safe, marketable drug. So it is not surprising that many over-the-counter drugs and some prescription drugs in common use have never been subjected to such trials. Many of them would fail under scientific scrutiny, yet individuals swear by them. Thanks to the placebo effect, many of us feel better after simply talking to a doctor, even before we swallow the first pill. Depending upon the disorder, our own judgments of effective "cures" for our various ills are often quite unreliable.

Unfortunately, there are many disorders for which there is no cure. In the absence of a real cure and in the presence of patients many of whom react favorably to *anything* which is done to help them, "treatments" tend to proliferate. If many treatments are in use for the same disorder, it is because there is no real treatment known for that disorder. If one treatment had ever been scientifically shown to be effective, it would have displaced all other treatments for that disorder. Yet people find it very difficult to accept lack of treatment. Even the most unorthodox and expensive treatments will always be glowingly recommended by some patient who preferred any action to none. Hair and skin clinics, for example, perpetuate a range of expensive treatments largely on a basis of "personal recommendation" from one patient to the next. Similarly, nonprescribed drugs, herbs, and "health" foods can be widely and profitably sold even where scientific testing would show them to be totally useless.

It should be obvious, from what I have said so far, that personal testimonials about a preparation are not worth the paper they are written on. Nor are endorsements from actors and athletes worth anything—they are paid to give them. And be careful about being taken in by television and newspaper advertising—the products concerned are nearly always expensive versions of already available and much cheaper drugs.

### Drug Regimens

Some drugs are taken occasionally as a single dose—for example, two aspirins for a headache. Others are taken daily as a single dose, such as a sleeping pill taken each bedtime. A few drugs are prescribed to be taken when necessary—nitroglycerin taken to relieve the pain of angina, or an antacid taken when indigestion is troublesome. But the majority of prescribed drugs are taken at intervals throughout the day, for several days, or even for weeks or years at a time. These specifications about amount and time are termed a "regimen."

Decisions about drug regimens, dosage, and the interval between doses are largely based on three considerations. First, the doctor must consider the length of time which this particular drug in this particular dosage takes to reach effective levels in the blood, and how quickly it starts to be eliminated from the body. Second, he must consider the therapeutic index (ratio of effectiveness to risks) for the drug. If the index is small and the therapeutic level in the blood is rather close to the toxic level, the dose will have to be carefully controlled to prevent adverse effects. If the index is large, there is more leeway. More than adequate doses can be given without much risk of adverse effects. Third, the duration of the illness being treated will affect the duration of drug treatment—for example, insulin treatment of diabetes is for life.

Some drugs, particularly antibiotics, can do their work properly only if the blood level is kept steady throughout the twenty-four hours. If the patient leaves a ten-hour gap between doses during the night, bacteria have a chance to reassert themselves. In such cases the doctor will probably prescribe the drug to be taken every six hours rather than four times daily.

Drugs with a long half-life—those which gradually build up and accumulate in the body—are much more difficult to control than drugs with a short half-life, which act rapidly and are readily excreted. Sometimes patients who are put on antidepressant drugs do not fully understand that the unpleasant side effects will appear almost at once, whereas the beneficial effects will be delayed for as much as two weeks. They decide that the drug is making them worse rather than better, and either abandon treatment or fail to stick to the regimen laid down by the doctor. Similarly, patients given phenobarbital for sedation may not realize that even while their regular dosage is producing the desired effect, the drug is accumulating in their bodies, being introduced faster than it can be excreted. When such a patient stops taking the pills, he will still have phenobarbital in his body for several days. The breakdown products of a major tranquilizer called chlorpromazine have been detected in the urine of patients up to six months after their last dose.

Obviously you should very carefully follow instructions about taking any drug, and check with your doctor or pharmacist before you alter either the recommended dosage or the interval between doses. The way in which drugs are taken can be important too. Most drugs, as we have seen, are absorbed better if they are taken when the stomach is empty. It makes sense therefore to take them before meals. But some drugs (for example aspirin and antirheumatic drugs) may irritate the empty stomach. They are better taken after meals. Most drugs are better absorbed if they are taken in solution. Soluble aspirin tablets taken in water will be effective more quickly than aspirin tablets taken dry. But many pills and capsules are not soluble and must be swallowed whole with a good drink of water. A few drugs, such as tetracycline, are ineffective if taken with milk. They may bind to substances in the milk and not be absorbed.

Many drugs are available in a wide variety of forms. Children may be given drugs in syrups and sweetened suspensions. People who suffer gastric irritation from drugs can often take the same medicine in the form of suppositories or specially coated tablets which protect the stomach from the drug until it reaches the intestines. The form is less important than the content—a suppository has just as much effect on the body as a pill does. Remember that some drugs should never be taken together, so that any doctor who is prescribing for you must be told of anything you are already taking—including alcohol. So must the pharmacist from whom you buy medicines over the counter.

Often a drug will appear to have made you better before you have taken the full course prescribed by the doctor. To stop taking it without consulting him may be harmful. The most usual example is probably antibiotics given to children. The child has a streptococcal sore throat and a high temperature; the doctor prescribes an antibiotic to be given for ten days. In two days the temperature is down and the child feels better, so the parents stop giving the drug and very probably put it away in the medicine cabinet for use without consulting the doctor the next time someone has a sore throat. The child may indeed be better because the disorder has cured itself, but on the other hand he may be better simply because the antibiotic has started its work, killing some of the bacteria but not all of them, and there may be a risk of producing rheumatic fever. The illness will then reappear in a few days, but this time with a possible added complication—bacteria may have become resistant to the antibiotic. At the same time, the bottle of medicine which has been stored away may well have such a short shelf life (the period during which it remains safe and effective) that it becomes useless or harmful after ten days.

Anyone who has a prescription filled or buys over the counter a drug he does not intend to use immediately should tell the pharmacist. The form in which the drug is dispensed may well affect its shelf life, and many formulations remain effective for only a short period of time. An ancient tube of antibiotic eye ointment dredged from the back of a medicine cabinet may well do more harm than good, because of the development of normal breakdown products. Similarly, anyone who suffers adverse effects from a prescribed drug should consider the form in which it is taken. An active drug ingredient is often mixed with other substances (called excipients or vehicles) to mask a bitter taste, for example, to give an ointment easy spreading properties, or to make it smell nice. Excipients in preparations to be given by mouth may alter the absorption of the drug and can themselves cause adverse effects, for instance diarrhea.

## ADVERSE EFFECTS OF DRUGS

Some experts believe that drugs are now prescribed out of all proportion to their need. Collections of unused drugs from patients' medicine cabinets indicate a tremendous wastage, but they also suggest that multiple drug use is now very common. Furthermore, increasing numbers of drugs are bought over the counter every year, and so the risk of adverse effects from drugs acting with or against each other is increased.

Any unintended reaction from a "normal" dose of a drug for one particular person with one particular disorder is an adverse effect. Most adverse effects of a drug have been observed and recorded; for example it is known that when a patient starts to take tricyclic antidepressants he may experience blurring of vision, dry mouth, constipation, and so forth. These are recognized adverse effects, which in this case luckily wear off after one or two weeks. Overdosage may produce enhanced side effects, and these may also occur over time with drugs that accumulate in the body and build up to a toxic level.

If any of the processes involved in the body's use of a drug (absorption, distribution, biotransformation, elimination) are altered, then a drug may have an excessive effect even when given in a "normal" dose. Some people may even become allergic to certain drugs and suffer hypersensitivity reactions. These reactions are idiosyncratic—that is, not common to everyone—but may also become recognized adverse effects of that drug over time. The commonest allergic reactions are skin rashes; there may also be fever, painful joints, a swollen face, wheezing, or increased sensitivity of the skin to sunlight. Very occasionally indeed a patient may drop dead from anaphylactic shock following the injection of a drug to which he has become allergic during previous treatment. (Death from a second bee sting is an example of this.) Other allergic reactions may result in jaundice.

Some rare reactions to drugs can be due to underlying genetic disorders which are not recognized until a drug touches them off. For example, barbiturates can trigger a first attack of a genetic disease called porphyria, which causes abdominal colic, polyneuritis, mental disturbances, and sometimes death. Genetic factors may also influence the effect of a particular drug on a particular patient. The drug isoniazid, which is used in tuberculosis, is used up quickly in most patients. But in a few it is broken down and excreted very slowly, so that such patients run the risk of harmful effects from it.

Many people believe that once they have been on a drug for some time without obvious ill effect, the appearance of adverse effects becomes unlikely. This is not true. The ill effects of a drug taken for a long time may be cumulative, as they are in the long-term consumption of compound pain-relieving preparations containing phenacetin, which have been shown to lead to kidney damage. Or ill effects may arise spontaneously even when the patient has been on a drug for years. Furthermore, certain drugs can produce serious adverse effects long after the patient has stopped taking them.

### Interactions Between Drugs

A drug interaction is the modification of the effects of one drug by another. Some drug interactions are used intentionally for therapeutic purposes, but most arise from unplanned combinations of drugs. Obviously the more drugs you take the more likely it is that some of them will react adversely with each other. The patient who takes over-the-counter drugs at the same time as prescribed ones, without advising the prescribing doctor or consulting the pharmacist, may be in danger.

Most drug experts oppose the use of medicines containing several active drugs because it is impossible to vary the dosage or time schedule of each drug separately. Also, if adverse effects arise it is difficult to know which drug is responsible for them. For example, phenacetin has been widely used for many years as one constituent in minor painkillers. A few patients who consumed such mixtures daily over a long period developed fatal kidney damage. Phenacetin is now considered to be the culprit, but it would have been indicted sooner had its consumption not been confused with the use of aspirin and caffeine and other ingredients in combined pain-reliever preparations. Even now, we are still unsure about the possible dangers of prolonged use of these combinations. Do not be impressed by advertisements which stress that products contain more than one active ingredient, and that they are approved by doctors. Several drugs are not necessarily more effective than one, and it would be surprising if such mixtures were not approved by doctors, since the drug companies employ doctors to advise them!

If the combined effect of two drugs is greater than the sum of each alone they are said to act synergistically. If the combined effect is less than the sum of the two they are said to be antagonistic. The combined effects of drugs with similar actions are usually referred to as additive.

The "normal" dose of a drug may become an overdose if it is given with another drug with which it interacts. For example the anticoagulant warfarin binds itself to the blood proteins. So does the antirheumatic drug phenylbutazone. If the two are given together, they compete for blood proteins to bind themselves to. The phenylbutazone takes over some of the protein from the warfarin, thus releasing free warfarin into the bloodstream, producing a dangerous level. Rather than receiving a beneficial anticoagulant action, such a patient may suffer severe bleeding. Overdosage may also arise from additive effects. Most of the mind-active drugs, for example, have additive effects with alcohol. The patient who drinks moderately when taking tranquilizers may unexpectedly become very drunk indeed. Drug interactions may cause adverse effects or simply make a drug ineffective. For example, the antibiotic tetracycline may interact with calcium salts (for instance in milk) or magnesium salts (as in many indigestion remedies) to form a chelate in the stomach. This interferes with the absorption of the antibiotic to a point where it cannot reach effective levels in the bloodstream.

Before starting to take more than one drug regularly, people should consider the possibility that their need for the second or third may in fact arise from their consumption of the first. All too often adverse drug effects result because patients and doctors try to deal with the ill effects of one drug by taking another.

## Vulnerability to Drugs

While all drugs are liable to produce some adverse effects, whether they are recognized or idiosyncratic, short-lived or long-term, the effects of single drugs or of drug interactions, some groups of people are particularly vulnerable.

### THE ELDERLY

"Aging" may be restricted to certain organs or tissues or may affect the whole body. Such changes may produce aging before the person is old in years. Whenever its onset, the aging process can alter the delicate physiochemical processes involved in drug action. Aging does not mean disease, although the older one gets the more chance he has of developing a disorder, particularly of the degenerative type (such as arthritis). In fact, older people are often found to have multiple disorders such as anemia, arthritis, and diseases of the arteries.

With advancing age, the body burns up energy more slowly, digestion may become affected, the acid in the stomach decreases, the gut wall may lose its muscular power, and the emptying of the stomach and movement of the bowels may become less efficient. Circulation may be affected, and the functions of the liver, kidneys, and brain may all be impaired.

Whether or not such actual deterioration has taken place, the diet of an old person may lack the basic elements essential to normal body functions and to the normal use of drugs by the body. So to give drugs to the elderly patient is not always without risk. Aspirin may cause bleeding from the stomach in anyone; in an elderly person such bleeding may be serious because dietary deficiencies have already led to anemia. Constipation caused by poor diet and weakened bowel action may become serious if the patient is given codeine, which slows gut action. Sleeping pills, sedatives, or tranquilizers in "average" doses may make the elderly person confused and unsteady; a barbiturate which would be excreted by most patients within eight hours may "hang over" the whole of the next day.

Clearly, then, fixed "average" doses and dosage schedules should not be applied to elderly patients. These patients, even more than the rest of us, need careful tailoring of drug dosages to their particular needs, current health, and social circumstances. Sometimes failure to provide this highly personal prescribing leads to difficulties. A patient who has become confused on tranquilizers may be considered senile and admitted to a psychogeriatric unit, where more drugs are given to control the confusion, beginning a vicious circle which may lead to the patient finishing his days on a hospital bed. The same kind of outcome may follow the prescribing of drugs to lower the blood pressure of elderly patients. These are seldom necessary, especially in elderly women, but nevertheless some doctors feel that high blood pressure must be lowered whatever the cost. In the elderly the cost can be high. The drugs reduce the volume of blood reaching the heart and brain, thus producing risks and mimicking symptoms of senility in someone who already has an insufficient supply of blood reaching these organs. Another group of drugs called diuretics make the kidneys pass out more water and salt in the urine. This makes the patient empty his bladder more frequently, and in the elderly patient often leads to incontinence. A drug-induced reaction may be the final straw to a harassed family, which promptly puts the elderly relative into institutional care.

In order to avoid such problems, the fewest possible drugs should be given to elderly patients, and in the minimum dosage which is effective for *them* even if this is far less than the "average." Furthermore, such patients, depending upon their disorder, should be seen and have their drug treatment assessed just as frequently and as thoroughly as younger patients—ideally every four to six weeks. Unless this is made routine, elderly people, especially when they are in homes or hospitals, are often left on numerous drugs indefinitely.

PREGNANT WOMEN

In the early weeks of pregnancy the placenta is developing. Until it is fully formed and able to protect the embryo, any drug circulating through the mother's body may enter the embryo. In later months the placenta does act as a barrier, protecting the developing baby from moderate doses of non-fat-soluble drugs. Fat-soluble drugs, and drugs given in high dosage, will continue to cross the placenta throughout pregnancy. Yet the baby's liver is not sufficiently developed to deal with the biotransformation of drugs, and its kidneys are not sufficiently developed to excrete them. Of course, the drugs do return to the mother through the umbilical vein for her to break them down and excrete them from her body.

From the moment the female egg is fertilized complex processes are set in motion. The egg embeds itself in the wall of the uterus (womb), and the cells of the fertilized egg start to divide and redivide; under chemical control they start grouping and organizing themselves. Cells destined to be part of the brain, the liver, the eyes, the kidneys, and so on position themselves, and the various organs start to develop. So the whole embryo baby is a group of cells, all dividing and being chemically organized.

We have already stated that while we know a good deal about the effects of drugs within the body, we know very little about how those effects are produced, how the drugs actually act on the cells. So we do not know much about how drugs act upon the cells that make up a developing baby either. We really know little more than that some drugs may produce abnormalities and that these are more likely when the drug is inadvertently given to the fetus at less than twelve weeks after conception.

Governments and pharmaceutical companies have increased and improved the testing of *new* drugs for possible dangers during pregnancy. But there are thousands of prescribed drugs and over-the-counter drugs on the market which have never been tested. Pregnant women take so many drugs, including tea, coffee, alcohol, cigarettes, aspirin, and antacids, that it is very difficult to discover the relationship between any abnormality in the baby and drugs used by the mother in pregnancy. There is some evidence that mothers of abnormal babies have taken more drugs than other mothers, but we do not know whether the abnormality is a direct result of the drug taking, or, if it is, whether it is the combinations of drugs or one specific one which causes the trouble. We do not even know whether prolonged drug use in both men and women of childbearing age may lead to some mutant change in the genes and thus cause abnormalities in the infant either at birth or later in life.

Only a few drugs are actually known to produce abnormalities. Heavy smoking, for example, leads to smaller babies; tetracycline can affect bone growth and stain teeth; anticonvulsant drugs are considered by some to increase the risk of clubfoot and cleft palate. Then there are a few drugs which can damage the baby by affecting its blood supply—excessive vitamin A, for example, affects the placenta. Yet others may damage the baby after it is fully developed: hormones may affect sexual development; iodine and antithyroid drugs may cause the baby to be born with a goiter. In Britain and Continental Europe and Canada in the late fifties, more than five thousand babies were born with gross defects traceable to their mothers' use during pregnancy of a sedative called thalidomide. (It was never sold in the United States.) Finally, of course, the baby may develop an overall reaction and even be born already dependent on narcotics or barbiturates.

What conclusions should we draw from this state of affairs? Without being alarmist, it is probably best to avoid taking any nonessential drugs in pregnancy or when anticipating pregnancy. If your doctor must prescribe drugs for you, he will choose among those which have been tested and shown to be safe.

BABIES AND CHILDREN

If you have read the beginning of this chapter you will realize that the way the body deals with drugs is very complex and relies on healthy, mature, and functioning organs. You will remember that the liver has to bring about the breakdown of drugs, so that the kidneys can excrete them. In babies, even after birth, the liver and kidneys are still immature. Some of the enzyme and other systems involved in drug breakdown and excretion are not fully developed. Ineffectively broken down or incompletely excreted, almost any drug may cause adverse effects.

Babies are also much more sensitive than older people to changes in the salt and water balance in their bodies. Drugs which alter this balance—such as drugs with a diuretic effect, or drugs which cause diarrhea—may produce serious adverse effects. Equally, any drug whose own effect is made worse by a change in salt and water balance may have adverse effects in babies.

Infants are growing and developing. Drugs which have few adverse effects in an adult may interfere with growth or development in a baby, or may have adverse effects on the infant's mechanisms for controlling his body temperature or on his newly developing muscle control or coordination.

All these factors apply also to toddlers and, to a lesser extent, to children too. Dosage is therefore absolutely critical. Infants and small children are not "small adults," and the simple scaling down of dosage on a weight and/or age basis can be extremely dangerous. There is urgent need for studies into the effects of drugs in the young.

Any liquid medicine should be administered using the 5-milliliter (ml.) spoon given to you by the pharmacist. If the instructions say "1 teaspoonful" they mean 5 ml. A domestic teaspoon may hold 4 or 7 mls., and such inaccuracy could be dangerous. Similarly, if any dilution of the medicine is required, this should be carried out by the pharmacist in the pharmacy; it should never be left to the mother to estimate the right quantity of a drug with a label saying, for instance, "Dilute in 5 parts of water."

On the whole, too many drugs are given to babies and children. Mothers have been led to expect a prescription or a shot every time they take their child to the doctor, and many doctors seem unable to resist prescribing antidiarrheal remedies, cough medicines, and antibiotics. Antibiotics in particular are often used inappropriately. The mother says, "Our doctor always gives Johnny an antibiotic when he gets these nasty colds." The very statement is a command. Many of those "nasty colds" are caused by viruses against which antibiotics are totally ineffective. In such a situation the only possible value of an antibiotic is in protecting the child against the possibility that the cold may be followed by a bacterial invasion of the chest, throat, or ears. With common colds and other virus infections of the nose and throat, secondary infections are the exception rather than the rule. Doctors ought to stop thinking that patients expect drugs at every consultation and try giving reassurance, explanation, and sound advice instead. Equally, mothers should not expect a prescription to relieve their child's every symptom.

DRIVERS

A high degree of mental and physical skill, coordination, and judgment are required to drive any motor vehicle safely. Most of us can manage these skills only when we are fully awake, alert, calm, and concentrating. Yet every day thousands of motorists drive while under the influence of drugs that are bound to affect their skills to some extent.

The drug most usually indicted after an accident is of course alcohol. The mechanisms by which alcohol affects the body are discussed in detail beginning on p. 25. Moderate amounts of alcohol impair driving ability to some extent. Often the driver himself does not notice this impairment. Because the alcohol has relaxed him and made him less inhibited than usual he may even feel that he is driving particularly well. In high doses alcohol produces disorientation and confusion, blurred vision, and poor muscle control. Such a driver is extremely lucky to get home without hurting himself or somebody else. Alcohol is not a suitable drug for drivers under any circumstances.

Many of the other drugs which impair driving ability do so to an even greater extent if they are combined with only a little alcohol. For example, many cough remedies and cold "cures" contain drugs which affect the nervous system. Because they have been bought over the counter, the patient may give little thought to their possible effects on his driving. Alone, they might not impair it seriously; but when he has a drink with his friends before driving home from work, the combination of cold medicine and alcohol may make him quite unfit to drive.

Even more dangerous are the many drugs which are prescribed by doctors without any warning to the patient about their possible effects on driving ability. These include many of the most commonly prescribed groups of drugs such as antihistamines, stimulants, sleeping drugs, sedatives, tranquilizers, antidepressants, slimming drugs, drugs used to treat blood pressure, bronchodilator drugs, antispasmodics, drugs used to treat nausea or vomiting in pregnancy or motion sickness, and insulin used to treat diabetes. Obviously in our society it would be impossible to prohibit any person taking any of these groups of drugs from driving a car. The effects depend on the person, the situation, the dose. What one can and must do is to point out the possible effects of all these drugs on driving skill, and above all the danger of combining them with alcohol and the steering wheel.

The rule is that any drug with an effect (whether intended or not) on the mind or the nervous system is likely to have some effect on driving ability. If a drug prescribed for you makes you feel drowsy, nervous, tense, dizzy, faint, or trembly, or makes it difficult for you to concentrate or blurs your vision, then you can be sure your driving skills are impaired.

PATIENTS ON LONG-TERM DRUG TREATMENT
Several groups of drugs discussed in detail in Part II may be responsible for very serious adverse effects when other drugs are given to the patient, or when he undergoes dental treatment, or when he requires emergency treatment, even for a minor injury at an outpatient department. The first rule for anyone undergoing long-term drug treatment is that he should tell any medical personnel with whom he comes in contact about his drugs. In most cases warning cards should be issued to such patients. They should always be carried. Then a patient can be sure that the hospital will have the information it needs in case he is admitted unconscious after an accident.

Corticosteroids, especially prednisone, are now frequently used to treat rheumatoid arthritis, allergic diseases, skin diseases, eye diseases, and asthma. During periods of anxiety, stress, or injury, the body requires and produces more corticosteroids. This natural response by the adrenal glands is blocked by the patient being treated with corticosteroids. His body is already living with large amounts of corticosteroids in the bloodstream, so the adrenal glands do not respond to stress by producing more. A patient having such treatment is therefore in danger of acute adrenal insufficiency if he has an accident, a surgical procedure, or even a severe infection. In such a patient, even the stress of an ordinary dental procedure can be enough to produce faintness, weakness, nausea, vomiting, and final collapse.

If you are on corticosteroids or have had treatment with them for even one month during the preceding two years, you should always carry your warning card with you.

Anticoagulants lessen the blood's ability to clot. They are most often used to prevent the extension or recurrence of a thrombosis (blood clot) in a vein or in one of the arteries of the heart. Patients taking these drugs tend to bleed easily, and bleeding, even from a minor injury, can be difficult to stop. They should always carry a warning card.

Any patient on antidiabetic treatment may experience a drastic fall in blood sugar (hypoglycemia), with weakness, faintness, or even collapse, if he skips a meal in order to have an anesthetic. Patients on antidiabetic pills must discuss any proposed dental anesthetic with their dentist and with their doctor. Those who are taking insulin, especially if the total dose is as high as 60 units a day, should be admitted to a hospital if they require dental anesthesia.

Those antidepressant drugs which belong to the group of monoamine oxidase inhibitors may produce adverse effects when taken with certain other drugs and with certain foods. Patients on these drugs should be given warning cards, and should carry them. Stimulant drugs, such as amphetamines, and pain relievers such as meperidine and morphine can be highly dangerous.

The other main group of antidepressants, the tricyclic compounds, make some patients sensitive to epinephrine and similar substances. A local anesthetic given for dental treatment or for minor surgery may make the heart race and send the blood pressure up. Dentists and emergency-room doctors should be told that the patient is on tricyclic antidepressants, so that they can give local anesthetic without epinephrine.

Many antihypertensive drugs may react with a general anesthetic to produce a severe drop in blood pressure. This can be very dangerous. If you are taking a drug to lower your blood pressure, make sure you carry a warning card.

Sedatives and tranquilizers may increase the depressant effects of general anesthetics on the brain, particularly on the breathing center. Make sure you carry a warning card.

Any patient on long-term drug treatment should have his treatment reviewed periodically.

## Warnings About Drug Use

1. Always know the name of the drug you are taking.
2. Always check its main effects and adverse effects.
3. Always tell the doctor or pharmacist about previous drug reactions and other allergies you or members of your family have had.
4. Always take the drug according to the instructions on the container.
5. Never take a drug daily for more than one or two weeks without checking on the benefits and risks.
6. Never share prescribed drugs with anyone else.
7. Never use drugs from an unlabeled container.
8. Never keep unwanted or unused drugs in the house—always flush them down the toilet.
9. Keep only a few household remedies on hand, and in small quantities.
10. Keep all drugs in one safety cabinet out of reach of children. Childhood poisonings are preventable.
11. Never mix the contents of one drug container with another.
12. Check with your pharmacist if you are not clear about:
    The expiration date of a drug and where you should store it.
    When you should take it (for example, before or after meals).
    How you should take it (for example, with or without milk).
    How frequently you should take it (for example, every four hours, every six hours, four times a day, or four times in twenty-four hours).
    For how many days you should take it.
13. Always ask the pharmacist for instruction leaflets when obtaining such medications as eye drops, nose drops, and vaginal tablets.
14. Ask what the doctor means when he states "as before," or "as directed," and ask about the maximum amount of one dose and the maximum amount allowable in twenty-four hours. Ask how often is "when necessary."
15. Be especially cautious when giving drugs to babies, debilitated and elderly patients, persons with impaired kidney or liver function, and patients with heart disease, chest disease, high blood pressure, glaucoma, enlarged prostate gland, peptic ulcers, history of allergy, and history of drug dependence.
16. If you are or think you may be pregnant, be extremely cautious about any drugs you take, particularly during the first twelve weeks.
17. If you are on steroids, anticoagulants, antidiabetic drugs, monoamine oxidase inhibitors, antidepressant drugs, or any other spe-

cial drugs, always ask for and carry a warning card with you. Be sure to advise your dentist before treatment.

18. Consider the possibility of a drug reaction if a new symptom (such as diarrhea or skin rash) develops while you are on drug treatment. If it is a prescribed drug, stop taking it and consult your doctor. If it is an over-the-counter drug, stop taking it, check its adverse effects, and report to your doctor or your pharmacist if the symptom does not clear up.

19. Remember the risk of adverse drug effects between drugs and also between drugs and certain foods. In particular, check on whether you can take alcohol while taking a drug.

20. Remember that many drugs may affect your ability to operate moving machinery and drive a motor vehicle.

21. If the patient is confused or depressed and/or drinks alcohol regularly, sometimes to excess, then take care to supervise the issue of tablets on a daily basis.

22. Never keep sleeping drugs at your bedside, particularly if you also drink alcohol. You may accidentally take an extra dose in the night.

## DEPENDENCE ON DRUGS

Most people think they know what a "drug addict" is. Yet they would be hard put to define drug addiction in a way that covered all the possible types of people who might be addicted and all the possible types of drug they might be addicted to. Because of such problems of definition and because of the extent to which the term "addiction" has been misused, most authorities are now in favor of substituting the general term "drug dependence" and then following it with a description of the type of dependence they mean.

In general, drug dependence can be defined as a psychological and/or physical state which results from the taking of a drug. The dependent person feels a compulsion to continue taking the drug either because of the "desired" effects it produces or because of the ill effects he fears will occur if he does not take it, or both.

Defined in this general way, it is clear that most of us are at least psychologically dependent on a great many substances we do not usually refer to as "drugs." Many of us feel we cannot start the day without coffee or a cigarette, cannot enjoy a rest without a cup of tea, or are deprived if we do not have a much more than adequate meal. And we are psychologically dependent on all kinds of other things in our daily lives too, from sex and sports to television and the newspapers. So psychological dependence is not *necessarily* a bad thing. What we have to decide is whether such dependencies are doing harm—mentally, physically, or socially—bearing in mind that different people will see different things as problems.

The person who is psychologically dependent may have such a craving for his drug, such a compulsion to continue taking it, that he goes on even when he knows full well that he is causing himself harm. Smokers and alcohol drinkers are often in this category.

Physical dependence is a condition in which repeated use of a drug leads to certain symptoms when that drug is stopped. Not all drugs that cause psychological dependence cause physical dependence, but all those that produce physical dependence produce psychological dependence also. The "withdrawal symptoms" that arise when a drug is taken from someone physically dependent on it can be extremely severe. Among the most usual are vomiting, convulsions, trembling, and confusion. Without the drug, the body goes to pieces. In serious cases, if no help is offered the patient may die. Physical withdrawal symptoms can always be instantly relieved by the administration of a dose of the drug which caused the dependence. In some cases one drug can replace another in this respect. Tranquilizers, for example, can relieve the symptoms of alcohol withdrawal. In instances like these, there is said to be cross-dependence between the two drugs.

Many of the drugs which can cause dependence also lead to tolerance in the user. The person's body becomes so accustomed to a drug that he has to increase the dose in order to achieve the desired effect. The double Scotch which makes a novice drinker feel pleasantly intoxicated will barely affect the seasoned drinker. Some drugs are capable of producing tremendous tolerance. Constant users of opium and morphine, for example, can take and tolerate doses which would be fatal to ordinary people.

Just as there can be cross-dependence between drugs, so too there can be cross-tolerance. A heavy drinker may need much more sleeping drug to "knock him out" than a teetotaler does.

A wide range of mood-altering drugs can cause dependence. But we are still very ignorant about who will become dependent on which drugs under what circumstances. Some drugs are highly likely to cause dependence, and some individuals are highly likely to become dependent. On the whole, dependence seems most likely to arise when three factors come together: a potential drug of dependence, a "vulnerable" personality, and some adverse aspect of the environment. Whether the risk becomes reality depends on many other complex sociopsychological factors affecting that particular individual.

## Alcohol Dependence

Alcohol is one of the most widely used and most misunderstood of drugs. In Western societies it is conventionally taken in social situations, where it is regarded as a stimulant. In fact it is not a stimulant at all but a sedative whose effect, as with so many other drugs, depends on the mood and the social circumstances of the taker. Its apparent stimulant effect arises from its ability to free us from some of the restraints which normally govern our behavior, relieving anxieties and releasing tensions. At a party such effects tend to give us a feeling of well-being and friendliness. The pretty girl seems more desirable, other people's anecdotes seem funnier, and one's own flow freely. Yet the same quantity of alcohol taken alone by an unhappy depressed individual will not lift his mood; it is more likely to remove his controls so that he weeps helplessly. Taken at bedtime, such a dose will simply make a person sleepy. Taken during a jealous quarrel, it may make one extremely aggressive. And even though the partygoer *feels* confident and therefore efficient, he is actually much less so than before. His increased sexual desire will not lead to a better sexual performance, his easy flow of conversation will be less intelligent than it is when he is sober, and if he goes home and tries to read or study he will find that his ability to concentrate is impaired.

The effects of alcohol on mood are not the only effects which are misleading. A drink of alcohol opens up the small blood vessels in the skin, so that it becomes warm and flushed and may result in sweating. The person who has taken alcohol therefore *feels* warmer than before but is, in fact, being cooled as more blood reaches the surface of the skin and therefore the outside air. To drink alcohol to make yourself feel warmer when you come in from the snow may be perfectly all right, but to drink it in preparation for going out into the cold, or to "keep you warm" while outside, can be dangerous.

Also, by increasing blood flow to the stomach, alcohol may give you a warm comfortable feeling inside, and temporarily banish uneasy feelings arising from indigestion or other stomach troubles. But in fact alcohol increases the secretion of gastric acid and may ultimately cause irritation and inflammation. It is therefore quite the wrong drug to put into a stomach that is already disturbed. Heavy drinkers often have chronic gastritis. People with peptic ulcers should abstain from alcohol completely, and above all, alcohol should never be taken with aspirin, which is an irritant to the stomach.

The effects of alcohol on the brain and nervous system are proportionate to the *blood alcohol level*. The effects are more marked when the level in the blood is rising than when it is on the way down again. They are very marked when a large amount of alcohol is taken quickly, because it is rapidly absorbed and the level in the blood rises very rapidly. The drug is absorbed from the stomach, small intestine, and colon. Absorption from the stomach is slowed by the presence of food or of milk; it is also slower when the alcohol is taken in the form of beer, since beer contains a lot of carbohydrate. Once the alcohol has left the stomach and reached the intestine, it is unaffected by the presence or absence of food. This is why patients who have had part of their stomachs removed absorb alcohol very rapidly and may easily become drunk.

Once absorbed into the blood, alcohol is distributed to all the body tissues, including fat; a thin person may experience greater effects from a drink of alcohol than does an obese person, because the alcohol is less dispersed. It is then burned up at the rate of about 10 ml. per hour. About 90 percent of it is used by the body, the rest being excreted in urine, sweat, tears, bile, gastric juice, saliva, and the breath. The alcohol excreted in breath has a fixed relationship to that which is present in the blood. It is therefore possible to estimate the blood alcohol level from the alcohol in expired air, and this is the principle used in breathalizer tests. Since the body can use and excrete only about 10 ml. of pure alcohol—two teaspoonfuls—per hour, during an evening's continuous drinking the drug is bound to accumulate in the body.

In high doses alcohol produces drunkenness, disorientation and confusion, blurred vision, slurred speech, poor muscle control, and often nausea and vomiting. As the dose increases, breathing becomes depressed; coma follows, and if some of the overdose is not eliminated in vomit, it may be followed by death. Intoxication with alcohol is followed by a "hangover" which makes one feel sick, weak, and dizzy, with aches and pains all over. Even moderate amounts of alcohol, and even a slight hangover, impair driving ability. Alcohol is a factor contributing to a large percentage of road traffic accidents. *Nobody should drive when he has been drinking.*

A great many of us are psychologically dependent on alcohol. We may associate a nightly drink with the end of the working day and the beginning of the evening's relaxation; or we may feel unable to face social occasions without it or use it to calm us down whenever we must face unusual stress. We use alcohol as a social prop and as a coping device.

The frequent use of alcohol that impairs health or adversely affects family or employment or other interpersonal relationships on a continuing basis can be termed "alcoholism."

Those who do become physically dependent on alcohol have usually passed through a period of many years of extreme psychological dependence and therefore regular daily drinking of increasing quantities. "Alcoholism" is thus a term used to describe a very wide range of disorders which may result from drinking alcohol. These end consequences include physical results of high alcohol intake and poor diet —alcoholic cirrhosis of the liver, disorders of the heart, circulation, kidneys, and brain. Others are the indirect results of alcoholism, caused by the neglect of personal care which is common among such patients. Malnutrition and other disorders resulting from it lead to a high risk of infections and other illnesses. The alcoholic is also liable to mental illness, convulsions, loss of memory, and sexual impotence.

While tolerance to alcohol may include learning to function apparently normally after heavy doses, it does *not* include being able to tolerate a lethal dose of the drug. Alcoholics often finally die of acute alcohol poisoning, although (as stated earlier) vomiting and coma often prevent the taking of a fatal dose.

The withdrawal of alcohol from a chronic heavy drinker who is physically dependent on the drug may produce nausea, agitation, anxiety, confusion, tremors, sweating, cramps, vomiting, rise in temperature, and hallucinations. These withdrawal effects are referred to as delirium tremens (the "d.t.'s").

If no alternatives are offered, such as tailing off the use of alcohol gradually or obviating the worse effects with tranquilizers, the patient may move on into convulsions, coma, and death.

In most alcoholics it takes years to produce the degree of physical dependence necessary for these extreme withdrawal effects. But this is at least partly dose-dependent. Extreme physical dependence can take place within a few weeks if the daily dosage is very high.

Alcoholism is often said to "run in families," but alcoholism itself cannot be inherited. What can be passed on from one generation to the next is whatever psychological genetic factors made the first victim turn to alcohol as a coping device in the first place, together with the stress and the example which come from living with an alcoholic and/or the stress of everyday life.

Cross-tolerance and cross-dependence occur among alcohol, sleeping drugs, sedatives, and tranquilizers. A man who tolerates a great deal of alcohol will need a larger dose of barbiturate than his teetotal brother. Unfortunately, this cross-tolerance does not affect the lethal dose of any of these drugs; it merely narrows the gap between the dose that is effective and the dose that is dangerous. Many deaths from overdosage arise from mixing alcohol with these drugs, and from taking more and more in an attempt to make them effective. Before giving such drugs to a patient, a doctor should find out about his drinking habits as well as investigating his symptoms.

## Tobacco Dependence

The main drugs in tobacco are nicotine and tar products. In addition, tobacco smoke contains more than five hundred other chemicals as well as appreciable amounts of carbon monoxide gas (which many consider to be a cause of heart disease). Smoking may give pleasure, relieve tension, or stimulate according to the personality of the user and the situation in which smoking occurs. Psychological dependence is common, tolerance occurs, and physical dependence is possible. There is an association between cigarette smoking and cancer of the lungs, chronic bronchitis, coronary artery disease, arterial diseases, and peptic ulcers. One of the greatest advances in this decade in the field of preventive medicine (and surely all health care services should aim at prevention) has been the discovery of the relationship between cigarette smoking and these diseases. To stop smoking is one of the most important steps you can take to ensure health. Yet, even knowing the risks, people continue to smoke—which shows how severe is the psychological dependence produced by tobacco.

The smoke inhaled from a cigarette may yield as much as 6 to 8 mg. of nicotine (cigar smoke has 15 to 40 mg.) and from 4 to 38 mg. of tar. (These quantities may, it is true, be considerably lower in newer brands advertised as being low in tar and nicotine.) About 90 percent of nicotine in inhaled smoke is absorbed into the body, compared with about 25 to 50 percent if it is not inhaled.

Because marked tolerance to nicotine develops rapidly once an individual begins to smoke regularly, few people realize that it is one of the most toxic of all drugs. The lethal dose may be as little as 60 mg. There is more than this quantity in ten cigarettes, even though this amount is not absorbed when the tobacco is smoked. (A toddler who eats a cigarette is in danger and should be treated with as much urgency as if he had taken pills from the medicine cabinet.)

In small doses, or in the tolerant individual, nicotine first stimulates and then depresses the functions and endings of certain nerves supplying the gut, heart, and circulation. It causes the tiny blood vessels of the skin to constrict, speeds up the pulse, elevates blood pressure, and increases bowel activity. It is readily absorbed from the lungs, the gut, and the skin, and it undergoes breakdown in the liver and excretion by the kidneys. Traces are also excreted in breast milk (0.5 mg. per l. in the milk of heavy smokers).

Nicotine poisoning leads to acute nausea, salivation, abdominal pain, vomiting, diarrhea, sweating, headaches, dizziness, confusion, weakness, and disturbances of hearing and vision. Untreated, these are followed by a dramatic rise in blood pressure, very rapid pulse, difficulty in breathing, and finally death.

The tars in tobacco smoke are probably responsible for producing cancer of the lung. They also irritate the linings of the bronchi, producing coughing and bronchitis. The use of tobacco by pregnant women can harm the unborn child.

## Barbiturate, Sedative, and Minor Tranquilizer Dependence

Sleeping drugs and sedatives, both barbiturate and nonbarbiturate types, and the minor tranquilizers all depress brain function. All are capable of producing drug dependence, although some are much more dangerous than others in this respect.

As with alcohol, many patients are psychologically dependent on such drugs, but comparatively few become physically dependent. Thousands of individuals take two sleeping pills every night and are sure that they would not sleep without them. Deprived of the pills, they might feel psychologically disturbed and would not begin sleeping properly until up to six weeks had elapsed. At the other extreme there is the true addict who is physically dependent on barbiturates and takes them by intravenous injection to maximize their effect.

All these drugs produce some degree of tolerance in the individual who takes them regularly. Indeed, the way to be sure that a sleeping pill will work for you when you really need it is to make sure that you don't get into the habit of taking it when you don't really need it. Habituation to such drugs means either that they are not useful when they are needed or that larger doses must be taken.

Tolerance to any of these drugs, especially the barbiturates, is dangerous because while the individual becomes tolerant to the sedative or intoxicant effects he does not become tolerant to the lethal ones. He may need a larger and larger dose to make him sleep, but it does not take a larger and larger dose to kill him. The bigger his regular dose, the smaller the gap of safety between that dose and a lethal dose.

Cross-tolerance occurs between all these drugs and between any one of them and alcohol. As already noted, many fatal overdoses arise from a combination of drinking and some of these drugs.

The symptoms of overdosage with any of these drugs show themselves most clearly in barbiturate intoxication. There is difficulty in thinking coherently, slurred speech, diminished concentration. The individual becomes emotional, irritable, suspicious—even paranoid. He may become depressed and suicidal. His gait may be unsteady and his vision blurred. In longstanding addiction there may also be skin rashes, and a poor state of general health and nutrition associated with the dependence.

If an individual does become physically dependent on any of these drugs he may suffer from withdrawal symptoms if they are suddenly stopped. These symptoms vary markedly in degree, depending on which drug is responsible, how long the individual has been taking it, and in what dosage. But they may include anxiety, restlessness, trembling, weakness, abdominal cramps, vomiting, hallucinations, delirium, convulsions, and even death.

## Amphetamine Dependence

The amphetamines are discussed in the section on stimulant drugs, p. 64. They may produce different effects in different people. Some individuals, after a moderate dose of amphetamine by mouth, feel alert, full of energy, and happy. Others feel very tense, anxious, and far from happy.

Amphetamines were widely used by the armed forces in World War II to combat fatigue. After the war this practice spread to students, night-shift workers, athletes, and long-distance drivers. In addition, doctors prescribed them freely in the treatment of obesity and depression. There is no doubt that the ability of amphetamines to lift mood and make you feel happy was one of the main reasons for their eventual widespread use and abuse, which reached a peak in the 1960s.

Tolerance to the amphetamines develops according to the drug used, the individual, the dose and frequency of use, and the purpose for which the drug is taken. For example, individuals who repeatedly use the drug to lift mood develop tolerance and have to increase the dose to produce the same desired effects. Tolerance also develops to the adverse effects, and addicts may use thousands of milligrams in a day —far above the toxic dose in "normal" individuals.

Withdrawal of amphetamines from chronic users does not produce the classical sort of withdrawal symptoms produced by, say, alcohol. Therefore it is claimed that amphetamines do not produce physical dependence. But withdrawal *does* produce fatigue, prolonged sleep, abdominal cramps, increased appetite, depression, and changes on electrical brain tracings (electroencephalograph). However, the important point is that amphetamines produce severe drug dependence and serious adverse effects, and show how psychological dependence can be a major factor in such abuse.

## Cocaine Dependence

Cocaine produces effects and adverse effects similar to those of amphetamines, even though the two drugs act very differently in the body. Marked tolerance to cocaine develops, so that addicts can tolerate huge doses. There is no cross-tolerance or cross-dependence with the amphetamines.

## Narcotic Pain-Reliever Dependence

Morphine and narcotic pain relievers are discussed on p. 115. The term "narcotic" in this book refers to drugs obtained from or pharmacologically related to those obtained from the opium poppy plant, *Papaver somniferum*.

The use of opium and opiate drugs goes back over thousands of years. The subjective effects produced by them vary considerably among individuals and under different situations. What may produce a warm feeling of peace in one person may cause nausea, drowsiness, lethargy, dizziness, and mood changes in another. They reduce the desire for sex and food and reduce aggression. Some regular users, for example doctors or other professionals, may lead "normal" lives with comparatively easy access to drugs, while others who steal to get the money to buy drugs on the black market may become social outcasts or criminals. Tolerance to the various effects of narcotics develops when the drugs are used so frequently that the addict who seeks a "kick" or "high" has to increase the dose continuously in order to achieve the same effects. Addicts are thus able to tolerate doses far in excess of those which could be tolerated by nonaddicts. However, tolerance is not the same for the different effects produced by these drugs; for example, an addict who tolerates very high doses of morphine may still exhibit the small pupils and constipation which a nonaddict has after a "normal" dose.

The development of physical dependence on narcotics is related to the size and frequency of dose taken, the length of time over which it is used, the particular drug, and the personality of the user. In some individuals, regular use of small doses over even a few days (perhaps following a painful accident) can cause some degree of physical dependence. Others in similar circumstances would not notice when the drug was withdrawn, provided that the pain it was given for had eased.

The severity of withdrawal symptoms is therefore closely related to all these factors. A baby born of a narcotic-dependent mother may be physically dependent himself and can die if his acute withdrawal symptoms are not recognized. The truly physically dependent individual whose drugs are withdrawn will experience an overwhelming desire to have the drugs restored. If he is unsuccessful, his first withdrawal symptoms will include watery eyes, a running nose, yawning, sweating, restlessness, and sleep. Later he will become irritable, develop tremors, and sneeze and yawn continuously while his nose and eyes run copiously. Later still there will be weakness, depression, nausea, vomiting, diarrhea, chilliness, sweating, abdominal cramps, pain in the back and legs, and kicking movements. At this stage the skin is cold and covered with "gooseflesh" (this is the source of the expression "withdrawing cold turkey"). Without treatment these symptoms burn themselves out in seven to ten days. But at any point they can be dramatically reversed by giving a dose of any narcotic, since cross-dependence occurs among them all.

This cross-dependence is the basis for the commonly used and often criticized methadone treatment of heroin and other opiate dependencies. There are two elements to the dependence on opiates: the taking of them for the pleasurable "high" they produce (a craving) and the taking of them to avoid unpleasant withdrawal symptoms, which in itself produces relief and pleasure without a "high." If methadone is substituted by mouth, these feelings are said to be decreased and the patient can be maintained over the long term with the hope of eventually weaning him from the methadone.But it is really just not that simple, since drug dependence is complex. Furthermore, methadone by injection may produce dependence effects similar to those of heroin.

## Marijuana

Marijuana is obtained from *Cannabis sativa* (Indian hemp), a herbaceous annual plant which readily grows in a variety of temperate climates. Under the single heading "marijuana" are a large variety of drug preparations made in different ways from different parts of the plant and known by different names in various parts of the world.

The crushed leaves, flowers, and twigs of the plant are called marijuana, often known as grass, pot, weed, tea, boo, or Mary Jane in various parts of the West, or as bhang or ganja in India, kif in Morocco, and dagga in Africa. Hemp is made only from the flowering tops of the plant. Hashish, known as hash in the West and charas in India, is made from the relatively pure resin of the plants; it is at least five times more potent than the highest-quality marijuana.

The use of marijuana in the East for its mood-altering effects goes back over many thousands of years. It spread to the West mainly after World War I, but was restricted to certain groups. It was only in the sixties that its use spread throughout the Western world. Following in its trail have come the usual governmental legislations and controls.

Marijuana is usually smoked in hand-rolled cigarettes, but both marijuana and hashish may be smoked by placing small pieces on the tip of a burning cigarette, or smoked through ordinary pipes or water pipes. The smoke is inhaled deeply into the lungs and held there for a while. Effects on mood start almost immediately, reach a peak in about three-quarters of an hour, and last for several hours. Marijuana resin can be taken by mouth in beverages or food, but it is less effective when swallowed than when smoked, and the effects produced by smoking may be more carefully controlled. Very little is known about the distribution, breakdown, and excretion of marijuana by the body. Our scientific knowledge of the effects and adverse effects of marijuana is, in fact, extremely scanty. It is not improved by the highly emotional and biased approach which many writers take to the subject. The difficulties in making objective studies of the effects of marijuana are numerous. The strength of preparations of the drug may vary widely, and varying quantities of inert "filler" may be added. The effects on mood obviously vary with the strength, but they also vary with the speed and method of administration, the personality, expectations, and previous drug experiences of the user, his mood and the mood and expectations of those around him. A controlled dose, smoked by a particular person at a specified rate in a laboratory, may therefore affect him quite differently from marijuana smoked at home or with friends.

The most frequently described subjective effects of the drug include a dreamy state or one of giggling happiness, feelings of timelessness and of increased awareness, feelings of great insight and the tapping of basic truth, free-flowing ideas, and feelings of deep inward joy usually known as a "high." Frequently described adverse effects include anxiety, impairment of concentration and memory, and unpleasant fantasies.

On the whole, desired subjective effects seem to arise most often when the drug is taken in pleasant supportive company by an experienced marijuana smoker. The markedly unpleasant effects described by inexperienced smokers who have taken large doses when alone include panic, fear of death, peculiar sensations in the limbs, suspiciousness, headaches, nausea, dizziness, confusion, depression, delusions, and loss of control. Such extreme reactions are apparently rare.

Marijuana is claimed by some (but denied by others) to produce an "amotivational syndrome" which is characterized by loss of interest and apathy. It has been claimed that it produces a loss of brain tissue similar to that seen in the elderly and in chronic alcoholics, that it produces deformity of the unborn baby and an increased tendency to miscarriage, and that its LSD-like effects may encourage experimentation with LSD. Furthermore, some people claim that the drug interferes with the white blood cells and their protecting role in virus infections. None of these claims is proven. They all require careful examination and further research.

Marijuana accumulates in the body. Tolerance to its effects is thought to develop, and withdrawal in heavy users may produce depression and anxiety, tremor, and insomnia. The long-term effects of marijuana on the individual are still undefined, its effects on motor driving ability have not been clearly stated, and its long-term social effects are still unrecognized.

## LSD

LSD (d-lysergic acid diethylamide), or simply "acid," produces incredible effects upon the mind with minor effects upon the body. It is active in minute doses. LSD is a semisynthetic derivative of lysergic acid, an ergot alkaloid produced by a parasitic fungus sometimes found on rye and other grain.

It was in the mid-forties that interest in its effects upon the mind gained publicity in scientific and medical circles. Because some of its effects were thought to resemble schizophrenia, LSD was called a psychotomimetic (mimicking psychosis) drug and was used by psychiatrists in the vain hope that it would enable them to understand this disorder more clearly. However, it was eventually realized that the mind effects of LSD are different from schizophrenia and it became known as a hallucinogenic (hallucination-producing) or illusinogenic (illusion-producing) drug. Subsequently in the fifties it was used in psychotherapy and became known by the general term "psychedelic" —mind-manifesting—a term which not only rapidly caught on but became a cant word during the early sixties.

Although psychedelic drugs have been used for thousands of years by various cultures in religious ceremonies, they received little real attention in the West until the 1950s, when a few academics and artists started experimenting with them. In the early 1960s the use of these drugs became almost a religion in itself. By the late 1960s governments had introduced legislation which made LSD possession a criminal offense. It is, however, almost impossible to detect this substance. It is tasteless, odorless, colorless in solution, and can be taken in minute doses. It may be taken by mouth, sniffed in powdered form, or injected in solution. A dose may be so minute that it is easily hidden and taken in sugar cubes or biscuits, from blotting paper, and so on. It is quickly absorbed from the gut and distributed around the body. In pregnant women it enters the unborn baby. Its physical effects on the body— while secondary to the mental effects—can include dilatation of the pupils, increase in blood pressure, rapid beating of the heart, tremor, nausea, muscle weakness, a rise in body temperature, sweating, headache, flushing of the face, goose pimples, chills, alertness, insomnia, decreased appetite, increased reflexes, and—very rarely—convulsions.

Like marijuana, the effects of LSD on the mind are not predictable and depend on many factors, such as the personality of the individual, what he expects and has been led to expect from the drug, the place where he takes it, and whether he is with friends who have had experience using it. The social setting in which he takes the drug may affect his response even more than the size of the dose. Larger doses prolong the duration of a "trip" but do not seem to alter its nature or intensity.

The experiences felt under LSD are very personal to the taker and may vary from one trip to another. However, there are recognized adverse effects. In a "freak-out," for example, the individual experiences panic, fear, hallucinations, and depression, symptoms just like those of an acute mental breakdown. Freak-outs are usually of short duration but may occasionally be prolonged. Other individuals under the influence of LSD may experience fear, illusions, and depression, and they may indulge in antisocial behavior. Others may relive past experiences and undergo severe emotional feelings as past conflicts are brought to the surface. Some may experience periods of "mad" thoughts. Others may have increased sensory perception with synesthesia, a "crossover" of sensations in which sounds may be seen, and colors and shapes may appear more beautiful. Some may feel joy and peace and a feeling of transcendence of time and space, or feelings of holiness, insight, and awareness. This "religious" experience occurs in only a minority of individuals and it does not last long. However, it has received much publicity.

Bad trips, in which there is often a fear of death or insanity, seem more likely to occur when the individual is on his own or not with friends who understand the use of LSD. However, they may sometimes occur in individuals who have previously had good trips, and even when the user is surrounded by experienced users. A tranquilizer such as diazepam (Valium) can terminate a bad trip, although most users feel that this may be harmful in that it does not permit the user to work out the trip with the help of understanding friends. Certainly one of the worst things that can happen to someone on a bad trip is to be put in an ambulance and sent to a hospital, an experience that can be absolutely terrifying. Users in this situation need to be "talked down" by friends, not subjected to questioning by men in uniforms and doctors in white coats.

LSD occasionally triggers a prolonged mental breakdown (psychotic episode) which can last for many months. It is impossible to predict which individual will respond to "acid" in this way; some claim that the drug merely triggers an underlying psychotic predisposition which would have developed anyway. Suicide is rare, but accidental deaths while on a trip are not rare. These accidental deaths generally occur because of delusions about being able to fly or feelings of indestructibility. "Flashbacks" or "echoes" of experiences under LSD may occur for many months. Although they are transient, they may be disturbing if the previous trip was a bad one.

Tolerance to the psychedelic effects of LSD develops with repeated use, although this is more related to the interval of time between dosage than to the actual dose. Paradoxically, experienced users may need a smaller dose than beginners to produce the same effects. Physical dependence does not occur, and psychological dependence is unlikely when the use of LSD is intermittent.

## Volatile Substances

Inhalation of volatile substances and gases for "kicks" has been known for many years. These intoxicants include glues, cements, dry-cleaning fluids, paints, lacquers, sprays, gasoline, kerosene, various petroleum products, lighter fuel, nail polish remover, aerosols, nitrous oxide, ether and chloroform used in anesthetics, and many other products. The general effects produced by these drugs are stimulation followed by sedation accompanied by floating, distant feelings, timelessness, and illusions. Frequently they are also associated with confusion, drunkenness, slurred speech, headache, nausea, and vomiting. Finally, the user goes into stupor and then unconsciousness. Some people may develop panic, fear, or acute mental breakdown, or exhibit antisocial behavior and aggression.

The use of these substances for "kicks" may produce ulcers on the nose and mouth, liver damage, kidney damage, blood disorders, gastroenteritis, loss of appetite, self-neglect and death due to overdose, inhalation of vomit, damage to lung tissue, or heart failure.

# OVER-THE-COUNTER DRUGS

There are numerous drug preparations which can be bought over the counter which no doctor would ever prescribe or be allowed to prescribe. Many of them are combinations of drugs, labeled with a brand name and sold at a much higher price than the drugs would cost if sold separately. Often these combinations contain doses of drugs which are too small to be effective. Others contain drugs which are considered useless or obsolete. The same drugs, in the same doses, under different brand names, may be widely advertised for the treatment of many different disorders. Extravagant claims are often made for the benefits of some over-the-counter drugs without any real supportive evidence. Yet we go on buying them, influenced in many cases by heavy sales promotion on television and in the press.

Despite the surplus of dubious over-the-counter drugs, there is a sufficient number of effective preparations available for most of our needs. I hope to see self-treatment become increasingly important in dealing with commonly occurring disorders. I should like to see self-prevention of disease increase too, with each person giving up smoking and overeating and driving under the influence of alcohol. But if self-treatment is to improve, people must know about the most appropriate preparations to buy. You need to be able to select drugs which will give you the most benefits for the least risks and the smallest expense. The best guide is to choose over-the-counter preparations which contain drugs which doctors do prescribe and in doses which are likely to be effective.

You can find out which drugs doctors prescribe for all sorts of different conditions by reading Part II of this book. Having decided that your particular disorder can probably be best treated with one or two drugs, you can then find out more about these drugs, their effects and adverse effects and recommended dosages, by looking them up under their generic names in the pharmacopeia in Part III. Those drugs available only on a doctor's prescription are marked with an asterisk.

The index to this book will tell you where to find discussions of various common categories of over-the-counter drugs. For example, antacids are treated in the section on Drugs Used to Treat Indigestion and Peptic Ulcers (p. 74).

## Warning

Always consult your pharmacist before buying an over-the-counter preparation for babies, young children, elderly and/or debilitated patients, or for yourself if you are pregnant or breast-feeding. Always consult a doctor or pharmacist before giving such a preparation to anyone with impaired liver or kidney function or other serious long-term disorders.

Always ask the pharmacist for a measuring spoon if you buy a liquid medicine.

Always ask the pharmacist for instructions if you buy a drug preparation in a form you do not fully understand—such as suppositories or prolonged-release tablets.

Remember that a drug bought under its generic name will almost always be cheaper than the same drug bought under a brand name, but it may vary in effectiveness because of the way it is presented. Read about bioavailability under "Absorption," pp. 5–6.

BABY MEDICINES. Read about the types of drug which may be included in preparations used to relieve pain, p. 113, indigestion, p. 74, and constipation, p. 82, to relieve cold symptoms, p. 132, and to treat skin disorders, p. 193. This should help you see that the use of such drug preparations in babies is usually unnecessary or ineffective—or harmful.

COLD REMEDIES. Read section Drugs Used to Treat Common Colds, p. 132.

COLD SORE TREATMENTS. See p. 208 in section Drugs Used to Treat Skin Disorders.

CORN AND WART REMEDIES. See pp. 208 and 210 in section Drugs Used to Treat Skin Disorders.

COUGH REMEDIES. Read section Drugs Used to Treat Coughs, p. 135.

DIARRHEA REMEDIES. Read section Drugs Used to Treat Diarrhea, p. 80.

EYE LOTIONS AND DROPS. It is advisable not to purchase any of these preparations. If you have any eye disorder which you feel needs treating, consult your doctor.

EAR DROPS. It is advisable not to purchase any of these preparations. If you have an ear disorder which you feel needs treating, consult your doctor.

HEMORRHOID TREATMENTS. Never diagnose hemorrhoids yourself—always consult a doctor. After getting a correct diagnosis, use what the doctor prescribes. For a change, you may also consult your pharmacist. Never use sprays. Read about astringents, p. 205, and local anesthetic applications, p. 204, in the section Drugs Used to Treat Skin Disorders.

LAXATIVES. Read section Drugs Used to Treat Constipation, p. 82.

MOTION SICKNESS REMEDIES. Read section Drugs Used to Treat Nausea, Vomiting, and Motion Sickness, p. 71.

MOUTH ULCER REMEDIES. Read about drugs used to treat mouth ulcers on p. 209 in the section Drugs Used to Treat Skin Disorders.

MUSCLE PAINS AND FIBROSITIS REMEDIES. Read about rheumatic liniments and rubs on pp. 202–3 and read section Aspirin, Nonnarcotic Pain Relievers, and Drugs Used to Treat Rheumatism and Arthritis, p. 118.

MENSTRUAL PAIN RELIEVERS. These usually contain one or more pain relievers such as aspirin, acetaminophen, codeine, salicylamide. You can learn about these by reading the two sections Morphine and Narcotic Pain Relievers, p. 115, and Aspirin, Nonnarcotic Pain Relievers, and Drugs Used to Treat Rheumatism and Arthritis, p. 118. In addition, they often contain an atropinelike drug to prevent painful spasms. Many of these nonprescription preparations contain such small doses of atropinelike drugs as to be ineffective. See atropine in Part III, and the section Drugs Which Act on the Autonomic Nervous System, p. 145. If menstrual pains are incapacitating, it is worth consulting your doctor.

HEALTH SALTS, RHEUMATIC SALTS, BACKACHE SALTS, ETC. Most of these contain saline laxatives; see p. 84. You do not have to belch and have loose bowel movements in order to be healthy.

BATH SALTS. Forget the salts and have a hot, soothing, relaxing bath.

LIVER PILLS, ETC. These contain laxatives; see p. 82.

ANTISMOKING AIDS. There is no convincing evidence that they work, but if you think they will, they may. Read about lobeline in Part III.

DIAPER RASH TREATMENTS. Read about drugs used in the treatment of diaper rash, p. 208, in the section Drugs Used to Treat Skin Disorders.

DRUGS USED TO CLEAR THE NOSE AND/OR STOP ITS RUNNING. Read sections Drugs Used to Treat Common Colds, p. 132, and Drugs Used to Treat Coughs, p. 135. In these sections you will learn about the drugs used to clear the nasal passages and about those used to dry up secretions.

SKIN TREATMENTS. Read section Drugs Used to Treat Skin Disorders, p. 193.

TEETHING PREPARATIONS. Any soothing application to the gums is quickly washed away in the saliva, and therefore teething applications are of little use. Among those used in the past, some have been very dangerous (e.g., those which contained mercury). Many now contain a local anesthetic; see p. 191.

THROAT REMEDIES. Read sections Drugs Used to Treat Common Colds, p. 132, and Drugs Used to Treat Coughs, p. 135.

VITAMIN PREPARATIONS. Read section Vitamins, p. 155.

IRON PREPARATIONS. Read section Iron, p. 152.

TONICS. Read section Tonics, p. 65.

WORM TREATMENTS. See piperazine and pyrvinium in Part III.

ANTIPERSPIRANTS. Read about antiperspirants on p. 206 in the section Drugs Used to Treat Skin Disorders.

DEODORANTS. Read about deodorants on p. 206 in the section Drugs Used to Treat Skin Disorders.

HAIR AND SCALP APPLICATIONS. If you have a persistent or recurrent scalp disorder, consult your doctor, particularly if it is worrying you. See "Dandruff," p. 208, and selenium in Part III.

ANTIHISTAMINE DRUGS. Read section Antihistamine Drugs, p. 127.

SEDATIVES AND SLEEPING DRUGS. Read section Sleeping Drugs and Sedatives, p. 43.

SUNBURN REMEDIES. See p. 196 in section Drugs Used to Treat Skin Disorders.

REDUCING AIDS. Read section Reducing Drugs, p. 68.

STIMULANTS. Read section Stimulants: Caffeine, p. 63.

# PART II

# GROUPS AND TYPES OF DRUGS

# PSYCHOTROPIC DRUGS

Drugs which affect the mood are called psychotropic drugs. Because so little is known about the causes of psychological disorders and the actions of psychotropic drugs, the various groups are usually classified according to their main effects. Hypnotics induce sleep, and sedatives calm a person without sending him to sleep. A small dose of hypnotic also sedates, and therefore this group of drugs is called hypnosedative. A tranquilizer calms a person without impairing consciousness. Tranquilizers are divided into two groups: *major* and *minor*. Major tranquilizers are of use in treating serious disorders such as mania and schizophrenia and are often called antipsychotic drugs. They also produce a neuroleptic state (see p. 53) and are sometimes called neuroleptics. The minor tranquilizers are so termed because they are not effective in serious psychological disorders, and also to distinguish them from sedatives. Some people call minor tranquilizers antianxiety drugs or anxiolytics because they are used to treat patients suffering from anxiety. Others talk about anxiolytic sedatives and include sedatives and minor tranquilizers under this group. Having given you sufficient indication of the confusion which exists, I will, for the purpose of this book, talk about hypnotics, sedatives, minor tranquilizers, and major tranquilizers.

The other two main groups of psychotropic drugs which doctors use are called antidepressants, which seems fine until you try to define depression (see p. 56); and stimulants (e.g., amphetamines), which lift mood.

## SLEEPING DRUGS AND SEDATIVES

### Sleep
Sleep requirements vary from person to person. "Normal" sleep is what suits you under ordinary everyday circumstances. The amount of sleep you need is as distinctive as your appetite or your conscience. If your sleep is disturbed for only a night or two, this is usually of no consequence; but if the disturbance persists for two or more weeks, you have a sleep problem and need to take action.

"Insomnia" means "sleeplessness," but nowadays it is a term used to describe most sleeping difficulties. These include difficulty in getting to sleep, inability to stay asleep, frequent wakenings, restless sleep with nightmares, early morning wakening, and sleep which is not refreshing.

There are many causes of sleep disturbance: social, physical, or mental. Among social causes are changes in environment—a strange bed or bedroom, variations in temperature, noise, or motion, or changes of routine, such as going on a night shift. Pain from any cause, irritation of the skin, discomfort from indigestion, and muscle cramps are some of the physical causes of disturbed sleep. Emotional disorders are a common cause of persistent insomnia. However, remember that social, physical, and mental factors are interrelated. Problems at work may produce anxiety, which may produce insomnia. Persistent noise at night may interfere with sleep which may cause you to worry about lack of sleep, which may then produce tension and irritability, resulting in further difficulty in sleeping. The death of a close friend or relative, the loss of a job, failure at work or in an examination, may trigger a depressive episode, a prominent symptom of which may be disturbed sleep.

Insomnia must always be regarded as a symptom of some underlying disorder. This is of particular importance in psychological disorders, especially in those patients who feel anxious, tense, and/or miserable. In such patients insomnia may be only one of a group of mental or physical symptoms experienced. It is, therefore, wrong to use sleeping drugs as the only form of treatment, particularly barbiturates, which only make you feel more tense and miserable when used over a period of time.

Drugs may even cause insomnia. For example, caffeine in tea, coffee, and cocoa may keep you awake, particularly as you get older. Regular alcohol drinkers may find themselves waking early, and people who take heroin or morphine may find their sleep impaired. Amphetamines, most reducing drugs, and some antidepressant drugs may keep you awake. So may some drugs used to treat rhinitis, colds, and asthma.

We really know very little about sleep and its function. It may be related to various anatomical structures in the brain and to certain chemical changes. It also produces electrical changes in the brain, eyes, and muscles (detected by electromyogram, EMG); eye movements (detected by electrooculogram, EOG); and brain waves (detected by electroencephalogram, EEG). From these tests two main kinds of "normal" sleep activity have been defined: a stage of nonrapid eye movements (NREM sleep) is followed by a stage of rapid eye movements (REM sleep). NREM sleep is called orthodox sleep and is the stage when we "think"; REM sleep is called paradoxical sleep and is the stage when we "dream." From these easily measured changes it seems that both stages of sleep are essential for health.

Tests have shown us that sleeping drugs disrupt normal sleeping patterns as recorded by these instruments. Most sleeping drugs suppress paradoxical sleep, but when these drugs are stopped paradoxical sleep increases, as if the body wants to catch up on it. Since paradoxical sleep is associated with dreaming, withdrawal of sleeping drugs (even after a few nights) may result in restless sleep with dreaming and nightmares. These withdrawal effects make the individual think that he is unable to sleep without sleeping drugs, while in fact the drug itself is responsible for the disturbed sleep. If you have been taking sleeping drugs nightly for weeks, months, or years and wish to stop them, you must reduce the dose very slowly over several weeks. It is better to consult your doctor, who will be able to give you a smaller dose preparation. Alternatively, he may change you to a drug which has less effect upon paradoxical sleep than do the barbiturates and other sleeping drugs. (Barbiturates also may lose their hypnotic power after several weeks of continued use.) A period of several weeks on one of these nonbarbiturate drugs (e.g., diazepam, flurazepam) in full dosage followed by a gradual reduction in dosage over several weeks may enable you to break a long-lasting sleeping drug habit. Even so, you are bound to have many restless nights until your brain gets used to sleep without drugs. It may take from one to two months.

## Hypnosedatives

These drugs depress brain function. In small doses they are used as sedatives and in larger doses as hypnotics. The barbiturates have been studied most, and much of what we know about their action and effects also applies to other hypnosedatives.

All hypnosedatives are habit-forming, so you can quickly become psychologically dependent upon them. The restless sleep which results when you stop these drugs also strengthens your psychological dependence. This is further complicated by the fact that four in ten patients sleep well on dummy sleeping tablets, which means that in addition to the drug's chemical effects upon the body there appears to be something "addictive" in the mere nightly ritual of *taking* sleeping tablets.

Like alcohol, they cause intoxication if taken regularly in a dosage above that normally recommended, and those which are long-acting may produce a hangover. Further, elderly and/or debilitated patients or those with impaired heart, kidney, or liver function may develop intoxication at "normal" dosage. Signs of intoxication are similar to those caused by alcohol—confusion, difficulty in speaking, unsteadiness on the feet, poor memory, faulty judgment, irritability, overemotion, hostility, suspicious and suicidal tendencies.

Physical dependence (see Dependence on Drugs, p. 23) may occur with all hypnosedatives, with resultant withdrawal symptoms when the drug is suddenly stopped. These include anxiety, trembling, weakness, dizziness, nausea, vomiting, convulsions, delirium, and sometimes death. However, considering the number of patients who take these drugs regularly, the incidence of physical dependence is low. Psychological dependence is, however, common. Tolerance (see p. 24) may develop to all hypnosedatives. This means that you will get less effect from the same dose over time, and therefore there is always the danger that you may increase the dose in order to make it work. With the barbiturates an increased breakdown in the liver may occur, producing a decreased sleeping time and an increase in the average dose required to maintain sleep. Yet it is surprising how many patients stay on these drugs for years and years without increasing the dose. Even so, tolerance is a danger, and if you find yourself having to increase the dose of your sedative or hypnotic to get the same effect, consult your doctor—you are in danger of becoming addicted.

If you drink alcohol regularly you ought not to take hypnosedatives regularly. This is because alcohol is also a depressant of the brain, and tolerance may develop to alcohol. It is quite easy to take an overdose of either, and the combination of alcohol with a hypnosedative may be fatal. Do not forget, therefore, that although you may be able to tolerate an increased dose of alcohol *or* hypnosedative the lethal dose of these drugs combined remains unaltered, and the combined dose can prove rapidly fatal. Another important point to remember is that hypnosedative drugs (especially barbiturates) can actually make you anxious, irritable, and depressed. Since your doctor probably put you on these drugs in the first place in order to control such symptoms, you or he may be tempted to increase the dose in order to control the symptoms further. Yet the increased dose will actually make you worse. This also applies to alcohol. So remember that if you are getting anxious and miserable despite the use of more alcohol and/or sleeping drugs or sedatives, it is probably the drugs themselves that are to blame. Many people have become trapped on this downward course. It may end in suicide. The deliberate taking of an overdose of barbiturates with suicidal intent accounts for most serious cases of overdose, but accidentally self-administered overdose is not uncommon as a result of what is called "drug automatism." If you take a dose of sleeping drug and fail to fall asleep you may reach out and take another dose. The effects of this increased dose may make you confused, and you may take further doses without knowing (or subsequently remembering). Therefore, never keep sleeping drugs by your bedside. Keep them locked in a drug cabinet in the bathroom or kitchen. Take only the recommended dose and leave the bottle in the locked cabinet. If you are responsible for, or live with, someone who is elderly, debilitated, or depressed and on sleeping drugs, supervise the administration of the drugs.

Don't forget that if you are tense or miserable, alcohol and hypnosedative drugs, although calming you at first, may eventually make you feel worse. You may sleep all right and awake feeling less tense, only to become tired, irritable, and bad-tempered later in the day. One more important point to remember about these drugs (especially barbiturates and alcohol) is that they may reduce the effects of antidepressant drugs.

Hypnosedatives impair learned behavior and interfere with your power to concentrate. Therefore, watch your driving. They may also decrease pain perception, making them useful when given along with pain relievers; but they should not be taken alone for this purpose because they may cause restlessness and confusion in the presence of pain. Hypnosedatives depress a wide range of functions in many vital organs, particularly nerves, muscles, respiration, and the heart and circulation. They may produce any state from mild sedation to confusion and unconsciousness. Like alcohol, they produce different effects according to the situation in which they are taken. At a discotheque they may produce excitement, while if taken on retiring to bed they may produce sleep. The combination of a strange environment (for instance, a hospital ward) and a dose of hypnosedative may make elderly patients very confused and disoriented. This is a warning against the habit of giving patients sleeping drugs as a routine just because they are in the hospital; although very convenient for the night staff, it is often not necessary and may lead to the development of the sleeping drug habit when the patient returns home. Also, there is some evidence that drug-induced sleep may interfere with the normal restorative functions of sleep. Barbiturates and other hypnosedatives must be used with special caution in patients with chest and heart disorders.

Don't forget that sleep produced by drugs is *not* natural. Remember also that most sleep studies have dealt only with brief periods of drug administration in "normal" subjects. The effects of long-term use of drugs in patients with impaired sleep rhythm are not known.

## The Use of Sleeping Drugs

It is perfectly sensible to take sleeping drugs now and again during periods of stress (for example, after a bereavement), or after periods of intense work when you just cannot relax, or intermittently through long periods of stress or when traveling or working shifts. In such circumstances they should be taken for a few nights in a row at most. It is accepted that the sleeping-drug habit is a real risk after several weeks of drug-induced sleep. If you have a persistent sleep problem, you ought to consult your doctor. Of course, sleeping drugs alone may not be the answer. Do not forget that emotional problems are a common cause of sleep disturbance, and these may produce many symptoms in addition to insomnia. They include frequent headaches, anxious or tense feelings, sadness, depression, weepiness, backaches, pains in the chest, indigestion, dizziness, lack of energy, fed-up feelings, touchiness, fears about your health or about going out by yourself, loss of appetite, loss of interest in sex, loss of weight, palpitations, feelings of guilt, unwanted feelings, or suspicions that people are talking about you. These are only some of the symptoms which should help your doctor diagnose a psychological disorder and organize appropriate treatment.

If you have a psychological disorder, the use of barbiturates or other hypnosedatives may aggravate your condition, especially if you are feeling miserable. It is important for your doctor to recognize what are labeled as depressive disorders because they produce characteristic sleep disturbances and because antidepressant drugs may be very effective in relieving the symptoms (see p. 56). These drugs not only help to restore your sleep rhythm, they also relieve many other symptoms which may interfere with your ability to cope with normal life when you are depressed. Once your symptoms have disappeared you will be able to cope, but you will still need support and advice. This again highlights the importance of the initial treatment of insomnia. You and your doctor need to consider together as many as possible of the factors that may be causing your insomnia.

What about those patients who have developed the habit of regularly taking sleeping drugs every night? They are often elderly, and many of them are widows. There may be no harm in letting them continue, provided they are not depressed, anxious, tense, or drinking alcohol regularly; and provided they do not increase the dose, show signs of intoxication, or have impaired kidney, heart, or liver function. They may come to little harm even if they are psychologically dependent. I think it would be wrong to give them guilt feelings about being on drugs, but it may be advisable to ask your doctor to change them slowly to a drug such as diazepam or flurazepam and then gradually to wean them from that. Perhaps in the future, with more careful understanding of insomnia, the long-term use of sleeping drugs may decrease.

In the treatment of insomnia there are many alternatives to sleeping drugs: a hot bath before retiring, reading a book, taking a walk, not having too large an evening meal, cutting down on coffee, tea, or cocoa in the evening, reducing smoking, reducing alcohol intake, trying to get some regular exercise and fresh air during the day, and probably most important of all—being taught how to relax. The ritual just before going to bed may condition you to go to sleep—undressing, washing, and so on. A milk-cereal drink may help you sleep more peacefully. A warm drink and a biscuit may help the older patient; but if you have pain, discomfort, or irritation of the skin you will need more specific treatment from your doctor.

## The Types of Hypnosedatives

### BARBITURATES

Barbituric acid was discovered in 1864. Its derivatives are called bar-biturates, and many of them can produce sleep. The first barbiturate sleeping drug (barbital) was introduced in 1903 under the trade name Veronal. The second-oldest barbiturate is phenobarbital, introduced in 1912 and marketed under the trade name Luminal. Since then hundreds of barbiturate sleeping drugs have been introduced. They are marketed in a multitude of shapes, colors, and sizes, as capsules, tablets, syrups, mixtures, and powders, and they are mixed with all kinds of other drugs from vitamins to antacids. Those used as sedatives or hypnotics have similar actions and effects, but some of them vary in their duration of action and in their methods of elimination from the body. Of those barbiturates used to produce sleep, duration of effect is usually about six or seven hours and the incidence of hangover is the same with all. Some of them may vary in intensity of effect, and, of course, there is always variation among individual responses to such drugs. Some barbiturates are broken down slowly in the body and excreted partly unchanged in the urine. They therefore have a long duration of effect (twelve to twenty-four hours). Such barbiturates include barbital, barbital sodium, phenobarbital, and phenobarbital sodium. These are often called "long-acting" barbiturates and are used more as sedatives than hypnotics. Another group is broken down fairly rapidly in the liver and only a small proportion is excreted unchanged in the urine. These drugs have a shorter duration of effect (about six or seven hours) and are referred to as intermediate-acting barbiturates. They include amobarbital, amobarbital sodium, butabarbital, pen-tobarbital sodium, hexobarbital, and secobarbital. The very short-acting barbiturates (e.g., thiopental sodium) are used as intravenous anesthetics.

Barbiturates produce tolerance, psychological dependence, physical dependence, and withdrawal symptoms (see p. 29). They increase the action of alcohol, and they are a common agent in accidental or intentional overdose. The signs of intoxication are similar to those produced by alcohol. Barbiturates are involved in complex chemical processes in the liver, and in patients suffering from a disease called porphyria (a rare congenital metabolic disease) they can trigger an acute attack resulting in abdominal colic, paralysis, confusion, and even death. They should be used with utmost caution by patients who are taking other sedatives, minor tranquilizers, major tranquilizers, alcohol, and antihistamines. They can affect the speed of breakdown of other drugs (e.g., oral contraceptives) in the liver, thus making those drugs less effective.

NONBARBITURATE HYPNOSEDATIVES

All nonbarbiturate hypnotics and sedatives depress brain function, and like the barbiturates they may produce tolerance or addiction, increase the effects of alcohol, interfere with ability to drive motor vehicles and operate moving machinery, and produce intoxication like alcohol.

BROMIDE was widely prescribed during the last half of the nineteenth century, and many patients developed bromide intoxication. Psychiatric wards often contained patients suffering from impaired memory, drowsiness, delirium, trembling, slurred speech, hallucinations, and skin rashes caused by bromide intoxication. Bromide, if taken daily, accumulates to reach a toxic level over several weeks. It should not be used, and yet it appears in some over-the-counter preparations.

CHLORAL HYDRATE is the oldest sleeping drug. It tastes horrible and irritates the stomach. It has less effect on paradoxical sleep than the barbiturates but may cause excitement and delirium if given to the patient in pain. Acute poisoning may occur from a mixture of alcohol and chloral hydrate—known as a Mickey Finn.

TRICHLORETHANOL is the active breakdown product of chloral hydrate, and a stable form of this is available as triclofos. PARALDEHYDE is a useful hypnotic but has an awful taste and makes the breath smell because a portion of it is excreted in the breath. It has to be given by injection or by enema. GLUTETHIMIDE has no particular advantage over other hypnotics which can be taken by mouth, nor has METHAQUALONE or METHYPRYLON or ETHCHLORVYNOL.

## Antihistamine Drugs Used to Produce Sleep

Antihistamine drugs (e.g., doxylamine, hydroxyzine, and methapyrilene) produce drowsiness as a side effect. This is sometimes promoted to produce sleep. An antihistamine may also be combined with a hypnotic drug to produce sleep because antihistamines increase the effects of hypnotics. Antihistamines which produce sedation are useful for promoting sleep in patients with skin irritations and in patients who may be kept awake by allergic symptoms. Some anticholinergic drugs (e.g., scopolamine) which act on the brain (see p. 147) are also promoted as sedatives, and so are some major tranquilizers. Many nonprescribed drugs contain methapyrilene, sometimes along with scopolamine, despite the fact that the hypnotic effect of methapyrilene is unreliable. There are great dangers in using these drugs to promote sleep, because sleep cannot be improved merely by increasing the dose. Rather the reverse happens, and after a large dose excitation occurs. This may result in restlessness, agitation, and convulsions. In young children, even the recommended doses can cause excitedness and restlessness.

### Benzodiazepines Used to Produce Sleep
The benzodiazepines are discussed under minor tranquilizers, below. They are the most widely prescribed antianxiety drugs, particularly chlordiazepoxide and diazepam. Any benzodiazepine in high enough dose will produce sleep, but the one marketed specifically for this purpose is flurazepam.

### Sleeping Drugs of Choice
To produce sleep for an occasional night or for several nights the choice of sleeping drugs is not critical. However, the benzodiazepines have several advantages over the barbiturates and nonbarbiturate hypnotics. They are fast becoming the drugs of choice, particularly if regular nightly use is considered necessary. They are especially useful if you are tense or anxious. In addition, benzodiazepines are significantly safer in cases of overdose. If your sleep disturbance is part of a depressive disorder, you would probably benefit more from a sedative tricyclic antidepressant drug taken at night. For this and other reasons, if you have a persistent sleep problem you ought to consult your doctor. Chloral hydrate is an alternative sleeping drug, particularly in children and the elderly.

## MINOR TRANQUILIZERS

Minor tranquilizers are primarily used to treat anxiety. They include the benzodiazepines (also widely used as hypnotics), meprobamate, and a miscellaneous group of related drugs.

### The Benzodiazepine Compounds
These, the most widely prescribed drugs in the Western world, include chlordiazepoxide, diazepam, oxazepam, clorazepate, and flurazepam. Compounds of this type were discovered in 1933, but it was not until 1960 that chlordiazepoxide was shown to produce "taming" in wild

animals. This taming effect was then shown to work on monkeys, and subsequent clinical trials carried out in human beings demonstrated that the drug suppressed anxiety.

The benzodiazepines produce four main effects. They sedate, combat anxiety, relax muscles, and act against convulsions. Flurazepam has been promoted as a sleep inducer, whereas chlordiazepoxide, diazepam, oxazepam, and clorazepate, have been promoted as antianxiety drugs. They are all anticonvulsants, but diazepam is the most popular for this purpose.

Most benzodiazepines are long-acting. All of them can interfere with driving ability and skills involved in operating moving machinery. They may sometimes increase the effects of alcohol. The most common adverse effects are drowsiness and lethargy. Drug dependence of the barbiturate/alcohol type, with withdrawal symptoms and convulsions, has in rare cases been connected with chlordiazepoxide and diazepam. They may cause a fall in blood pressure and stimulate the appetite. Sometimes paradoxical excitement may be set off by these drugs, so that instead of becoming calm, patients become excited and look and act as though they are drunk.

## Meprobamate

Meprobamate was developed in 1954, and it soon became widely prescribed as an antianxiety drug. It produces less drowsiness than the barbiturates. It has slight muscle-relaxant and anticonvulsant properties. Meprobamate, like the barbiturates, affects the metabolism of other drugs in the liver. Tolerance and psychological and physical drug dependence with withdrawal symptoms of the barbiturate/alcohol type occur. Other drugs related to meprobamate are tybamate, carisoprodol, and ethinamate.

## Miscellaneous Antianxiety Drugs

These are numerous and include hydroxyzine, chlormezanone, mephenoxalone, and oxanamide. Increasingly, antidepressant drugs which possess sedating properties are being used to treat anxiety, and several major tranquilizers (see facing page) are marketed in small doses as antianxiety drugs.

## Drugs of Choice in Anxiety

The barbiturates are dangerous in overdose, cause drug dependence, aggravate tension and depression, and interfere with certain enzymes in the liver. The benzodiazepines offer more flexibility between the dose required to produce relief of anxiety and the dose required to produce sleep. They are relatively safe in overdose. The difference between the dose of a barbiturate used to produce sedation and that used to produce sleep is small, and thus drowsiness is always a problem when barbiturates are used as sedatives.

Considering all the problems involved in defining, recognizing, and treating anxiety, it seems reasonable to recommend benzodiazepines as drugs of choice if you and your doctor feel that drug treatment is necessary. They should be used intermittently if they are to produce their most desired effect. This is because tolerance to their beneficial effects develops and the severity of anxiety fluctuates, so it is better to push up the dose when you are very tense and decrease a step when you feel better—provided of course that you do not exceed the recommended dose and that your doctor is aware of what you are doing.

## MAJOR TRANQUILIZERS

The major tranquilizers are drugs used to treat serious psychological disorders (often labeled psychoses), such as schizophrenia and mania, and acute confusional states, dementia, behavior disorders, and personality disorders. Since they may also produce a state of emotional quietness and indifference called neurolepsy, they may be called neuroleptics. In addition, they are frequently prescribed (in small doses) for the treatment of anxiety, tension, and agitation, and some of them are used to treat dizziness, nausea, and vomiting.

The main groups of major tranquilizers are phenothiazines, rauwolfia alkaloids, thioxanthine derivatives, and butyrophenones.

PHENOTHIAZINES are the most widely used major tranquilizers; between twenty and thirty products are available. About half of them are used to treat psychological disorders and to treat nausea, vomiting, and dizziness. Others have antihistamine properties, some relieve itching, and some are used to treat Parkinsonism. All phenothiazines share a common chemical structure, but because of minor variations there are three principal groups: aliphatic (e.g., chlorpromazine); piperidine (e.g., thioridazine); and piperazine (e.g., fluphenazine, trifluoperazine, perphenazine, and prochlorperazine).

These compounds are very similar in their effects and uses. Chlorpromazine, the first to be discovered (and still one of the most useful), will be discussed here. It produces considerable sedation, but it differs from that produced by the barbiturates in that the patient on chlorpromazine may be easily awakened. It impairs the ability of animals to make a conditioned response (for instance, a response to a learned signal such as an electric buzzer) but not an unconditioned response (such as escape). Barbiturates affect both conditioned and unconditioned responses. Sustained attention is impaired by chlorpromazine.

It also diminishes spontaneous aggressive activity, and thus may be used to tame wild animals. It produces changes in all parts of the nervous system. It generally produces muscle relaxation but may cause muscle rigidity and trembling (Parkinsonism). By causing dilation of the blood vessels in the skin and by acting on control centers in the brain it may cause the body temperature to drop. It may increase the effects of all depressant drugs—alcohol, hypnotics, sedatives, and anesthetics. It affects the heart and blood vessels, producing a fall in blood pressure and changes in heart rate.

Chlorpromazine controls overactive and manic patients without impairing consciousness. It relieves many symptoms of schizophrenia and modifies behavior, making the patient more socially compliant. It calms agitation and is useful in the treatment of drug- or disease-induced vomiting but is of no value in treating motion sickness. It produces many adverse effects, including liver damage. (Read about these in Part III.)

Other phenothiazines resemble chlorpromazine but differ in the amount of sedation they produce, in their effect on blood pressure, and in adverse effects such as Parkinsonism and other changes in muscle tone. The piperidine group (e.g., thioridazine) produce strong atropine-like effects (see p. 146), and thioridazine in high dose may cause pigmentation of the retina and impaired vision. Members of the piperazine group have a stimulant effect and cause less liver damage, but they may produce serious changes affecting muscular movements and coordination, which may be crippling and permanent.

The phenothiazines have revolutionized the symptomatic treatment of serious psychological disorders and have enabled patients to be treated in the community rather than being locked away in a psychiatric hospital. They are not curative, but they do relieve distressing symptoms such as thought disturbances, paranoid symptoms, delusions, loss of self-care, social withdrawal, anxiety, and agitation. Patients may need to take a daily maintenance dose for many years, because it has been observed that failure to take a regular dose may lead to relapse and the necessity of hospitalization.

A high proportion of those patients who have been labeled schizophrenic can stop using the drugs after a year or two without relapse. It is therefore important that they are seen regularly by a psychiatrist. Note also that relapse may not occur until two to eight weeks after stopping the drugs.

Chlorpromazine is the drug of choice if sedation is required, and a piperazine phenothiazine (e.g., fluphenazine, perphenazine, trifluoperazine) if stimulation is required. It is important that any doctor prescribing phenothiazines get to know one of each group well. He should not let himself be confused by the number of new drugs which are appearing faster than they can be compared with already established drugs. Long-lasting injections of fluphenazine are now available and have improved the management of some schizophrenic patients in the community. If you are a patient receiving such injections, you should carry a warning card and be seen regularly by your doctor, because the drug given in this way can affect the heart and circulation and also cause severe depression. Remember that the toxicity of phenothiazines is more pronounced in children.

RAUWOLFIA ALKALOIDS and related drugs are no longer in use, with the rare exception of reserpine (used to treat high blood pressure). These were prescribed enthusiastically throughout the fifties but have now been replaced by the phenothiazines. Rauwolfia alkaloids come from the roots of an Indian climbing shrub *(Rauwolfia serpentina)*. Used to treat psychoses and also high blood pressure, reserpine was soon discovered to have a most serious adverse effect—it produced mental depression, sometimes leading to suicide. It is now agreed that these drugs should not be used to treat psychological disorders. For their use in treating blood pressure, see the section Drugs Used to Treat Raised Blood Pressure, p. 108.

THIOXANTHINE DERIVATIVES such as thiothixene and chlorprothixene appear to offer no advantages over the phenothiazines.

BUTYROPHENONES (for example, haloperidol) resemble in their effects the piperazine phenothiazines. Haloperidol, the most frequently used, depresses the brain and has marked antivomiting properties. It is long-acting and is useful in the treatment of mania and excitement, delusions, hallucinations, and paranoia. It is also useful in treating a severe tic disorder in children called Gilles de la Tourette's disease. Trembling and muscle rigidity (Parkinsonism) occur frequently but are dose-related.

## The Use of Major Tranquilizers in Nonpsychotic Disorders

Phenothiazines and haloperidol are marketed in small-dose preparations for the relief of anxiety. Since major tranquilizers reduce drive and energy, most anxieties do not respond well to them. They may be useful to relieve anxiety and agitation in the early stages of treating depression, free-floating anxiety (anxiety coming on without apparent cause) in some patients, and confusion and agitation in elderly patients.

Some of them are also used to relieve nausea and vomiting and are often prescribed to treat dizziness and vertigo. They have been used in the treatment of alcohol and drug dependence, but most of them increase the tendency to convulsions, and so their use in the treatment of withdrawal symptoms (which often include convulsions) is not usually recommended. Toxic confusional states resulting from infections or metabolic disorders are sometimes helped by phenothiazines, as are certain dementias. Major tranquilizers may also be of use in disturbed mentally subnormal patients and in patients with involuntary movements. They can be used to increase the effects of pain relievers in patients with terminal cancer. The use of major tranquilizers in restraining overactive children and captive individuals (e.g., prisoners and inmates in psychiatric and geriatric hospitals) requires more critical analysis and assessment than it has so far received.

In conclusion, the major tranquilizers are useful and versatile drugs. They are, however, complex and potentially dangerous. If you are taking one of these drugs regularly, learn about it from Part III of this book and discuss your treatment with your doctor.

## ANTIDEPRESSANTS

Antidepressant drugs are prescribed to patients who are labeled by their doctors as suffering from "depression." But what is depression? We can all feel sad or happy, and some of us at times may feel very happy or very sad. These feelings are part of everyday life, so why do doctors talk about depression and why do some patients need drugs? Why can't they "just pull themselves together"? The fact is that many patients who go to their doctors for help have got sick of trying to pull themselves together. They may complain of various mental and/or physical symptoms and not feel or recognize that they are suffering from a psychological disorder.

Of course it is impossible to separate social, physical, and mental factors, but it is possible to recognize a group of symptoms which for want of a better term doctors now call "depression." Admittedly there is a continuum from feeling blue to feeling severely depressed and suicidal, and from feeling tired and fed up to possessing symptoms which interfere seriously with one's capacity to cope with everyday life. Feeling sad and miserable for long periods is not merely "feeling blue." Doctors would call it "depression." There can be many reasons for depression: social factors (for example, unemployment or bereavement); physical factors (the aftermath of virus infections such as influenza, continuous pain, irritation, or discomfort, surgery or a heart attack); or reactions to drug treatment (for instance, reserpine for blood pressure, cortisone for arthritis, and certain sulfonamide drugs). You may feel severely depressed after childbirth, during the menopause, or just before a menstrual period, or if you have vitamin deficiencies. But you may also be severely depressed for no "obvious" reason.

That last sort of "causeless" depressive episode is labeled endogenous (meaning "from inside"). Other depressive episodes may be termed reactive, meaning that there appears to be cause, such as a bereavement or loss of a job. However, let me state quite clearly that these are arbitrary labels. You cannot separate the social from the mental from the physical. But because of antidepressant drugs, doctors may now relieve painful physical and mental symptoms and enable patients to cope with everyday problems of living.

Along with feelings of depression (sad, miserable, weepy, suicidal), patients may develop changes in behavior. They may stop wanting to mix socially or go out in the evenings. They may develop physiological changes—alterations in sleep rhythm (particularly difficulty in getting to sleep or early morning wakening), alteration in appetite, weight, or sex drive, and loss of energy. They may develop physical symptoms —headaches, dizziness, chest pains, palpitations, dyspepsia, diarrhea, or backache. These symptoms may provoke fears that they have some physical disease such as cancer, heart disease, or tuberculosis. They may develop mental symptoms and feel unreal, divorced from themselves, as if they are looking from outside at themselves; they may have difficulty in concentrating or thinking; their memory may be affected, and they may keep thinking morbid thoughts about death, dying, and suicide. They may become very tense and anxious, as if something dreadful is going to happen all the time. Some develop fears, such as the fear of seeing people or the fear of going out. They may become very agitated and irritable or very withdrawn and quiet. Some become obsessive, some feel guilty, and some brood over all sorts of episodes from their past lives.

This is a very sketchy description of what doctors call depression. Patients may experience a few or many of these symptoms. Some symptoms may be mild and some intense, and according to his upbringing, his culture, his personality, and his environment, the patient will exhibit them in different ways. Certainly in Western society the puritan ethic of "being firm and standing on one's own two feet" may produce awful feelings of guilt and unworthiness in which suicide appears to be the only way out. The whole problem is far too complex to be merely labeled "depression." Some patients may need individual or group psychotherapy; others may respond to counseling or to drugs; some just want a new house and a check for $5,000; others want a new husband; others need to be taught how to relax; some may need electroshock therapy. Having stated some of the alternative types of therapy, since this book is about drugs I must discuss their use for these disorders.

The antidepressant drugs introduced since 1958 have greatly improved the treatment of depression. This has resulted in an impressive relief from suffering for patients and their relatives, a reduction in hospitalization and in electroshock treatments, and an involvement of family doctors in the treatment of such disorders. We must remember that drugs do not "cure" depressive disorders. Fortunately, however, many of the disorders are self-limiting, yielding to what is called spontaneous remission. Why give antidepressant drugs then? Doctors prescribe these drugs because within a few weeks of treatment, crippling symptoms may be relieved: the patient may start to sleep better, his energy and appetite return, his interests revive, his depression lifts, and he may begin to see how dreadful he has felt for months or years. But as the patient begins to sort himself out, a new problem arises for the doctor; having relieved the patient's symptoms he must not now forget to treat the patient. The duration of treatment may be short or long and may require the help of a clinical psychologist, psychotherapist, or psychiatrist. However, because the patient's symptoms are relieved, he may respond that much better to such therapy. This does not mean that all depressed patients need drugs—the decision to use antidepressants should be taken only after careful consideration of all the facts by the doctor.

Some of us can tolerate physical pain better than others, and some of us can tolerate mental pain better than others—but at some stage we all may need help. Some may respond better to one drug and not to another or to one doctor and not another. Some will respond to individual therapy and others to group therapy. We all vary. It is, therefore, as wrong to say that all depressed patients should receive drug therapy as it is to say that they should all have psychotherapy. What is certain, however, is that doctors within the limits of their present knowledge must aim at giving maximum benefit with minimum risks to the maximum number of patients. At present the responsible and rational use of drugs appears to offer the best hope of accomplishing this end.

There are two main groups of antidepressant drugs. The *monoamine oxidase inhibitors* (MAO inhibitors) were popular toward the end of the fifties. They have now fallen out of favor because of their potential for causing adverse effects. The *tricyclic compounds* were introduced in 1958 and are now the most widely prescribed antidepressant drugs.

Before the introduction of these two drug groups, amphetamines were the principal and most popular drug treatment for depression. But because they produce an initial lift in mood followed by a letdown, and because they became widely abused drugs of dependence, most authoritative medical opinion now opposes their use for the treatment of depression.

### The Monoamine Oxidase Inhibitors

Members of this mixed group of drugs share the ability to block the breakdown (by the enzyme monoamine oxidase) of naturally occurring chemicals (amines) in the body. These amines (such as epinephrine and norepinephrine) are chemicals produced in response to emotion, fear, and exercise. They have an effect on mood—if their levels are high, we may feel "high"; if they are low, we may feel "low."

The MAO inhibitors block many other enzymes in addition to monoamine oxidase and produce numerous other effects unrelated to their enzyme activity. They raise mood and lower blood pressure (some have been used in the past to treat high blood pressure). Their action also affects the way the body deals with a whole range of drugs such as barbiturates, alcohol, analgesics (e.g., meperidine), anticholinergic drugs, particularly those used to treat Parkinsonism, and antidepressant drugs, especially imipramine, and chemicals in foods. The breakdown of these products is blocked, and their concentration in the body increases. The MAO inhibitors are probably present in the body for only a short time, but they produce long-lasting effects by inactivating enzymes. It may take several weeks before these enzymes regenerate.

The adverse effects of MAO inhibitors are greater and more serious than those of any other drugs used in the treatment of mental illness. Some of the earlier MAO inhibitors produced liver damage either from hypersensitivity (allergy) or by activating a virus infection (infectious hepatitis, infectious jaundice). The risk of liver damage with currently used MAO inhibitors—phenelzine, isocarboxazid, and tranylcypromine—is low. But these drugs may excessively stimulate the brain, causing trembling, insomnia, sweating, agitation, hallucinations, confusions, and convulsions. A fall in blood pressure is usual, and dizziness, headaches, delayed or inhibited ejaculation, difficulty in passing urine, weakness, fatigue, dry mouth, edema, and skin rashes may occur.

Interaction with other drugs may produce serious effects. What is called a hypertensive crisis may occur when certain drugs or foods are taken with MAO inhibitors. This is caused by a sudden increase in blood pressure, which may lead to severe headache, bleeding into the brain, heart failure, and death. The foods which may produce this interaction all contain an amine called tyramine which may affect the blood pressure. The MAO inhibitors prevent the breakdown of tyramine in the liver and allow it to work at the nerve endings, releasing a chemical (norepinephrine) which elevates the blood pressure. Tyramine is present in cheese and various other foods. Patients taking

MAO inhibitors should carry a warning card which lists the prohibited foods and drugs. See phenelzine in Part III.

## Tricyclic Compounds

These antidepressant drugs, because they share a basic chemical structure which includes three benzene rings, are known as tricyclic (three-ring) compounds. They include amitriptyline, desipramine, doxepin, imipramine, nortriptyline, and protriptyline. The antidepressant properties of the parent drug (imipramine) of this group was discovered in 1958. Since then, chemical variations of the tricyclic structure have produced a continuous supply of antidepressant drugs sufficiently similar to confuse even the experts, let alone the family doctor.

Although these drugs lift mood, they do not produce the same kind of "lift" as pep pills or the euphoria produced by the MAO inhibitors. In fact imipramine, one of the more stimulating tricyclics, produces fatigue, dry mouth, blurred vision, palpitations, and retention of urine in "normal" people. Continued use leads to an increase of these symptoms along with difficulty in concentrating and thinking. Some of them, such as amitriptyline and trimipramine, produce a marked drowsiness. Nevertheless, the tricyclics are extremely useful drugs for treating depressive symptoms, and they lack the abuse potential of the amphetamines.

The manner in which tricyclic drugs relieve the symptoms of depression is not understood, but it is thought that they may produce an increased quantity of stimulating chemicals (amines produced by the body) at nerve endings by blocking the re-uptake of these stimulants. They do not produce a "high," even though there are reports of imipramine producing manic excitement in some patients. Like the anticholinergic (atropinelike) drugs (see p. 146), they block certain nerve endings, some more so than others, to produce blurred vision, dryness of the mouth, constipation, and difficulty in passing urine. Because these drugs may affect the eyes, doctors should give them with caution to patients with glaucoma. Similarly, their effect on the bladder should make doctors cautious when using them to treat depression in patients who have an enlarged prostate gland, since the patient may develop retention of urine. Some tricyclic drugs may affect sexual function. They may produce rapid beating of the heart, palpitations, and a fall in blood pressure. Furthermore, they may produce changes on the electrocardiogram, and therefore they should be used with caution in patients with heart disorders.

Tolerance develops to some of the adverse effects (dry mouth, blurred vision, etc.), and within one or two weeks patients notice these symptoms less and less. At the same time their mental and physical symptoms start to disappear and they begin to feel better as each day goes by. This knowledge is important to anyone prescribing or taking antidepressant drugs. Their beneficial effects are slow to develop (from two to five weeks from the time of starting), whereas adverse effects begin immediately. It is during these first few weeks of treatment, when adverse effects are more pronounced than the desired effects, that patients need much reassurance from their doctor and those around them that they are going to improve. Depending upon the circumstances of the patient, it may be better to start with large daily doses and then reduce the dose steadily to a maintenance dose as the patient improves. This is fine if the patient is in a hospital. Alternatively, one may start with a small daily dose and slowly increase it.

The tricyclics are useful because they offer a choice in dealing with different depressive symptoms. For example, imipramine is relatively nonsedating and is of use in treating depressed patients who are slow and withdrawn (melancholic). Amitriptyline has a more pronounced sedative action and is therefore useful for depressed people who are tense, anxious, or irritable. Amitriptyline and trimipramine are particularly useful to patients with sleep disorders, since the whole daily dose may be given at night and helps to improve sleep. The other antidepressant drugs come somewhere between imipramine and trimipramine with respect to sedative properties, and some have reduced adverse effects, but often at the expense of reduced desired effects.

## Precautions When Using Antidepressant Drugs

*Monoamine oxidase inhibitors* should not be prescribed by doctors for children under twelve years of age or to patients with a history of liver disease, with heart failure, or a previous thrombosis or hemorrhage in the brain. They should not be given to patients with epilepsy or with a disorder of the adrenal glands which may cause episodes of high blood pressure (pheochromocytoma). Patients should always be warned about diet and issued a warning card. During treatment and for two weeks after stopping an MAO inhibitor, patients should not be given meperidine, amphetamines, ephedrine, or tricyclic drugs such as imipramine. The MAO inhibitors also increase the effects of antihistamines, barbiturates, and drugs taken by mouth to treat diabetes. They may produce sensitivity to insulin. They may also interact with alcohol, opiates, cocaine and procaine, anesthetics, reserpine, antihistamines, diuretics, dopa, caffeine, various drugs in over-the-counter cough medicines, cold remedies, and reducing drugs. Before taking *any* additional drugs, consult your doctor or pharmacist.

*Tricyclic drugs* should be prescribed with caution for patients with heart disease, glaucoma, thrombophlebitis, or overworking of the thyroid gland, or on drug treatment for thyroid disorders, epilepsy, enlargement of the prostate gland, or pyloric stenosis (narrowing of the stomach outlet). Doctors and dentists should give local anesthetic solutions containing epinephrine (adrenaline) with care to patients taking tricyclics (p. 21). Tricyclics should preferably not be given within two weeks of stopping MAO inhibitor drugs. Alcohol and barbiturates may decrease the blood level of tricyclic drugs, and thus directly relate to the degree of improvement. As a patient, you should preferably not take barbiturates when being treated with tricyclic drugs, and if you drink regularly you should attempt to reduce your daily intake of alcohol. Tricyclic drugs may reduce the effectiveness of some blood pressure drugs such as guanethidine.

## Choice of Antidepressant Drug Treatments

The tricyclics are the drugs of first choice for any depressive disorder. The selection of a particular tricyclic depends upon the degree of sedation required. Use imipramine if sedation is not required, and amitriptyline if sedation is needed, especially at night to produce sleep. If the patient drives a motor vehicle or operates moving machinery, the dose of sedative tricyclic should be watched and the patient may need a few days off work. Instead of taking the drug in divided doses throughout the day, a larger dose may be taken about one hour before going to bed. Desired sedative effects, stimulant effects, and adverse effects must be balanced to obtain maximum benefit. Daily dosage must be worked out between patient and doctor and then continued for at least two weeks. If there is no improvement the daily dose should be increased for a further two weeks before changing to an alternative drug. However, if one tricyclic drug does not work, another one seldom will, although adverse effects may be less.

The MAO inhibitors are now used by a minority of psychiatrists and very rarely by family doctors. They are occasionally useful in patients who have failed to respond to tricyclics, in certain "neurotic" depressive disorders, and in patients with phobic anxiety disorders. Sometimes it is necessary to combine an antidepressant drug with a major tranquilizer (a phenothiazine) or with a minor tranquilizer.

Once a patient feels better he should keep taking the drug on a maintenance basis, by slowly reducing the regular daily dose while keeping the symptoms under control. This minimum dose for maximum response should be continued for three months, after which the dose should be slowly reduced over a period of two weeks. If the symptoms do not recur, stop the drug; if they do, then go back to a maintenance dose.

Some patients may be able to stop the drugs after six weeks to six months of treatment, and some may need to take a daily maintenance dose for much longer. Others may need to take a course of drugs intermittently (for example, for cyclical depression). Some patients are able to recognize the early warning symptoms of depression. If they feel an episode developing, and this may be nothing more than a reduction in energy and/or sleep disturbance, they start their own drug treatment. There appears to be little dependence on tricyclic antidepressant drugs in common use, and rather than desiring to increase dosage, patients on antidepressants seem on the contrary to want to bring down the daily dose to its minimal effective level.

## Lithium Salts

Lithium salts are now used to prevent and treat manic-depressive episodes. Lithium competes for sodium salt in the body and changes the composition of the body fluids. It is accumulative, and adverse effects, related to dosage, include nausea, trembling, weakness, thirst, and frequent urination. At high blood levels, lithium causes unsteadiness on the feet, trembling, confusion, diarrhea, drowsiness, and slurred speech. When these appear, the drug must be *stopped* immediately. Lithium should be given only under hospital supervision and with weekly blood tests to estimate the plasma level. When the dosage is stabilized, the tests can be reduced to once every two to four weeks.

## STIMULANTS: CAFFEINE

Coffee contains the drug caffeine, plus certain oils; tea contains caffeine, theophylline, and tannin; cola contains caffeine; and cocoa contains caffeine, theobromine, and tannin. Caffeine is also present in numerous over-the-counter tonics, "pickups," and pain relievers. The drugs caffeine, theophylline, and theobromine are usually referred to as xanthines. They produce stimulation of the nervous system, make the kidneys produce more urine, stimulate heart muscle, relax the muscles of the bronchial tubes, and have various effects on blood pressure and blood vessels. Caffeine is used as a stimulant, and theophylline is used in the treatment of bronchial spasm, as in asthma. The xanthines also possess other properties which affect the heart and circulation: they increase the blood supply to the heart, dilate blood vessels to the skin, and constrict blood vessels which supply the brain. Theobromine produces less of these effects than caffeine or theophylline.

The use of caffeine (as in a strong cup of tea or coffee) to wake you up or to help you deal with a hangover is a well-founded tradition. Caffeine stimulates the brain and all parts of the central nervous system. It stops tiredness and makes you think clearly. It lessens fatigue and increases muscular power to do physical work. After a dose of caffeine typists are said to type faster and with fewer mistakes. The dose of caffeine adequate to produce stimulation varies from 100 to 300 mg. The caffeine content of a cup of tea or coffee varies according to how strong a person likes his drink, but the average in a cup of tea or coffee is 100 to 150 mg. and in cocoa from 50 up to about 200 mg. per cup. An average-sized bottle of a cola drink contains 35 to 55 mg. of caffeine.

The effects of caffeine vary from person to person, but a dose of 1,000 mg. or more will produce adverse effects such as difficulty in sleeping, restlessness, excitement, trembling, rapid beating of the heart with extra beats, increased breathing, desire to urinate, ringing in the ears, and flashes of light in front of the eyes. Caffeine increases the production of acid in the stomach, and therefore patients with indigestion or stomach ulcers should restrict their intake of tea, coffee, cola, or cocoa. They should preferably drink their tea or coffee with meals and add milk to their drinks. The oils in coffee may cause irritation of the gut, and the tannin in tea may produce constipation.

Psychological dependence and tolerance to caffeine obviously develop, and it must be accepted that the majority of us are dependent upon our daily supply of tea, coffee, cocoa, or cola.

## STIMULANTS: AMPHETAMINES

The term "stimulant" generally refers to a drug which stimulates the brain, producing increased activity and alertness. Amphetamines are the principal group of drugs used. Other drugs used to produce mental stimulation include methylphenidate.

AMPHETAMINES are synthetic compounds. They produce actions and effects that are in many ways similar to those produced by the body's own stimulant, epinephrine, a hormone secreted under conditions of fear, emotion, or physical exertion. It lifts you up ready for what has been called "fight or flight." It makes you "high." The amphetamines include amphetamine, dexamphetamine, and methamphetamine.

Amphetamines were previously used to treat depression, as tonics, to treat overactive children and bed wetters, and to treat patients who kept falling asleep (narcolepsy). They were also used to treat alcoholism and drug dependence. Psychiatrists even used them to get patients to talk. In addition, doctors issued millions of prescriptions each year to people who wanted to lose weight. Patients were (and some still are) allowed to pick up repeat prescriptions for months and even years, even though after only two or three weeks the drugs cease to have any appetite-reducing effects. However, as the result of alarm and warnings about the widespread abuse of amphetamines, many doctors have reduced their use of these drugs.

The effects produced by amphetamines vary with dose and the route of administration. Children also respond to them differently—amphetamines have been used to calm hyperactive children. In moderate dosage they increase heart rate, blood pressure, and blood sugar. The pupils dilate, respiration increases, and the appetite decreases.

Depending on the person, the effect on mood varies tremendously, and is influenced by many factors. In some people there is increased wakefulness and alertness, with greater physical and mental activity and a delay in fatigue; their thinking gets clearer and they become more responsive and aware of their surroundings—in effect, more sociable. Other individuals, however, may become restless, irritable, and anxious.

Amphetamines may cause nausea, headache, dry mouth, trembling, difficult urination, rapid heartbeat and chest pains, diarrhea, and inability to concentrate. Higher doses may produce panic, confusion, aggression, hallucinations, mental breakdown, and heart irregularities.

On stopping the use of moderate doses, the individual becomes fatigued, drowsy, and depressed. He feels "let down" and has a strong desire to take another dose to lift himself back up. Drug dependence to amphetamines is discussed on p. 30.

The medical use of amphetamines should be restricted to treating narcolepsy, a rare disorder. Their use in treating hyperactive children has been rightly challenged. So too has their use in treating bed wetting. You should not use them as reducing aids, and if you are depressed they will do you more harm than good.

METHYLPHENIDATE is a mental stimulant. It increases activity, delays fatigue, lifts mood, and has little effect on appetite or blood pressure. Its widespread use to treat overactive children needs thorough investigation.

# TONICS

Millions of dollars are spent every year on pick-me-ups and tonics, and yet most doctors accept that there is no single substance which may be called a tonic. Pharmacologists are highly critical of the whole concept of tonics, and their criticism has influenced prescribing doctors. However, although medical fashions can change quickly, patients' expectations often do not. Doctors' prescribing habits so influence patients' demands that patients often expect what they have been led to expect. For decades many doctors prescribed tonics for everybody and everything yet are now critical of patients who ask for a tonic even though they accept the use of a placebo. Some doctors who cannot come to terms with prescribing an inert substance or a tonic prescribe vitamins, iron, and other remedies just to reassure themselves that their treatment may be pharmacologically active. They thus strengthen the belief in the value of vitamins and iron for nonspecific symptoms.

For obvious reasons some drug companies have not rejected tonics; they spend millions each year in persuading us that we need this or that product. But instead of being purely placebos, some of these tonics contain substances such as strychnine which may be harmful if taken over a prolonged period of time.

A tonic is something that we hope will help us to feel better. However, drug tonics are usually taken because the individual is feeling persistently run down, physically or mentally. They are often and quite wrongly taken for a multiplicity of mental and/or physical symptoms, the cause of which may be fairly straightforward, such as convalescence from an attack of influenza, or quite complex and due to a serious underlying physical or psychological disorder. The reasons which make a person feel in need of a tonic are complex and include social, physical, and mental factors: someone who is anemic will require a blood test and specific treatment; someone who is depressed needs specific treatment, as does someone with an underlying physical disease. If you feel persistently run down and/or fed up, see your doctor.

Many over-the-counter tonics are based on the principle that if you belch and have your bowels opened then you are living life to the full. Some tonics are very expensive foods containing malt, wheat germ, or bone marrow. Iron salts are often included in tonics because many individuals have been successfully led to believe that anemia is a common cause of feeling run down. You may develop iron-deficiency anemia because your diet is low in iron and/or because you are losing blood regularly through, for example, heavy menstrual periods, a bleeding peptic ulcer, or bleeding hemorrhoids. However, iron deficiency is only one cause of anemia, and doctors cannot recognize the type of anemia from which you may be suffering without carrying out blood tests. Incredible variations have been reported when a group of doctors were asked to *estimate* the degree of anemia in a particular patient. Yet patients still believe that a doctor has some magical power to diagnose anemia without blood tests. One reason is that in the past doctors frequently spoke to patients of anemia and the need for iron when in fact they were simply administering a placebo for its psychological effect. As a consequence many patients will say to their doctor, "I think I am anemic. Can I have some iron, please?" Of course, drug companies and health stores cash in on this belief.

The same applies to vitamins. There is an optimum daily intake to prevent vitamin deficiency disorders, and there is a recommended dose for treating these disorders. However, as far as these drugs are concerned, some practice the principle that if 100 units will make you feel good, 1,000 units will make you feel even better. And so we are seeing an increasing number of disorders produced by taking too many vitamins.

Many decades ago it was found that nerve cells contain glycerophosphates. Because of this, the manufacture and sale of "nerve" tonics containing glycerophosphates and hypophosphates has proved an extremely lucrative business, despite the fact that the use of these drugs is based entirely on a misconception. It has never been shown that the taking of hypophosphates by mouth produces any benefit over and above that which would be produced by an inert substance. However, hypophosphates are harmless and therefore useful as a placebo. Unfortunately, they are mixed with all sorts of bitters (appetite stimulants), laxatives, and stimulants. Some of these may produce adverse effects if taken regularly over time. Tonic wines contain hypophosphates and vitamins, but people who take tonic wines should not fool themselves. It is the wine that makes them feel better.

Yeast is the basis of many tonics. Again, it can do you no harm on its own, and it supplies you with a few vitamins. However, it is often combined with other drugs such as caffeine (you would get the same degree of stimulation from a cup of coffee), with obsolete drugs, and with rarely used pain relievers.

Bitters, which appear in many tonics, stimulate salivation and the production of gastric juice by taste and smell. Certain alcoholic drinks are used for this purpose (apéritifs); but persistent loss of appetite is not the sort of symptom you should treat yourself.

Over-the-counter remedies containing digestive enzymes such as pepsin and pancreatin, liver salts, and bile salts are valueless. Some contain small amounts of obsolete laxatives. Health salts have nothing to do with health, and honey can make you feel beautiful if you think it will. There is also no evidence that if you take vitamin E you will be more sexy or prevent or treat heart disease or any other human disorder, except possibly those which interfere with the absorption of fat and fat-soluble vitamins.

There is no substitute for a good balanced diet and reasonable exercise and sleep. If you feel you really need a tonic, you ought to see your doctor. Otherwise take the least harmful and least expensive tonic (but only for a short period of time). Remember, the only part of a tonic that is really guaranteed to make you feel better is your belief that it is going to work.

# REDUCING DRUGS

Obesity or fatness may be divided into two main types: that due to glandular disturbances, which is very rare, and simple obesity, which is very common. Actually there is nothing very simple about obesity, and most of us prefer to talk about being overweight. This, however, implies that there is a range of normal weights to which we should conform. Because of these and the relationship between weight and diet, being overweight is said to be the commonest nutritional disorder in the Western world. In order to persuade us that this is true and in order to help us conform to these "normal weights," a multimillion-dollar reducing industry has developed since the last world war.

"Overweight" may simply be a result of a big frame, but it is usually due to fat. Stand naked in front of a mirror—if you have rolls that shake when you jump up and down then you are fat! Being fat is mainly due to eating more food, particularly foods containing a large number of calories, than we require for our everyday needs. This results in the storage of fat in some of us. Lack of physical exercise also predisposes to the accumulation of fat. Women have more fat cells than men, and there is a relationship between the size and number of fat cells and being overweight. Hereditary factors may influence the number of fat cells we have (fat parents may have fat children, but children may also "inherit" the parents' eating habits). The number of our fat cells may also increase up to about the age of twenty as a result of overeating in childhood, and thus fat children may become fat adults. We may also become overweight if our fat cells store a lot of fat and increase in size. This is because of the way we use up fats and sugars and is related to diet and exercise. Glandular influences which make us put on weight must be regarded as normal; for example, women may gain weight in their early teens, after pregnancy, and during the menopause. These may be short-term increases in weight, but we must not forget that everyone tends to gain weight with age. Women tend to acquire fat on their buttocks and breasts and men around their abdomens.

Our appetites and the foods that we eat often have little to do with our requirements and are more determined by the eating habits we have acquired since childhood. These are related to family and environmental factors, economic status, various customs, and social requirements. Further, overeating may be as much a problem of habit as alcoholism, drug taking, or smoking, and as such is as much related to our personality as it is to social and family factors.

## The Use of Reducing Drugs

Doctors consider that obesity requires treatment when fat deposits have raised the body weight by 10 percent or more above the standards for people of the same age, sex, and race. They point out the possible hazards of being fat: flat feet, varicose veins, osteoarthritis, gall bladder disorders, high blood pressure, bronchitis, diabetes, complications after surgical operations, degenerative changes in heart muscle, and a shortening of life. Doctors have certainly been successful in giving some of us the motivation to lose weight, although much of their evidence may not stand up to very close scrutiny.

Since the commonest cause of being fat is the eating of more food than required, the only sensible way to reduce weight is to reduce the amount of food you eat or to alter your eating habits so that you eat a balanced diet and take in fewer calories. You should also take more physical exercise.

Four groups of drugs are used to aid reducing:

### DRUGS WHICH CAUSE LOSS OF FLUIDS

Some patent reducing medicines contain laxatives such as cascara, rhubarb, or phenolphthalein. These cause a loss of water from the bowel and therefore from the tissues, resulting in weight reduction. The body immediately replaces this water loss the next time you drink, and so such medicines are useless. They could be harmful if taken regularly.

Some doctors prescribe diuretics—drugs which interfere with the body's storage of salt and water. They act on the kidneys to make them excrete more salt, which takes water with it. The loss of water and salt results in a fall in body fluids and a subsequent temporary reduction in body weight. Diuretics also alter the body's excretion of other salts. They may be harmful and should be taken only under medical supervision for the treatment of an excess of body fluids caused by certain kidney, liver, or heart diseases. Similarly, diureticlike laxatives that cause a loss of salt and water from the bowel are of no use. The body quickly restores the balance and the weight goes back to what it was.

DRUGS WHICH INCREASE THE BULK OF FOOD

Many patent reducing remedies contain methylcellulose in tablet form or as biscuits or granules. Methylcellulose absorbs water from the stomach, swells, and is supposed to make you feel less hungry if taken before meals. It is not absorbed, and it increases the bulk of the bowel motions, taking some water with it. As reducing aids these preparations have not been proved to be of any value at all.

THYROID EXTRACTS

Thyroid extracts given to increase the speed at which the body burns up calories are ineffective in small doses and dangerous in high doses.

DRUGS WHICH SUPPRESS THE APPETITE

Most reducing drugs prescribed by doctors are amphetamines or related compounds. They have been widely used in the past because they suppress hunger, but they lose this effect after a few weeks. They do stimulate you, give you more energy, and make you feel happy, but only for a short period of time. These effects cause some people to increase the dosage, which may eventually lead to abuse and drug dependence.

*Diethylpropion, phentermine, chlorphentermine, phendimetrazine, phenmetrazine, mazindol.* These are also commonly used to suppress appetite. Their toxic effects are similar to those of the amphetamines, but they have less effect upon the heart and circulation. Their power to suppress appetite soon wears off, and they may produce drug dependence of the amphetamine type.

*Fenfluramine.* Fenfluramine has some chemical resemblance to the amphetamines but does not produce stimulation. It suppresses the appetite and has an effect upon the way the body utilizes certain fats and glucose.

Overall, the value of drugs in reducing appetite must be regarded as completely trivial when compared with diet control.

Occasionally, being overweight may be due to a psychological disorder. If you are a compulsive eater, excessive nibbler, or night eater, consult your doctor for more specific treatment for your problems, which may be psychological. However, if your doctor uses certain tranquilizers or antidepressant drugs, these can in fact increase your appetite and make you put on more weight. Certainly reducing pills are not indicated, because they will only make you feel more "nervy" or depressed. The oral contraceptive pill may also make some women put on weight. If diet fails to control this increase, it may be worth trying a lower-dose pill.

In conclusion, reducing drugs are no long-term substitute for will power and motivation. The tendency to obesity is a life-long problem. Although drugs may help you lose weight initially, they have no effect on your motivation or will power, and thus you will soon regain your weight when treatment is stopped. There is no evidence that they recondition you to a low-calorie diet. The hard fact is that you must reeducate yourself to accept a change in eating habits for life.

# DRUGS USED TO TREAT NAUSEA, VOMITING, AND MOTION SICKNESS

Nausea and vomiting are symptoms. They may occur with all kinds of physical disorders, some of which are quite simple and short-lasting, such as food "poisoning," some very serious and long-lasting, such as cancer of the stomach or a brain tumor. Drugs such as morphine, digitalis, and estrogens often cause nausea and vomiting, and so may motion, pregnancy, and emotion (for instance, the sight of a severely injured person). Nausea and vomiting may serve a useful purpose in food poisoning, but usually they are distressing symptoms which call for relief.

There is a vomiting center in the brain which responds to stimulations from the stomach and gut and also from the brain. Another part of the brain seems to respond to chemical stimulation. It is thought that this area is stimulated by certain drugs (e.g., morphine) and also by chemicals produced in the body, as in diabetes or kidney failure. Two groups of drugs help to prevent vomiting and are thought to work on the vomiting center. These are the anticholinergic (atropinelike) drugs (see p. 146) and antihistamines (see p. 127). A third group, the phenothiazines (see p. 53), are useful in preventing vomiting when it is due to drugs or toxic reactions in the body. However, there is an overlap between the effects produced by these drugs. Antihistamines resemble anticholinergic drugs in some respects, and some phenothiazines work like antihistamines.

## Motion Sickness
Movement can affect the organ of balance, which has associations with the vomiting center. For example, motion produced by traveling in a car, on a boat, or on a merry-go-round stimulates the organ of balance.

This may stimulate the vomiting center, resulting in a feeling of nausea (sweating, salivation, rapid beating of the heart, and the feeling you are going to vomit) and vomiting. Motion sickness is more common in children. Certain movements, such as swinging, will make some people sick, whereas others may become sick at sea. Numerous physical, social, and psychological factors are involved in motion sickness; fortunately, tolerance to motion develops over a period of several days.

The aim of drug use should be to prevent an attack of motion sickness from developing. A short-acting drug should be taken for a short journey and a long-acting one for a long journey. Many drugs are effective, provided the right dose is taken at the right time. Unwanted adverse effects are drowsiness, blurred vision, and dry mouth. *When taking such drugs, alcohol should be avoided. They also may interfere with your ability to drive a motor vehicle.* There are two main groups:

ANTICHOLINERGIC DRUGS may produce blurred vision, dry mouth and rapid beating of the heart (see adverse effects of atropine, page 146). They should not be used if you have glaucoma or a tendency to develop retention of urine (e.g., men with enlarged prostate glands). They are short-acting and are therefore useful for relieving motion sickness on short journeys (up to half a day). Their prolonged use for this purpose is not satisfactory because of troublesome adverse effects. They usually contain atropine or scopolamine.

ANTIHISTAMINE DRUGS. There is a marked variation between individuals in their response to antihistamines (see adverse effects in section on Antihistamines, p. 130). The most common adverse effect is drowsiness, but in infants and young children antihistamines may produce stimulation, making them nervous and unable to sleep. Some antihistamines may actually cause nausea and vomiting. Do not drink alcohol on the day that you have taken an antihistamine drug. Antihistamines may interfere with your ability to drive a motor vehicle, and they may increase the effects of other depressant drugs such as sedatives, tranquilizers, and sleeping drugs.

The antihistamines most frequently used to treat motion sickness are cyclizine, dimenhydrinate, diphenhydramine, meclizine, and promethazine.

## Vomiting of Pregnancy

Vomiting of pregnancy is probably due to the rapidly increasing production of estrogens which occurs between the fourth and eighth week of pregnancy. In addition there are numerous psychological, social, and dietary factors. Excessive vomiting may lead to an alteration in blood chemistry, which then causes further vomiting. Although all unnecessary drugs should be avoided during early pregnancy, doctors continue to prescribe a great variety of drugs to control vomiting of pregnancy. These include anticholinergic drugs, antihistamines, and phenothiazine tranquilizers.

Because deficiency of vitamin $B_6$ (pyridoxine) can occur in severe continuous vomiting, it is widely used to treat vomiting of pregnancy, although there has been no proof that a deficiency of pyridoxine occurs in this particular disorder. It is usually taken in combination with an antivomiting drug. The main considerations should be: How much distress is being caused by the vomiting and what effects may these drugs have upon the unborn child? A decision in the light of these considerations is not easy. Vomiting of pregnancy is extremely distressing. You need sound advice, understanding, and careful support, preferably from someone who knows you and your family—the ideal person is your family doctor.

DRUGS USED TO TREAT VOMITING OF PREGNANCY include: *Anticholinergic drugs* (for adverse effects, see p. 146), such as dicyclomine. *Antihistamine drugs* (for adverse effects, see p. 130): cyclizine, meclizine, promethazine. (Note that though they are widely used there is still a *suspicion* that cyclizine and meclizine in high doses may produce abnormalities in the unborn baby.) *Phenothiazine drugs* (for adverse effects, see p. 53): chlorpromazine, prochlorperazine, trifluoperazine. (Note that for vomiting of pregnancy phenothiazines are best avoided except in severe cases.)

## Other Vomiting Disorders

Drug-induced vomiting, postanesthetic vomiting, vomiting due to disease, and radiation sickness are best treated with phenothiazine drugs such as chlorpromazine or an antihistamine such as cyclizine or promethazine. Anticholinergic drugs are of little use.

## Dizziness (Vertigo)

Vertigo—sensations of movement within the head or in the environment—is always accompanied by a disturbance of balance. If severe, it can be associated with sweating, pallor, nausea, vomiting, and occasionally diarrhea and fainting. It may be caused by disorders of the eyes, brain, organ of balance, and ears. The organ of balance may be disturbed by infections (labyrinthitis) and by drugs such as streptomycin, quinine, or aspirin. Dizziness and giddiness are much more vague. They are highly subjective feelings and may be associated with all manner of disorders, although most elderly patients wrongly persist in thinking that dizziness is due to anemia or blood pressure.

An incredible mixture of drugs is used to treat vertigo. These include the antivomiting drugs (anticholinergic drugs, antihistamines, and phenothiazines); drugs which constrict blood vessels and others which dilate blood vessels; sedatives; tranquilizers; antidepressants; and vitamins. As often stated in this book, if there is no specific treatment for a disorder there are numerous treatments.

### Ménière's Disease

This most unpleasant disorder is characterized by recurrent attacks of vertigo associated with noises in the ears (tinnitus) and progressive nerve deafness. Men get it more often than women, and more attacks develop between the ages of forty and sixty than at any other age. It is self-limiting, and spontaneous recovery occurs at any stage. Patients with Ménière's disease get very anxious and depressed and therefore need a lot of sympathy and understanding.

The drug treatment of Ménière's is as confused as the drug treatment of vertigo and dizziness, and it is often a matter of trying different products at different times. In an acute phase the patient is unwilling to move his head because he may vomit, and therefore an injection or suppository of promethazine or prochlorperazine may help.

# DRUGS USED TO TREAT INDIGESTION AND PEPTIC ULCERS

The middle and upper parts of the stomach act as a reservoir for food: the part near its outlet into the duodenum contracts and relaxes to churn and mix the food. The rate of emptying the stomach varies with the volume of contents; the greater the volume the faster the rate of emptying. So you are not going to go longer without feeling hungry just because you eat a large meal. A fatty meal delays emptying; so does an increase in stomach acidity. Some drugs increase and some decrease the rate of emptying of the stomach. Another important function of the stomach is to make digestive juice. This contains hydrochloric acid (about one and a half liters are produced every day), mucus which protects the surface of the stomach, and an enzyme called pepsin which helps to digest protein in food.

The stomach can get "upset" if its lining is irritated by substances such as aspirin or alcohol, by eating too much, by eating unusual food, or by viral or bacterial infections. The lining of the stomach can also become irritated or inflamed (gastritis). This may be caused or aggravated by many things; for example, certain foods (pickles, fried food), alcohol, and smoking. Gastritis may produce such symptoms as discomfort, nausea, pain, loss of appetite, and heartburn. These symptoms are usually referred to as indigestion or dyspepsia. Sometimes the surface of the stomach may ulcerate to produce a peptic ulcer. A peptic ulcer may occur in the esophagus (gullet), stomach (where it may be called a gastric ulcer), or duodenum (duodenal ulcer).

Relatively little is known about the factors which cause peptic ulcers, but there is evidence that acid and pepsin are partly responsible. However, "normal" stomachs do not develop ulcers. Therefore, the "normal" lining of the stomach must be protective, and it may be something affecting this protection that causes ulcers. This may be related to the mucus that covers the surface, the ability of the mucus cells to renew themselves every few days, the nutrition of the stomach itself, its blood supply, and various chemical factors. There are other factors, such as heredity (there is often a family history of ulcers), seasonal factors, diet, smoking, alcohol, and worry and stress.

The symptoms of peptic ulcer usually start with "indigestion," but may start with acute pain, or bleeding or perforation. Indigestion going on for more than a few days may be due to a peptic ulcer, particularly if the episodes keep recurring and if accompanied by pain rather than "discomfort." Pain from a duodenal ulcer often comes when you are hungry and it wakes you in the night, whereas gastric ulcer pain may come on fairly soon after eating. Food, antacids, or vomiting may relieve peptic ulcer pains.

You should always consult your doctor if you have indigestion lasting more than a few weeks or recurring at intervals—you may have a peptic ulcer. The treatment of a peptic ulcer includes taking a well-balanced diet and frequent, regular, small meals. You should avoid alcohol and any foods which you know give you pain. You should stop drinking coffee and not take any drugs known to irritate the stomach —for example aspirin, corticosteroids (e.g., prednisone), and most drugs used to treat rheumatism and arthritis (e.g., phenylbutazone and indomethacin). You should also stop smoking. There is no point in filling yourself full of indigestion mixture while continuing to smoke and drink alcohol. If you are worried, anxious, or tense, you need help and advice on sorting out the stresses which are affecting you; in addition, a drug to calm you down for a short period of time may help.

The main drugs used to treat peptic ulcers fall into two groups: drugs which neutralize the acid in the stomach (antacids) and drugs which reduce the production of acid by the stomach cells (anticholinergic drugs).

### Antacids (Alkali Mixtures)

Antacids neutralize the acid in the stomach contents, and this process relieves pain. This is a specific action, and yet antacid preparations are swallowed in huge amounts by millions of people for the relief of numerous minor symptoms of indigestion totally unrelated to acid production. However, some antacids which contain aluminum, bismuth, or calcium also possess antipepsin activity (which may prevent the pepsin from enlarging the ulcer), and those that reduce acidity sufficiently also damp down the production of pepsin by the stomach cells. Unfortunately, the presence of antacids in the stomach may actually increase the amount of acid produced, so an antacid like calcium carbonate may leave the patient with more acid in his stomach than before he took the antacid. This is often called an acid rebound —initial relief is followed by a flare-up of pain.

Remember: antacid drugs relieve the pain of a peptic ulcer but they do not alter the rate of healing or prevent its recurrence.

The benefits of antacid consumption are difficult to evaluate, because according to advertisements we are all apparently suffering from "acid indigestion." Of course, this is not true, but the carefree use of antacids distorts their real value in the treatment of disorders such as peptic ulcers, for which they are highly effective if taken in appropriate dosages.

Antacids usually consist of mixtures of various base salts of sodium, magnesium, calcium, aluminum, and bismuth. The amount needed to neutralize stomach acid depends upon the rate of acid production by the stomach, the presence or absence of food, and the rate of emptying of the stomach. Antacids may be classified according to whether they produce an effect upon the rest of the body (systemic effect) or produce only a local effect in the stomach (nonsystemic). A systemic antacid is absorbed into the blood stream and produces changes in the chemistry of the blood. This effect is often of no consequence because the kidneys quickly restore the chemical balance, but in patients with impaired heart or kidney function it may be serious. Repeated use of these antacids (e.g., sodium bicarbonate) may also cause kidney stones. Nonsystemic antacids form insoluble compounds in the stomach which are not absorbed.

SODIUM BICARBONATE relieves pain rapidly, but its effects quickly wear off and it may cause changes in the blood chemistry. It releases carbon dioxide gas into the stomach, causing belching, which makes some people think it is working effectively, but it may also cause an unpleasant distension of the stomach. It is useful for quick relief, but there is nothing to recommend its continued use. Patients with impaired heart or kidney function should not use it. Also, it should not be used in patients with fluid retention problems (as in edema due to congestive heart failure) because it increases the blood salt level and may cause further retention of water by the kidneys. When taken with milk, which contains calcium, it may give rise to the milk-alkali syndrome (see below under calcium carbonate).

MAGNESIUM HYDROXIDE is slow to act, but its effects are fairly long-lasting. *Magnesium oxide* is converted to magnesium hydroxide in water, but it may not react completely with water or acid before it is emptied from the stomach. *Magnesium carbonate* is fairly slow to act. *Magnesium trisilicate* is slow to act but neutralizes the acid and absorbs pepsin; it has a prolonged action. *Magnesium salts* may cause diarrhea, and some magnesium may be absorbed into the bloodstream—they should not be used in patients with impaired kidney function.

CALCIUM CARBONATE acts quickly and effectively. Some calcium is absorbed into the bloodstream. Many patients with peptic ulcers are put on milk diets which contain calcium, and therefore patients who take milk and calcium carbonate regularly for long periods of time may develop a high blood calcium which may cause a group of symptoms —loss of appetite, nausea, vomiting, headache, weakness, abdominal pains, constipation, and thirst. This is often called the milk-alkali syndrome ("syndrome" being the term used to indicate a group of symptoms). Temporary or permanent kidney damage and an increase in blood pressure may occur. Calcium salts tend to cause constipation; they are, therefore, often given mixed with magnesium salts.

ALUMINUM HYDROXIDE is slow to act but quicker than magnesium trisilicate. It does not alter the blood chemistry, because it forms insoluble complexes in the stomach. It also forms these complexes with certain antibiotic drugs (tetracyclines), and it may interfere with the absorption of vitamins. Excessive use of aluminum salts may sometimes cause weakness due to a fall in blood phosphates caused by its formation of complexes with phosphates in the stomach. In the presence of a low-phosphate diet this may result in kidney damage and lead to rickets and bone softening. Aluminum hydroxide is no more effective than other insoluble alkalis, and differences in antacid effects may vary tremendously between different commercial preparations of aluminum antacids. Aluminum compounds cause constipation; for example, aluminum silicate (kaolin) is used to treat diarrhea. *Dihydroxy-aluminum aminoacetate* is an alternative but has not been shown to be more effective. *Bismuth salts* are not very effective.

Antacids relieve the pain of uncomplicated peptic ulcer, but as previously stated, they have not been shown to speed healing or delay recurrences. They are also useful in relieving the pain of hiatus hernia. They are less effective in gastritis, in which acid production is often reduced. None of the available antacids is ideal. They vary in their rate and duration of action and in the amounts required to neutralize the acid contents of the stomach. Liquid preparations and powders mixed with water are more effective than tablets. Tablets should be sucked slowly between meals; their routine use after meals to prevent symptoms is of no use. Because no specific antacid can be recommended, mixtures are generally used. Mixtures also help to avoid bowel complications such as diarrhea from magnesium salts and constipation from calcium or aluminum salts.

Recently introduced antacid mixtures contain agents which are said to coat the surface of the ulcer, spread the antacid over the surface of the stomach, and disperse it. These include co-dried gels, complexes of silicates, and alginic acid derived from algae. The latter is also used as a tablet disintegrant. The latest fashion is to include these spreading agents into antacid mixtures. These could represent an advance, but we need to have much more objective evidence that such additions really serve any useful purpose.

For repeated use, preparations containing systemic (absorbable) antacids such as sodium bicarbonate should be avoided. The choice is wide, but be cautious about terms like peptic inhibition, demulcent properties, dispersant agents, and what have you. For cheapness, ordinary unadulterated calcium carbonate (chalk) takes some beating. Comparative preparations are not necessarily equivalent in their ability to neutralize the acid, and unless they are given in sufficiently high doses at frequent intervals, it is doubtful whether they reduce the activity of pepsin. Do not forget that the speed of action of antacids depends upon their ability to neutralize the acid in the stomach. This depends principally upon the speed with which they dissolve and the rate of emptying of the stomach. The choice is really what suits you, and the right dose is what relieves *your* symptoms. Money will not buy you the best. Calcium carbonate, magnesium carbonate, magnesium oxide, and magnesium hydroxide are more effective antacids than magnesium trisilicate and the aluminum salts.

## Drugs Which Reduce Acid Production by the Stomach

These drugs are called anticholinergic because they block cholinergic nerves (see p. 146). They are used to treat peptic ulcers because cholinergic nerves supply the stomach and their stimulation leads to an increased production of gastric juice. These nerves also increase muscle movement in the stomach and gut to produce pain. Anticholinergic drugs, therefore, reduce acid production and reduce movement of the stomach wall, which in turn reduces pain. They are discussed on p. 146.

There are many anticholinergic drugs on the market, and some of them, such as the belladonna alkaloids, have been very popular for the treatment of peptic ulcer symptoms. However, these preparations tend to produce adverse effects such as blurred vision, dry mouth, rapid heartbeat, retention of urine, and constipation. These are called atropinelike effects because they are classically produced by atropine and are not very pleasant. Other anticholinergic drugs are available which do not produce so many of these adverse effects: for example, propantheline, poldine, glycopyrrolate, clidinium bromide, and methscopolamine bromide.

Anticholinergic drugs may be of use in treating peptic ulcers if given in high dose at night; this helps to reduce the acid production which occurs during sleep. However, despite the fact that such drugs are widely prescribed and appear in all kinds of mixtures, authoritative medical opinion remains divided about their value. Because of their adverse effects they should not be taken by patients with glaucoma. They should be prescribed with caution by doctors to patients with enlarged prostate glands and to those with heart disease. In patients with coronary heart disease, the rapid beating of the heart which these drugs produce may cause angina. They should not be given to patients taking MAO inhibitor antidepressant drugs. Antihistamines, phenothiazine tranquilizers, and tricyclic antidepressants may increase the atropinelike effects of these drugs.

Anticholinergic drugs should be taken separately and not in mixtures containing sedatives and/or antacids. In this way the smallest effective dose may be worked out. This is simple common sense, because with such mixtures you cannot alter the dose of one drug without altering the dose of the others. So if you want to push up the dose of antacid you also increase the dose of anticholinergic drug. No wonder patients on these mixtures may develop a dry mouth, blurred vision, and constipation. Also, increasing the dosage of mixtures containing a minor tranquilizer may prove quite dangerous to drivers of motor vehicles and people who operate machinery.

A promising new drug for peptic ulcers may soon be available. Cimetidine, an antihistamine which inhibits the stomach's secretion of hydrochloric acid, appears to be superior to current drugs in promoting ulcer healing and in reducing stomach and upper-small-intestine bleeding.

# DRUGS USED
# TO TREAT DIARRHEA

An acute attack of diarrhea, frequent passage of watery bowel movements, is unpleasant and can be exhausting. It results from increased bowel activity caused by inflammation, infection, irritation, or emotional factors. If associated with vomiting in infants it may be very dangerous because of the risk of dehydration, and therefore any baby or infant who develops an acute attack of vomiting and diarrhea should be seen immediately by a doctor. Similar precautions apply to very elderly and debilitated patients. In most of us, apart from typhoid fever and certain bacillary and amoebic dysenteries, an attack of diarrhea is usually self-limiting and of no consequence. It may be regarded as the body's way of getting rid of a noxious substance; and so some regard its treatment as unnecessary and possibly harmful. Others regard diarrhea as an unpleasant symptom warranting drug treatment. Certainly, if it goes on for more than a day it can be exhausting. It may also ruin a holiday. In addition to plenty of fluids and a bland diet it is therefore worth taking one of the popular remedies.

Drug treatment of diarrhea includes drugs which reduce the number of bowel movements by acting on the contents of the gut or the wall of the gut, and anti-infective drugs which are used to treat bacterial or amoebic infections. These are often given in various combinations. Finally, correction of fluid and salt loss is important and lifesaving in certain cases.

## Drugs Which Alter the Bowel Contents
Inert powders are used to absorb noxious substances in the bowel. Such powders include bismuth salts; activated charcoal; aluminum salts (e.g., kaolin); pectin (a purified carbohydrate product obtained from citrus fruits); activated attapulgite (a hydrated magnesium aluminum silicate); calcium carbonate (chalk); and methylcellulose.

## Drugs Which Act on the Bowel Wall
OPIUM ALKALOIDS
Opium alkaloids (see p. 115) and related drugs slow down movement of the bowel wall. They are still the most effective agents for treating diarrhea. They are often mixed with kaolin or chalk. One of them,

codeine phosphate, is very useful on its own. Fortunately, with these drugs, the dose to stop diarrhea is much less than the dose which produces adverse effects.

Lomotil, a frequently prescribed proprietary preparation for the treatment of diarrhea, contains diphenoxylate and a very small dose of atropine. Diphenoxylate is related to meperidine and is used to treat diarrhea because of its constipating effects. It should not be used in patients with impaired liver function. Do not take it casually. It has caused serious adverse effects in children, either from overdose or from idiosyncratic reactions to a normal dose.

ANTICHOLINERGIC DRUGS

Belladonna alkaloids and related drugs (see p. 146) reduce the movements of the bowel and the spasm of bowel muscles. They may produce atropinelike effects such as dry mouth, dizziness, and blurring of vision. In mild diarrhea they may relieve pain and reduce the number of bowel movements. They are not much use in severe diarrhea or in the chronic diarrhea of ulcerative colitis and similar disorders.

ANTI-INFECTIVE DRUGS

Numerous antidiarrhea remedies contain antibiotic drugs mixed with absorbent powders such as kaolin, or with mixtures which contain anticholinergic drugs. But after decades of excessive use of antibiotic drugs in patients suffering from diarrhea, most authoritative opinion is now against their widespread use except in specific infections such as typhoid fever and certain dysenteries. However, many doctors still cannot resist the temptation to prescribe an antibiotic drug to a patient at the onset of an acute episode of diarrhea.

Antibiotic drugs may alter the normal bacterial content of the gut and result in a superadded fungal infection (moniliasis). With some bacterial infections antibiotic drugs may prolong the period when the patient can pass on the disease as a carrier. They may also increase the risk of relapse, interfere with subsequent bacterial diagnosis, promote the development of resistant organisms, and cause rashes. They should not be used routinely, nor should they be provided to travelers wishing to avoid an attack of diarrhea while visiting foreign countries.

Iodochlorhydroxyquin is an antiseptic and was originally marketed in a dusting powder for skin wounds and ulcers. Subsequently it was found to be effective in amoebic dysentery. It was widely promoted for the prevention of travelers' diarrhea, under the name Entero-Vioform. It is an iodine compound and is partly absorbed into the bloodstream. It increases the level of iodine bound to proteins in the blood, which may give false values on iodine laboratory tests of thyroid function. These may remain high for up to three months after taking the drug. It may cause itching of the anus and skin rashes in people sensitive to iodine, and it should not be used by patients with impaired liver function. Furthermore, Entero-Vioform may cause toxic effects on the central nervous system. This drug is no longer being manufactured but may still be available in some regions.

### Choice of Drugs in the Treatment of Diarrhea

Babies and infants need urgent replacement of any fluid loss and it is advisable to seek the advice of a physician. Drug treatment is often not necessary in older children, whose diarrhea usually responds to clear fluids given in frequent small quantities. For adults, codeine phosphate is the drug of choice (and in tablet form is easy to carry). Alternatives are kaolin and kaolin mixed with an opium alkaloid (kaolin and morphine mixture or paregoric mixture) or a chalk and opium mixture. Diphenoxylate with atropine is also an alternative. Mixtures containing kaolin and an anticholinergic drug are useful for mild diarrhea where there is pain due to spasm of the gut.

# DRUGS USED
# TO TREAT CONSTIPATION

Drugs used to treat constipation are called laxatives. They are extensively misused, in the mistaken belief that there is some relationship between regular daily emptying of the bowels and health. It does not matter if your bowels empty two to three times a day or two to three times a week. If you only go a day or two over the normal for you, this doesn't matter either. Only if you develop a radical change in bowel habits should you be concerned.

We usually talk about laxatives when we wish to produce a soft, formed, easy-to-pass stool, and a cathartic or purgative when we wish to produce fairly quick and fluid emptying of the bowel. Laxatives are harmless when taken infrequently, but their continued use over long periods of time may lead to such complications as loss of fluid, salt, and fat. This may make you feel tired, weak, and thirsty. Calcium loss may occur and lead to bone softening, and the bowel wall may become permanently damaged or inflamed.

The taking of laxatives is only occasionally necessary—for example, after childbirth, after an operation for piles or some other condition around the anus, after some abdominal operations, after a coronary thrombosis (when a patient should not strain), and in elderly or debilitated bedridden patients. Apart from these situations, the use of a laxative is seldom indicated.

The most natural treatment for simple constipation is to increase the amount of indigestible waste products in your diet, an increase easily achieved by eating more fruit and leafy vegetables or by adding bran in the form of a processed cereal or as bread or biscuits. For children, simply increasing the amount of water in the diet may do the trick. If you have a longstanding problem, then in addition to diet make sure that you drink plenty of fluids and take regular exercise. Also, develop a habit of trying to empty your bowels just after a meal, when food entering the stomach stimulates the large bowel to empty its contents into the rectum, thus producing the urge to eliminate. Never neglect a feeling that you want to empty your bowels. The same advice applies if you have developed a laxative habit. In addition, slowly try to reduce the dose over time.

Laxatives should never be taken regularly, nor should they be taken to relieve abdominal pains, cramps, colic, nausea, or any other symptom, whether associated with constipation or not. You may have, for instance, acute appendicitis, in which case the taking of laxatives could cause the appendix to rupture and lead to peritonitis. If in doubt you should always consult your doctor, particularly if you pass blood in the stool, if you are developing the laxative habit, or if you develop a change in bowel habits.

The occasional use of laxatives is not harmful, but repeated use may lead to the laxative habit. When you have taken one dose of laxative, your rectum will be empty and it may take several days for it to fill and give you the urge to go again. Unfortunately, some patients cannot wait that long before taking another dose. A regular routine develops, the bowel action becomes so abnormal that it is unable to function properly, and the person is totally reliant upon the use of drugs. This warning applies to all laxatives, from health salts before breakfast to the numerous patent remedies. In fact, many of these contain irritant purgatives now regarded as dangerous.

Four main groups of drugs are used to treat constipation: stimulant, saline, lubricant, and bulk-forming.

## Stimulant Laxatives
These include senna, cascara sagrada, danthron, phenolphthalein, bisacodyl, and castor oil. Preparations containing aloe, podophyllum, or aloin should not be used; they have a higher degree of toxicity. There are so many preparations on the market which contain stimulant laxatives that it would be impractical to list them—you need to know only one. Stimulant laxatives increase large bowel movements by irritating

the lining and/or stimulating the bowel muscles to contract. They may cause cramps, increased mucus secretion, and excessive fluid loss. Response to dosage varies tremendously, and what may produce stomach cramps and diarrhea in one person may have no effect in another.

Senna, cascara sagrada, and danthron may color the urine and feces red and cause excessive loss of fluids; if taken for a long time, they may cause patchy pigmentation of the colon. This is not serious and is reversible on stopping the drug. Phenolphthalein may cause allergic skin rashes and color the urine pink and the feces red. Bisacodyl is related to phenolphthalein. It may be used as a rectal suppository as well as taken by mouth. Another popular rectal suppository contains glycerin, gelatin, and water. Castor oil differs from the other stimulant laxatives in that it works on the small bowel and therefore produces an effect in about three hours. The others work on the large bowel and act in six to twelve hours. Bisacodyl suppositories act in one-half to one hour.

## Saline Laxatives

These are salts of magnesium, sodium, and potassium in various mixtures. They are incompletely absorbed and increase the bulk of the bowel contents by causing it to retain water. Some of them are made fizzy by adding bicarbonate of soda and weak acids such as citric and tartaric. These salts, which may take fluids from the body and cause dehydration, should be taken with large amounts of water. They include magnesium sulfate, magnesium hydroxide, sodium sulfate, potassium sodium tartrate, and potassium bitartrate. They are commonly called health salts, which is reasonable enough if health is defined as bowel movements and belching. Their prolonged use may be harmful. Health salts containing sodium salts should never be taken by patients with congestive heart disease because they may increase the amount of fluids in the tissues. Likewise they should never be taken by patients on diuretic drugs, which eliminate salt from the body. Also, magnesium-containing health salts should never be taken by patients with impaired kidney function, since some magnesium is absorbed from the gut. As it is excreted by the kidneys, any impairment may lead to an accumulation of magnesium in the blood, resulting in magnesium intoxication (sharp drop in blood pressure and respiratory paralysis).

## Lubricant Laxatives

There are three types of lubricant laxatives: mineral oils, dioctyl sodium sulfosuccinate, and poloxalkol. Mineral oil softens and lubricates bowel motions. Its habitual use should be avoided, since it interferes with absorption of carotene (preformed vitamin A), vitamin A, and vitamin D. In pregnancy it may reduce the absorption of vitamin K and produce a disorder of blood clotting. When young, elderly, or debilitated patients swallow mineral oil, they may inhale a few drops into their lungs, and this may cause a type of pneumonia. Mineral oil may also be absorbed from the gut and cause swelling of lymph glands in the gut wall, liver, and spleen. It may leak from the anus in the night and cause irritation. Dioctyl sodium sulfosuccinate and dioctyl calcium sulfosuccinate lower surface tension and are used in the pharmaceutical industry as emulsifying or wetting agents. They soften the feces in 24 to 48 hours and are present in numerous laxative preparations. They are also used to soften wax in the ears. Poloxalkol, another surface-active agent, is marketed as a lubricant laxative for children.

### Bulk-forming Laxatives

These are substances which increase the bulk of the bowel content and stimulate the bowel muscles to become active. In addition they dissolve or swell in water to form a soft mass which helps to lubricate bowel movement. They usually take twelve to twenty-four hours to work, although their full effect may not be achieved until the second or third day of medication. Some bulk-forming laxatives are naturally occurring substances such as mucilaginous seeds, psyllium seeds, and gums such as agar, tragacanth, and karaya. These are present in numerous proprietary laxatives. Others are semisynthetic—methylcellulose and sodium carboxymethylcellulose compounds. They must be taken with plenty of fluids because of the risk of obstruction in elderly or debilitated patients. Gums may cause hypersensitivity resulting in skin rashes and asthmalike symptoms. Bran, a by-product of the milling of wheat, contains about 20 percent indigestible cellulose. It is an effective bulk laxative and may also help to prevent certain bowel disorders such as diverticulitis.

### Which Laxative to Take

For the occasional attack of constipation which you feel needs treating after diet has failed, use a stimulant laxative (e.g., senna, cascara, or bisacodyl) or a saline laxative (e.g., magnesium sulfate). For bedridden, elderly, or debilitated patients, a simple bulk laxative such as bran may be effective. If this does not work, try a semisynthetic compound like methylcellulose, but make sure that the patient, provided his bladder control is normal, drinks plenty of fluids. After operations on the anus, after childbirth, or when you don't want to have to strain, a lubricant laxative such as dioctyl sodium sulfosuccinate is probably the best.

It is better not to take preparations containing mixtures or differently acting laxatives. Always take the smallest effective dose of any laxative as infrequently as possible.

# DRUGS USED TO TREAT HEART FAILURE AND HEART RHYTHM DISORDERS

### Digitalis and Related Drugs

These drugs have been used for centuries to treat heart failure. They are called cardiac glycosides and are found in a number of plants. From the leaves of *Digitalis purpurea* (purple foxglove) are prepared digitoxin, gitoxin, and gitalin, and from the leaves of *Digitalis lanata* (white foxglove), digitoxin, gitoxin, and digoxin. Prepared digitalis is a crude mixture obtained from both types of foxglove. Strophanthus is extracted from the seeds of the plants *Strophanthus kombi* and *S. gratus*. Ouabain is also extracted from *S. gratus*. Squill, another cardiac glycoside, is obtained from the fleshy bulb of the sea onion, *Urginea maritima*.

Digoxin is the most commonly used of the digitalis group. The drugs all have similar actions and effects, differing in the rate at which they start to act and the duration of their effects. Digitoxin is slower-acting than digoxin, and ouabain acts most rapidly. They act mainly on the heart, increasing both the force of contraction of the heart muscles and the work done by the heart, without increasing its oxygen consumption.

In the failing heart the volume of blood in the heart chambers during relaxation of the muscle increases. This causes the chambers to stretch, which in turn interferes with their pumping capacity when they contract. More blood accumulates in the chambers, causing a back pressure to build up in the blood vessels returning blood to the heart. This back pressure may cause congestion of the lungs and produce breathlessness and disorders of respiration. If the back pressure affects the right side of the heart, to which blood from all over the body is returned, then the pressure builds up in the veins and back to the tissues. This produces an increase of fluids in the tissues called edema (dropsy). Edema may also be due to other causes, such as impaired kidney or liver function, and so one usually distinguishes this form of it as cardiac edema or congestive heart failure.

In heart failure, digitalis and related drugs cause the heart muscle to work more efficiently, causing increased output from the heart, reduction of back pressure, decrease in the size of the heart, and reduction in blood volume. The latter is produced by the effects of a more efficient circulation of blood to the kidneys resulting in increased urine. The drugs are therefore used principally to treat heart failure. They also commonly reduce heart rate secondary to the above-mentioned circulatory improvement by stimulating the vagus nerve, which is normally responsible for slowing the heart. In addition they slow down the rate at which electrical impulses pass from the heart's pacemaker (the part of the heart where electrical impulses start) to the rest of the heart. They are equally effective in treating edema and/or respiratory complications caused by heart disease. They are also used to regulate disorders of heart rate.

When taken by mouth, digoxin, digitalis, and digitoxin are adequately absorbed, although significant variation in absorption among different brands (particularly with digoxin) has been demonstrated. Digoxin should *not* be taken with antacids or kaolin-pectin mixtures, which substantially reduce its absorption. Ouabain is poorly absorbed and should *not* be taken by mouth. Variations in speed of absorption occur, but this is not important in influencing their effects upon the heart, which are more related to differences in transportation of the drugs in the blood and their rate of penetration and accumulation in the cells of the heart muscle. They are broken down very slowly in the body, mainly in the liver, and are eliminated by the kidneys. In patients with impaired kidney or liver function, dangerously high blood levels may occur. Digitalis and digoxin are slowly excreted and are accumulative; traces have been detected in the urine up to six weeks after stopping these drugs.

Digitalis and related drugs cause signs and symptoms of intoxication when taken in high doses, and can produce dangerous adverse effects which may prove fatal.

Many doctors adjust the dose carefully, but intoxication may still occur because of variations in patient response. Even measuring the blood levels may not give an indication of the most appropriate dose, that is, the dose that achieves the most benefits with the least toxic effects.

Loss of appetite, nausea, and vomiting are the early indications of overdose from digitalis and related drugs. Nausea is an important warning, and vomiting can be most distressing to a patient with heart failure. They may also cause diarrhea and abdominal discomfort or pain. These symptoms disappear in a few days, but by using smaller starting doses they are generally avoidable. They must be distinguished from similar symptoms which occasionally develop in heart failure and which are quickly relieved by the correct dose of drug.

Headache, fatigue, drowsiness, and yellow-green vision may also occur, and elderly patients may become confused.

*OD*

The most frequent and well-recognized adverse effect on the heart is the appearance of extra heartbeats. Extra heartbeats occurring after each regular beat are called "coupling" and are a good clue that the patient has been overdosed. Toxic amounts interfere with the passage of electrical impulses from the heart's pacemaker down to the main transmission paths between the upper chambers and the lower chambers. This leads to missed or dropped heartbeats and sometimes to partial or complete heart block. It means that the pacemaker has lost control and the upper and lower chambers of the heart are beating independently. This dangerous adverse effect should be suspected if the heart rate drops below sixty beats per minute. However, an *increase* in rate is sometimes the first evidence of poisoning, because of excitatory effects upon heart muscle. This is a particular hazard in patients

*poison ?wl*

who are also receiving diuretics—these may reduce the blood potassium, and such a reduction sensitizes heart muscle to the effects of digitalislike drugs. In these patients the heart rate may increase even in the presence of heart block. The rapid beating of the heart may become quite irregular, and if it affects the lower chambers (ventricles) it may cause sudden death.

Dosage with these drugs involves two problems: the amount required to produce the desired effects as quickly as possible in someone not previously on the drug (initial digitalization) and the amount required to maintain the good effects with minimal adverse effects (maintenance dosage). There is a wide variation in individual response, and therefore the solution of these two problems requires skill and care. The "right" dose for an individual patient is that which proves right for him.

Digoxin is the drug of choice among the digitalislike drugs. Lanatoside-C (a natural digoxin precursor) has been used as an alternative if the patient vomits on digoxin.

## Drugs Used to Treat Disorders of Heart Rhythm

A large number of unrelated drugs act on the heart and are used to treat disorders of heart rhythm. A disorder of heart rhythm is called an arrhythmia, and drugs used to treat the condition are called antiarrhythmic drugs. The normal heart beats fast (tachycardia) during exercise, during fevers, if you are scared or anxious, and if your thyroid gland overworks. The heart may also beat fast due to disorders of the blood vessels and/or heart. Many drugs increase heartbeat. Slowing of the heart (bradycardia) also has many causes—physical training, obstructive jaundice, drugs, underworking of the thyroid, and heart disorders. Extra heartbeats may occur with anxiety and tension, drinking too much coffee or tea, smoking, and drinking alcohol. Certain drugs such as digitalis and amphetamines may cause extra beats (ectopic beats); so too can disorders of the heart.

## QUINIDINE

Quinidine is related to quinine and comes from cinchona bark. Its main use is restricted to the treatment of disorders of heart rhythm. Since the advent of direct electric current stimulation (DC shock therapy) of the heart in cases of acute disorders of rhythm, quinidine is much less used than previously, but it is still valuable in preventing attacks of arrhythmia. Quinidine depresses excitability of the heart muscle and therefore suppresses extra beats. It reduces the rate of passage of electrical impulses through the heart and depresses the ease with which it contracts. It also prolongs the period of rest between contractions of the heart and prolongs the action of the slowing nerve of the heart (the vagus nerve). It is rapidly absorbed from the gut; its maximal effect occurs in about one to three hours and lasts up to eight hours. However, there is a wide individual variation in response.

Quinidine is also used to prevent recurrent attacks of rapid beating of the heart (paroxysmal tachycardia) and to control extra beats. Most authorities now say it should never be given by injection, and its use by mouth is often preceded by a test dose, since patients may be hypersensitive to it.

## PROCAINAMIDE

Procainamide is related to procaine (a local anesthetic) and has actions on the heart similar to those of quinidine. It is used to regulate disorders of heart rhythm. A large proportion of it is excreted unchanged by the kidneys, and therefore it should be used with caution in patients with impaired kidney function and congestive heart failure. Cumulative effects are more likely to occur in these patients. The metabolism of procainamide is complex and highly variable, so dosage must be calculated to suit the individual patient.

As with quinidine, procainamide may cause a rapid increase in contraction rate of the lower heart chambers when it is used to treat disorders of rhythm arising from the upper chambers. This rapid increase may be dangerous, and treatment with digoxin before using procainamide may reduce the danger.

## LIDOCAINE

Lidocaine, a local anesthetic, was first shown to have an effect on disordered heart rhythm in 1950. It can be given only by injection because of its brief duration of action. It is, therefore, of no use for maintenance treatment. It is used principally to treat disordered rhythm in the lower heart chambers, where it may be used in conjunction with electric heart shock therapy. Reports of convulsions are relatively common, and therefore an intravenous preparation of an anticonvulsant drug should always be available.

### PHENYTOIN (DIPHENYLHYDANTOIN)

Phenytoin has been used to treat epileptic convulsions for many years. In the 1960s it was found to be useful in treating disorders of heart rhythm. It is thought to work on the walls of heart muscle cells, making it easier for sodium and potassium to pass in and out. These elements are involved in causing the heart muscle to contract and relax. When given intravenously it may cause heart block and slowing of the heart rate. Occasionally it may prevent the patient from breathing.

### BETA-RECEPTOR BLOCKING AGENTS

These are discussed in the section on drugs used to treat angina and also in the section on drugs which act on the autonomic nervous system. They include propranolol.

### OTHER DRUGS

Other drugs used to treat disorders of heart rhythm include isoproterenol (of use in complete heart block), atropine (of value in treating slow heart rates), and antazoline (in certain disorders which do not respond to other drugs). Bretylium, reserpine, and guanethidine, which reduce blood pressure, have also been used. Mephentermine and metaraminol, which raise the blood pressure, have been used, and intravenous magnesium sulfate used to be popular for certain disorders of rhythm affecting the lower heart chambers. Recently, edrophonium has been tried.

# DRUGS USED TO PREVENT
# BLOOD FROM CLOTTING

Drugs used to prevent blood from clotting are called anticoagulants. We do not completely understand how these drugs work, partly because of the complexities involved in the process of clotting. Twelve known factors have been recognized as contributing to the eventual formation of a blood clot, and anticoagulant drugs interfere with these various processes.

Anticoagulant drugs are principally used to treat patients who have already developed a thrombus, a clot which develops on the inside wall of a blood vessel. A thrombus may be related to damage or changes in the surface lining and also to changes in the blood. The relationship between blood clotting (as tested outside in the laboratory) and the development of a thrombus inside a blood vessel is not known.

Anticoagulants are used to treat an acute thrombosis (e.g., coronary thrombosis) in hopes that they may reduce further thrombosis. They may also prevent pieces of the thrombus from coming loose and being carried by the flow of blood to other organs; if a clot reaches the lungs or the brain the consequences can be serious and sometimes fatal. This process of a clot coming loose and passing along the bloodstream is called embolism. The piece of clot which ends up wedged in and blocking a blood vessel is called an embolus. Embolism is one of the great dangers of thrombosis, particularly if the thrombosis affects the veins in the abdomen or legs after injury, surgical operations, or childbirth.

The degree to which a certain dose of anticoagulant drug alters the rate of blood clotting in a specimen of a patient's blood is only a guide (but a most important guide) to the possible benefits to the patient and the risks of adverse effects due to bleeding. Prolonged clinical experience of the use of anticoagulant drugs in millions of patients has shown that they are of great benefit in treating thromboses—if used appropriately.

Prolonged anticoagulant treatment may be used in order to prevent recurrence of a coronary thrombosis and in certain other disorders affecting the coronary arteries. They greatly reduce the risk of death in patients with thrombosis affecting deep veins and in those patients who have developed an embolus in their lungs. They may help to prevent deep-vein thrombosis, particularly in elderly patients confined to bed after a surgical operation. Anticoagulant drugs are also used to treat thrombosis of the vessels supplying the eyes and to treat thrombosis occurring in other arteries. They are used to treat patients with rheumatic heart disease who develop irregularities of heart rhythm and who run the risk of "shooting off" an embolus when the rate is controlled by drugs. Anticoagulants are also used after heart operations. Their value in patients who have had a thrombosis in one of the arteries in the brain is not clear, but in certain patients they may be of help.

Anticoagulant drugs may be divided into two groups: those that act directly by interfering with the process of blood clotting and have to be given by injection, and those that act indirectly and may be given by mouth. The latter act by interfering with the production of factors involved in blood clotting. Those drugs which act directly are rapidly effective, whereas those that act indirectly take up to three days to work. The principal direct-acting anticoagulant is heparin. Indirect-acting anticoagulants (oral anticoagulants) include the coumarin derivatives (dicoumarol [bishydroxycoumarin], acenocoumarol, and warfarin sodium) and the indanedione derivatives (diphenadione, phenindione, and anisindione).

Heparin does not work when given by mouth; it is best given by injection into a vein. It works immediately, but its effects quickly wear off and it has to be given every four or six hours—although, more recently, for *preventative* purposes, it has been used effectively in low doses given every eight to twelve hours. The drug may also be given by injection (mixed with a dispersing agent) under the skin or into a muscle. The normal time taken for the blood to clot on glass (known as the clotting time) is about five to seven minutes. If heparin is to be effective, the dose should be adjusted to keep the clotting time above fifteen minutes. Adverse effects to heparin therapy are bleeding into various sites and, in rare cases, fever and allergic reactions. Signs of overdose are nosebleeds, bruising, and red blood cells in the urine. Slight bleeding due to overdosage can usually be treated by stopping the drug. Severe bleeding may be reduced by giving a slow intravenous injection of protamine sulfate.

Coumarin derivatives are anticoagulants that prevent the production of certain clotting factors. They may be taken by mouth and are slow to act. Dicoumarol is irregularly absorbed from the gut and takes 24 to 72 hours to work. Its effects may last for up to five to six days after the last dose. Because of its slow onset, unpredictable response, and dangers of bleeding, dicoumarol is now seldom used, having been replaced by warfarin sodium. Acenocoumarol is rapidly absorbed from the gut. It works in 36 to 48 hours, and its effects wear off within 36 to 48 hours of the last dose. Warfarin sodium is readily absorbed from the gut and is equally effective by mouth or injection into a vein or muscle. It works in 36 to 72 hours and its effects may last up to four to five days after stopping the drug. (It is also used as a rat poison.)

Phenindione takes up to 24 or 48 hours to reach its desired effect, which wears off one to four days after stopping the drug. Its metabolites color the urine red-orange. Early signs of overdosage are bleeding from the gums or elsewhere and red blood cells in the urine. Deaths have occurred in people allergic to phenindione; a sore throat may be an early sign of such an allergy. Diphenadione is far less toxic than phenindione. However, its long duration of action (15 to 20 days) complicates the management of bleeding in "overdoses." Anisindione appears safer than phenindione, though more clinical studies are necessary to verify this. Rashes have been reported, and it colors the urine red-orange.

## The Use of Oral Anticoagulants

Because of their delayed action, a loading dose of oral anticoagulants was given initially, in the past. But this technique has largely been discontinued due to the danger of hemorrhage. Therefore, in order to start patients off on a course of anticoagulants in emergency situations, heparin is given at the same time, usually for the first two days. Maintenance doses of oral anticoagulants are calculated according to a blood-clotting test (called the prothrombin time). The aim of treatment is to keep the prothrombin time at two to three times the normal value of twelve seconds. Daily estimates are made initially, and once a steady prothrombin time is achieved, the frequency of tests may be reduced. Since these drugs are accumulative, the dose should not be changed more frequently than every five or seven days. Bleeding is the most common adverse effect; it may be reduced by administering vitamin $K_1$ in about four hours by an intravenous injection or by mouth in about twelve hours. Vitamin $K_3$ (menadione) is of no value in this circumstance.

Oral anticoagulants should be used with caution in patients with impaired kidney or liver function and in patients in whom there is a risk of hemorrhage. (They may be used during menstruation.) They should not be used within three days of childbirth or a surgical operation. Mothers on these drugs should not breast-feed, and the drugs should not be taken in the last few months of pregnancy.

Many drugs interact with oral anticoagulants. For example, the effects of phenindione are increased by clofibrate and by anabolic steroids (e.g., nandrolone). Its anticoagulant effects may be reduced by haloperidol. The effects of warfarin sodium are increased by, for example, aspirin and other salicylates, clofibrate, dextrothyroxine, disulfiram, oxyphenbutazone, phenylbutazone, and possibly by anabolic steroids, antibiotics, and quinidine.

If you are on an oral anticoagulant drug you should carry a warning card and carefully check the list of drugs which may interact with anticoagulants. If there is an unexpected change in your prothrombin time, check any drug you have been taking to see if it interferes with the effects of your anticoagulant drug. In general, avoid taking any other drugs until you talk to your doctor or pharmacist.

Because of the risk of severe hypersensitivity reactions from the indanedione derivative phenindione, it is better to use the coumarin derivative warfarin sodium. Acenocoumarol is an alternative.

# DRUGS USED TO TREAT DISORDERS OF CIRCULATION

**Drugs Used to Increase Circulation to the Limbs**

The blood supply to the arms and legs may be affected by anything which obstructs the flow of blood through the arteries. This may be a blockage within the artery—a thrombus, for example, if recognized very quickly, may sometimes be removed by surgery. (However, most thrombi are treated with drugs which stop the blood from clotting.) The flow of blood may also be reduced by narrowing of arteries. This may be the result of hardening and loss of elasticity of the artery walls (arteriosclerosis). Such hardening occurs with advancing age, especially in patients with high blood pressure, in whom arteriosclerosis may be found not only in medium-sized and large arteries but also in the smaller arteries which supply the various tissues and organs of the body. Medium and large arteries may also be affected by atherosclerosis, the process of depositing fatty materials on the inside walls of arteries. Such deposits narrow the artery and reduce the blood flow, and may affect the coronary arteries supplying the heart, the circulation to the brain, or the circulation to the limbs. Atherosclerosis appears to be related to blood fat levels. The artery walls may also be affected by inflammation (as in syphilis) or by allergic reactions. A disorder called Buerger's disease (thromboangiitis obliterans) occasionally affects the arteries of the legs, particularly in men who are heavy smokers. Children may also suffer from disorders of circulation because of damaged arteries produced by certain immunological diseases.

The amount of blood flowing through an artery may also be reduced because its walls close up (go into spasm) due to some fault in the control mechanisms which normally govern the supply of blood to a particular tissue or organ. Blood flow to any part of the body (e.g., skin or muscle) is controlled by a balance between the pressure of blood within the arteries and the amount of resistance the flow meets when it gets to the blood vessels supplying the tissues. This resistance can vary. The body itself controls the resistance by monitoring the degree of spasm of the terminal vessels and smaller arteries. Nerves in the vessel walls respond to three mechanisms: first, stimulation that produces constriction; second, the natural tone of the blood vessel muscles, which makes them "want" to constrict; third, reaction to a variety of chemicals produced by the body in response to certain influences.

There are two types of nerve receptors in blood vessels. Alpha receptors cause constriction, and beta receptors cause dilation.

Drugs which improve the circulation act by blocking the stimulation of the alpha receptors, by stimulating the beta receptors, or by acting directly upon muscles in the vessel walls. Unfortunately, most disorders of circulation are due to changes in the artery walls (arteriosclerosis, atherosclerosis) which have made the wall hardened and unresponsive to stimulation. Also, if a medium or large artery supplying an arm or leg is hardened or narrowed, the branch arteries (collateral circulation) are usually working to maximum capacity and cannot be stimulated to dilate further. In such cases the use of drugs may be harmful. It may, for example, divert an already poor blood supply from the skin to the muscles instead, leading to further damage to the skin.

Drugs used to improve circulation are often referred to as vasodilator drugs, and the patients who may benefit from the use of these drugs are those with disorders due to spasm of arteries (vasospasm). For example, there is a vasospastic disorder called Raynaud's syndrome which usually affects women under fifty. In these patients exposure to cold, and sometimes emotion, may cause the fingers to "go dead." All fingers are affected and sometimes the toes. The patient experiences pins and needles, numbness, burning, and pain. The fingers go pale, bluish, and then red. Vasodilator drugs may benefit persons with mild symptoms, but severe and longstanding symptoms are usually associated with irreversible changes in the vessels which may make vasodilator drugs ineffective.

Vasodilator drugs are of limited value in other vasospastic disorders. Their benefit to patients with chilblains is very doubtful, and their use to prevent frostbite has been disappointing. This is because exposure to low temperatures closes up the blood vessels supplying the local areas of skin and makes them unresponsive to vasodilator drugs. Other conditions such as acrocyanosis (blueness of the fingers, hands, ears, and nose on exposure to cold) and erythrocyanosis (a bluish red discoloration of the legs) are not helped by such drugs. A disorder characterized by red, burning feet (erythromelalgia) may occasionally be helped by vasodilator drugs.

In patients with diseases of artery walls (arteriosclerosis, atherosclerosis, Buerger's disease) vasodilator drugs may not work. But they may increase blood flow to the skin and be of use in treating ulcers of the skin caused by poor circulation. They may also be useful in treating gangrene.

Poor circulation may cause pain in the muscles after exercise (intermittent claudication), but, unfortunately, this is not much helped by vasodilator drugs.

There are several groups of vasodilator drugs:

ALPHA-RECEPTOR BLOCKERS

These drugs block the alpha receptors and, therefore, cause the peripheral blood vessels to dilate. Their effects are most marked on the blood vessels in the skin of the arms and legs. The blood vessels supplying muscles are less affected. Drugs belonging to this group include phenoxybenzamine, phentolamine, tolazoline, and azapetine. Azapetine is an alpha-receptor blocker but also acts on the artery muscles.

Doctors should prescribe phenoxybenzamine with caution to patients with high blood pressure, impaired kidney function, or coronary artery disease, and never to a patient in whom a fall in blood pressure may be harmful. Phentolamine should be given with caution to patients with coronary artery disease. Tolazoline should also be given with caution to patients with coronary artery disease or heart disorders, and since it increases acid production by the stomach it should not be given to patients with peptic ulcers. Azapetine may also cause a fall in blood pressure.

BETA-RECEPTOR STIMULANTS

These cause dilation of the arteries by stimulating the beta receptors. Since beta receptors are mainly present in blood vessels supplying muscles, these drugs are principally used to improve the blood circulation to muscles. They stimulate the heart, increase its rate and output, and are likely to cause a fall in blood pressure. They include nylidrin and isoxsuprine.

Nylidrin may cause palpitations and should be given with caution to patients who suffer from episodes of rapid beating of the heart or overworking of the thyroid gland. It increases production of acid by the stomach and should not be given to patients with peptic ulcers. It should not be given to patients with coronary artery disease or severe angina. Isoxsuprine should be given with caution to patients with low blood pressure and a fast heart rate.

DRUGS WHICH ACT DIRECTLY UPON ARTERIAL MUSCLES

These drugs cause arteries to dilate by a direct unknown action upon the artery walls. They include: cyclandelate, nicotinyl, and niacin (nicotinic acid).

This vasodilatation increases the blood flow to muscles and skin.

The changes in the skin circulation are more marked in the face and neck (where you blush) than in the arms and legs.

In addition to the vasodilator drugs mentioned above, ethyl alcohol by mouth has also been used because it has a direct action on blood vessels and also works on the center in the brain which controls the tone of arteries. Reserpine has this effect, and an ergot preparation (dihydroergotoxine) has been shown to block alpha receptors and have vasodilator effects.

*Topical* application of a newly marketed nitroglycerin ointment may be of some use in the treatment of Raynaud's syndrome and of slowly healing ulcers with reduced blood supply.

### Choice of Vasodilator Drugs

Mild adverse effects with vasodilator drugs are common, and when given in effective dose they usually cause rapid beating of the heart and a fall in blood pressure. Patients may complain of flushing of the face and stuffiness of the nose. Some of the drugs may cause gastrointestinal symptoms—nausea, vomiting, diarrhea. Some patients complain of feeling excitable. Vasodilator drugs should not be used in patients with coronary artery disease, congestive heart failure, peptic ulcers, overworking of the thyroid, or glaucoma. They should be used with caution in patients with impaired heart function and by those with diabetes or impaired kidney function.

They may be of some use in disorders of arterial spasm, but their use in arterial diseases which damage vessel walls is doubtful. There is no one drug which may be recommended over the others in the various groups. They are sometimes prescribed for chilblains, but warm surroundings, warm clothes, and exercise will be of more benefit than any drug available.

### Drugs Used to Increase the Circulation to the Brain

No drug has a special effect upon the blood vessels which supply the brain. Those that are used are general vasodilators. Their effectiveness in treating disorders produced by changes in the arteries supplying the brain, though of help in some patients, has never been clearly evaluated because of the complexities involved. Furthermore, there are risks involved in the use of such drugs—fall in blood pressure and redistribution of blood supply away from areas that may require more oxygen as the result of an already diminished blood supply.

Cyclandelate, isoxsuprine, papaverine, and dihydroergotoxine have been used and have been heavily promoted for the treatment of forgetful elderly people. Their usefulness in such patients, who are labeled as suffering from arteriosclerotic cerebrovascular disease, has not been satisfactorily proved.

# DRUGS USED TO
# TREAT ATHEROSCLEROSIS

Atherosclerosis refers to the thickening of the walls of arteries caused by deposits of fats and other substances. It causes the vessels to become narrow and the lining surface roughened, producing a serious impairment of blood flow. Atherosclerosis of the coronary arteries has been directly related to angina and deaths from heart attacks due to coronary thrombosis. When it affects the arteries supplying the brain it may cause impairment of mental function and thrombosis leading to paralysis. In the legs it may cause pains in the muscles during exercise, poor circulation to the skin, and many other serious consequences.

In recent years it has become apparent that many factors are involved in coronary artery disease. We should all know the risks of smoking, overeating, and not taking enough exercise. But one fairly constant factor which has been observed is the relationship between high "blood fat levels" and coronary artery disease in some patients. I use "blood fat levels" to cover the blood levels of a complex group of fats and other chemicals (including cholesterol)—five different chemical compositions classed into four groups which are called lipoproteins. The importance of the relationship between blood fat levels and atherosclerosis has repeatedly been demonstrated. In families who suffer from high blood fat levels and in patients with such disorders as diabetes (in which blood fat levels are increased) the incidence of coronary artery disease is markedly increased. In countries where diets are different than in Western countries and where it has been found that blood fat levels are lower, the incidence of coronary artery disease is less. Also, in World War II the incidence dropped in some European countries, probably because of changes in diet. Animal experiments have also shown a relationship between diet and atherosclerosis.

Drugs are available which lower blood fat levels, but the need to use these drugs is not clear. Different drugs lower different blood fats, and yet the part played by each is not fully understood. Certain high-risk patients may benefit from the use of these drugs—patients in whom high blood fat levels run in the family; patients with high blood fat levels and high blood pressure; and patients who have survived a coronary thrombosis. But, obviously, the most sensible approach to treatment of high blood fat is to control the diet.

Obesity may be related to a high blood fat level; so may the amounts of carbohydrates or fats in the diet. The type and ratio of different fats in the diet can also influence the blood fat level, particularly the ratio of what are called unsaturated fatty acids (in vegetable and fish oils) to saturated fatty acids (in animal fats and dairy produce). A source of unsaturated fatty acids was shown over twenty years ago to be beneficial in preventing coronary artery disease. However, recently there have been reports linking premature aging with consumption of unsaturated fatty acids, and "oxidized" vegetable oils (a condition produced when vegetable oils are reused and reheated in frying) may be harmful.

The answer is to eat a well-balanced diet, exercise regularly, keep your weight down, and cut out smoking. Eat margarine instead of butter and fry in oil instead of lard. Those with high blood pressure should be treated.

## Drugs Which Lower Blood Fat Levels

Clofibrate is effective in lowering certain of the blood fats, although its mode of action is not fully understood. It may affect enzymes in the body and produce a group of symptoms which include muscle cramps, stiffness, weakness, and muscle tenderness. It should not be given to patients with impaired kidney or liver function or during pregnancy.

Large doses of nicotinic acid (of the vitamin B group) may reduce blood fat levels but can produce flushing and itching. This usually clears after a few weeks in most patients. Such large doses may cause liver damage and jaundice.

Cholestyramine also reduces blood fat levels. It works in the gut by exchanging chloride ions for bile salts (which are formed in part from blood fats), which it binds into an insoluble complex that is excreted in the feces, thus preventing the reabsorption of bile salts. This causes further conversion of fats to bile salts, which eventually may lead to a reduction in blood fat levels. It may also interfere with the absorption of other drugs (chlorothiazide, phenylbutazone, phenobarbital, various digitalis preparations, tetracyclines, thyroid hormones, and many others). High doses interfere with the absorption of fat and fat-soluble vitamins, such as vitamins A and D. Therefore, any other drug should be given one hour before or three hours after a dose of cholestyramine. Extra vitamins A and D that are mixable with water and also vitamin K should be given to patients on prolonged treatment.

Blood fat levels are low in disorders which cause overworking of the thyroid gland, and they are high in disorders which cause underworking. Drugs related to thyroid hormones, although lowering blood fat levels, also push up the frequency and severity of anginal attacks. They may also produce disorders of heart rhythm and other adverse effects and therefore are not suitable for lowering blood fat levels.

Estrogens (female sex hormones) when given to males reduce their blood fat levels, but only in high doses which cause men to develop breasts, become impotent, lose their sexual desires, and (not surprisingly) become depressed. Needless to say, these drugs are not used. Some oral contraceptive pills may produce a rise in certain of the blood fats.

### The Choice of Drugs to Lower Blood Fat

Obviously the future must lie in attempting to prevent atherosclerosis by controlling diet and taking more exercise. In the meantime drugs are of use in treating selected patients who have been shown to have raised blood fat levels, although as yet conclusive proof of the long-term value of such drugs is needed. The three drugs discussed—clofibrate, nicotinic acid, and cholestyramine—work on different blood fats. The decision to use one or the other must depend upon detailed and repeated tests of blood fat levels.

Remember also that heavy smoking appears to be a causative factor, along with raised blood fat levels and high blood pressure, in producing diseases of the arteries.

# DRUGS USED
# TO TREAT ANGINA

*Angina pectoris* is the term used to describe attacks of pain from the heart of short duration and without evidence of lasting damage to the heart muscle. It is caused by a constriction in some of the coronary arteries which supply the heart. This results in a deficient supply of blood to part of the working heart muscle, and a consequent shortage of oxygen. A heart attack results when the blood supply to part of the muscle is actually cut off as a consequence of a spasm or blockage in one of the coronary arteries or its branches. A thrombus (clot) is one of the commonest causes of this blockage. Narrowing and closure (coronary occlusion) may produce a similar effect.

Angina usually occurs during effort and stops during rest. This is because during exertion the heart has to do more work and the heart muscle requires more oxygen. If the coronary arteries are not healthy enough to supply the extra oxygen, the muscle starts to ache. As soon as the patient rests, the heart has to do less work, oxygen demand falls, and the pain ceases. Many factors can trigger an attack of angina, and people vary tremendously in their response to treatment. For these reasons the assessment of drugs in relieving angina is very difficult. Most of these drugs are aimed at improving the blood supply and therefore the oxygen supply to the heart muscle.

Drugs used to treat angina include those used to treat an acute attack or to prevent an attack over the short term, and those used to prevent attacks over the long term. They belong to two major groups: organic nitrates and nitrites, and inorganic nitrites; and beta-receptor blocking drugs.

## Nitrites and Nitrates

Amyl nitrite and nitroglycerin (glyceryl trinitrate) have been used for over one hundred years. Organic nitrites and nitrates and inorganic nitrites have similar actions and effects. Their basic action is to relax involuntary muscles, particularly those in the walls of blood vessels. This results in dilation of blood vessels and various other effects. High doses of these drugs reduce the return and output of blood to and from the heart—so much so that a "normal" individual may faint if kept standing up. They lead to a reduction of workload for the heart, so less oxygen is needed. In addition, these drugs improve the flow of blood through the coronary arteries.

The choice of a nitrate or nitrite is not an important one. Amyl nitrite has to be sniffed up the nose and it smells, whereas nitroglycerin is available as small tablets which act quickly when sucked slowly under the tongue. These drugs decrease electrocardiographic evidence of reduced oxygen supply to heart muscle, they increase the amount of exercise a patient can do before getting an attack of angina, and they relieve or prevent pain.

## Beta-Receptor Blocking Drugs

The principal beta-receptor blocking drug is propranolol. Many patients develop angina in response to an emotional upset or physical exercise. The heart beats faster in response to fear, panic, tension, anxiety, excitation, or aggression, increasing its workload (called psychomotor stimulation), and in the presence of a deficient coronary artery blood supply, anginal pain will develop. The rapid beating of the heart is caused by stimulation through beta receptors, and thus drugs which prevent such stimulation protect the heart. Blocking beta receptors will also prevent stimulation that occurs during exercise.

Beta-receptor blocking drugs in present use have a marked effect when the heart is being stimulated by exercise, emotion, or epinephrinelike drugs. They reduce the effects of such stimulation to produce slowing of the rate and force of contraction of the heart. Some of them reduce the rate of conduction of impulses through the conducting system of the heart and some have a quinidinelike action. The overall result from beta-receptor blockers is a reduction in the volume of blood pumped out by the heart during each contraction and a decreased oxygen consumption because the heart has to do less work.

They are used to treat angina, to lower blood pressure, and to correct abnormal rhythms. Beta-receptor blockers may also be used to treat patients who develop heart symptoms in response to stress or tension —for example, in patients who, because of anxiety, develop rapid heartbeat and/or extra beats before going on stage or just before a public lecture. They are also used for treating some patients with anxiety who develop heart symptoms and then worry about their heart. Such patients have had numerous labels placed on their condition: effort syndrome, disorderly action of the heart (DAH), hyperkinetic heart syndrome.

However, beta-receptor blocking drugs can trigger heart failure in patients who are near to such a state. They should be given to patients with heart failure only when they have been fully digitalized (see p. 86). They may make heart block worse, and they should not be used in pregnancy. In patients with asthma, bronchospasm, and bronchitis they may cause constriction of the bronchial tubes. Note that discontinuance of beta-blocking drugs after long-term therapy in patients with angina must be done *gradually* and under careful supervision of a doctor. Sudden discontinuance has caused heart attacks.

## Other Drugs Used to Treat Angina

Monoamine oxidase inhibitor antidepressant drugs (see p. 59) have been tried, but they provide relief only of the symptoms of angina. They do not affect the abnormal readings shown on the electrocardiogram. This means that in relieving the pain they may mask the danger, and the patient may do more exercise than is good for him. Their use is not recommended. Dipyridamole increases coronary blood flow but has been found to be ineffective in treating angina. Prenylamine also increases coronary blood flow but like dipyridamole has been found not to prevent electrocardiogram changes produced during an attack.

Patients with angina who suffer from anxiety or tension may benefit from intermittent use of an antianxiety drug. All such patients should stop smoking, take regular moderate exercise, eat a well-balanced diet, and watch their weight.

Coronary artery disease may be related to blood fat levels in certain patients. The use of drugs to lower blood fat levels is discussed on p. 99.

## Choice of Drugs in the Treatment of Angina

Nitroglycerin is the drug of choice in the treatment or prevention of individual attacks of angina. You should learn your own dosage regimens. Relief of pain takes about two minutes. Many patients take a tablet just before the onset of exertion which they know will produce pain—e.g., going up stairs or engaging in sexual intercourse. It protects them for twenty to thirty minutes. What is important about the nitrates and nitrites is that not only do they increase the amount of exercise you can do before developing angina and relieve pain if taken when an attack develops, but they also produce evidence of their good effects on the electrocardiogram. Some of the longer-acting nitrates such as erythrityl tetranitrate and isosorbide dinitrate may produce relief for up to two hours.

The aim of long-term treatment of angina is to try to get a more steady drug effect without having to anticipate or experience an attack. The beta-receptor blockers delay both the onset of pain and the appearance of exercise changes on the electrocardiogram. However, the relationship between pain and oxygen requirements is not quite as straightforward as it is with nitroglycerin. The use of these drugs has been shown to reduce the number of anginal attacks and the consumption of nitroglycerin, but we do not yet know the consequences of their long-term use. In any case, propranolol is the only beta-receptor blocker available at the present time in the United States.

# DIURETICS

The term "diuretic" refers to a drug which acts on the kidneys to produce an increased output of sodium salt and water in the urine. It is generally restricted to those drugs used to treat disorders of the heart, kidneys, or liver which result in an excessive retention of fluids in the body, so much so that swelling may be visible. Such swelling is called edema and used to be called dropsy. Swelling of the tissues is usually more obvious in the feet and ankles because of the effect of gravity. In a patient confined to bed the fluid gravitates to the lower part of the back. Excessive fluid inside the abdominal cavity is called ascites.

Some weak diuretics are used to decrease the fluid pressure inside the eyeballs, as in glaucoma, where the drainage of the eye fluid is impaired. Diuretics are also used to treat certain lung disorders in which fluid accumulates in the lung tissue (pulmonary edema)—this is a serious medical emergency. However, it must be remembered that the underlying disease process in all of these disorders is not affected by diuretic treatment. Diuretics are also used in the treatment of high blood pressure, both to enhance the effects of other drugs and to counteract the salt and water retention produced by certain other drugs. In addition, because they increase urinary output, they are used to treat overdose with certain drugs that are excreted by the kidneys.

The kidneys exercise a most delicate and complex control over the body's salt and water balance. Salt at first enters the urine but is subsequently reabsorbed into the bloodstream according to the body's needs. The amount of salt in the urine governs the amount of water passed out by the process known as osmosis (the tendency of fluids, separated by a membrane which is partly permeable, to mix). The process of osmosis takes the direction from the weaker to the stronger solution, and therefore, if there is a lot of salt in the urine, a lot of water will pass out and be excreted in the urine. In addition, there are also other rather complex chemical and hormonal processes which affect the amount of salt and water passed out in the urine.

The great majority of diuretics in use today act directly upon the kidneys by depressing the reabsorption of various salts from the urine back into the bloodstream, thus producing an increased output of salt and water from the body. Some diuretics not only interfere with the reabsorption of sodium salt (ordinary salt) but also with potassium salts. This produces a low blood potassium level, which may produce muscle weakness, constipation, or loss of appetite; more seriously, a low blood potassium level sensitizes the heart to digitalis drugs, which are frequently used to treat heart failure and disorders of rhythm (see p. 86).

There are several groups of diuretic drugs:

## Thiazide Diuretics and Related Drugs

These drugs vary greatly in potency and duration of effect. They are well absorbed when given by mouth, and they increase the excretion of sodium chloride by the kidneys. When used in effective dosage they all increase the excretion of potassium. They are widely used alone or in combination with drugs used to treat high blood pressure.

They include: bendroflumethiazide, benzthiazide, chlorothiazide, hydrochlorothiazide, chlorthalidone, clopamide, clorexolone, cyclopenthiazide, hydroflumethiazide, methyclothiazide, metolazone, polythiazide, quinethazone.

All thiazide diuretics have effects similar to chlorothiazide, which may cause nausea, dizziness, weakness, numbness, pins and needles, skin rashes, allergic reactions, blood disorders, and sensitivity of the skin to sunlight. Thiazide diuretics may cause alterations in water and salt balance—reduced sodium and potassium blood levels and sometimes increased blood calcium. They may elevate blood sugar and cause sugar to appear in the urine in diabetics and other susceptible individuals. They may also cause an increase in blood uric acid level and trigger an attack of gout in some people. They should be used with caution in patients with impaired kidney or liver function or diabetes. They may reduce blood potassium levels and thereby increase the toxicity of the digitalis drugs. The blood-pressure-lowering effects of certain drugs (e.g., guanethidine, methyldopa, reserpine) are increased by thiazide diuretics.

If you are on a thiazide diuretic and have impaired liver or kidney function, you should restrict your salt intake. You will need to be advised about low-salt diets. Patients with congestive heart failure may benefit by eating a normal diet, but they should avoid *adding* salt to their meals. In order to compensate for any potassium loss caused by thiazide diuretics you should eat a diet containing foods such as fruit that are rich in potassium. A satisfactory diet can usually do away with the need for potassium supplements. Potassium supplements are frequently prescribed, but some are unpleasant to take Liquids and tablets of potassium may cause stomach pains. Specially coated tablets may produce ulcers of the gut and should not be used.

The practice of adding potassium to tablets of diuretics has never been convincingly shown to be of benefit in preventing a fall in body potassium levels. Some doctors consider that it is better to use the diuretic intermittently (every other day or twice a week) and maintain a good diet. If potassium levels fall, the addition of a potassium-retaining diuretic may help, or supplements of potassium salts given separately from the diuretics (e.g., on different days) will help. Potassium chloride is the best salt to use because of the loss of chloride which diuretics produce. Effervescent potassium chloride tablets are satisfactory. Slow-release potassium chloride tablets may cause ulcers of the gut, though less often than specially coated tablets. Liquid preparations of potassium chloride are safest.

Because of the effect of thiazide diuretics on blood sugar, they may sometimes trigger an attack of diabetes in a person predisposed to develop diabetes. If you are on long-term treatment with one of these drugs you ought to get your urine tested for sugar periodically. Similarly, if you have a family history of gout it may be worth asking your doctor to check your blood uric acid levels at intervals. Your blood salt levels should also be checked at intervals.

Diuretic drugs have revolutionized the treatment of congestive heart failure. Yet they are not infrequently prescribed in inappropriate dosage for too long a time and without sufficient advice to the patient about frequency of dosage and diet and warnings of adverse effects.

## Ethacrynic Acid and Furosemide

These are more potent than the thiazide diuretics. They increase the excretion of salt, and although they are chemically different they have similar effects. They are sometimes combined with other classes of diuretics, particularly those which conserve potassium, in the management of hard-to-treat edema. They act quickly when given by injection, and their duration of effect is short. Dosage must be controlled with caution, since high doses may produce a massive output of urine, leading to a fall in blood pressure and a decreased production of urine by the kidneys. Furosemide is somewhat easier to adjust to the individual patient's needs. These drugs are of particular use when urgent diuresis is required, as in edema of the lungs, and where thiazide diuretics have failed. They should be used with caution in elderly men with enlarged prostate glands, since the increased production of urine may lead to retention. Both drugs may cause potassium loss (sometimes severe), and some patients may require potassium supplements.

## Mild Diuretics Used to Treat Glaucoma

In the early 1950s a group of diuretics was introduced which blocked the action of an enzyme involved in the kidneys' control of water and salt balance. The enzyme is responsible for exchanging hydrogen ions for sodium ions in the urine so that body sodium is conserved. The diuretics block this action and cause the sodium not to be absorbed. This group of drugs includes acetazolamide and dichlorphenamide. Acetazolamide causes mild adverse effects fairly frequently. The body's potassium and sodium level may fall after prolonged use. Patients with impaired liver function may become confused and disoriented. Dichlorphenamide produces adverse effects similar to those described under acetazolamide, but no blood disorders or kidney damage have been reported (see these drugs in Part III). In the treatment of glaucoma, both drugs reduce the formation of fluid inside the eye and reduce the pressure. Tolerance quickly develops to the diuretic effects, and they should be given only intermittently.

## Osmotic Diuretics

Any substance which passes out of the blood in the kidneys and into the urine may interfere with salt reabsorption, resulting in increased salt in the urine, which then takes water with it by a process of osmosis. The ones used for this purpose are called osmotic diuretics, and they must produce no other action in the body. They include mannitol, urea, and glycerin (glycerol). Mannitol is a type of alcohol which passes from blood to urine in the kidneys and is not reabsorbed.

Glycerin is another type of alcohol and works in a fashion similar to that of mannitol.

Urea may be used as an osmotic diuretic. When given by mouth it may cause nausea and vomiting, while intravenous injection may cause headache, nausea, vomiting, and a fall in blood pressure. It may also produce phlebitis at the site of the injection. It should not be used in patients with impaired kidney function.

Osmotic diuretics may be used to keep urine flow going after severe injury, to prevent kidney damage, to eliminate certain drugs after overdose (e.g., aspirin), and to reduce the pressure from fluid accumulation inside the eyes in glaucoma and inside the skull after head injury. They are rarely used to treat edema.

## Diuretics Which Conserve Potassium

Aldosterone is a hormone produced by the adrenal glands. It plays a role in the body's salt and water balancing mechanisms. An excess of it may be produced by a tumor of the adrenal glands or in response to certain disorders such as severe congestive heart failure or cirrhosis of the liver associated with the collection of increased fluid in the abdomen (ascites) It works on the kidneys, where it increases the reabsorption of sodium and the excretion of potassium. There are drugs which block these effects, thus increasing the excretion of sodium (which takes water with it) and reducing the excretion of potassium.

Spironolactone is such a drug. It is of some use in treating ascites due to cirrhosis of the liver, but in treating other disorders not primarily due to overproduction of adrenal hormone, it is best combined with a thiazide diuretic. It is absorbed from the gut, is slow to act (up to three days), and is excreted slowly. Because of the risk of causing a high blood potassium, spironolactone should be given with caution to patients with impaired kidney function.

Triamterene reduces sodium reabsorption and reduces potassium loss in the urine. It was originally thought that it blocked the effects of aldosterone on the kidneys like spironolactone, but animal experiments have not confirmed this. Triamterene is not a very potent diuretic, and it is usually combined with a thiazide diuretic. It increases urate excretion rather than decreasing it like the thiazide diuretics (see Drugs Used to Treat Gout, p. 124). It may also cause an increased excretion of calcium in the urine and other disturbances of salt and water balance. It should be used with caution in patients with impaired liver or kidney function and in those with diabetes. Amiloride has effects and uses similar to triamterene.

The principal use of triamterene and amiloride is in combination with a thiazide diuretic in order to reduce potassium loss in the urine. There are rare reports of deaths caused by high body potassium levels in patients treated with such combinations. This risk is increased in patients with impaired kidney function. Since the dangers from a high body potassium are greater than from a low body potassium, some authorities do not recommend these mixtures as routine.

### Xanthine Diuretics
This group includes caffeine, theophylline, and theobromine. They are present in tea, coffee, cola drinks, and cocoa. They are mild diuretics and work by increasing the rate of salt excretion. They were used for this purpose until the thiazide diuretics were discovered in the 1950s.

### Choice of Diuretic
Thiazide diuretics are taken by mouth and are suitable if you are being treated at home and are not bedridden. They are useful for long-term treatment, and the choice is not critical. Potassium loss may be reduced by taking them every other day or twice a week and by following a diet containing fruit or other foods high in potassium, or by taking potassium supplements on different days and not adding salt to the diet. In urgent cases of edema, furosemide or ethacrynic acid by injection is indicated, but opinion is divided about their prolonged use once the patient has got over the acute episode. Spironolactone is of use in treating disorders in which there is considered to be an increased production of aldosterone hormone. The combination of a potassium-retaining diuretic (triamterene, amiloride) with a thiazide diuretic may be helpful in certain patients. But remember, any combination of diuretics should be used with caution because of the risks produced by an increase or decrease in body potassium level.

# DRUGS USED TO TREAT
# RAISED BLOOD PRESSURE

The blood is driven around the body under pressure from the contractions of the heart. This blood pressure depends principally upon the amount of blood being pumped out by the heart and the resistance it meets as it enters smaller and smaller blood vessels.

The range of "normal" blood pressure varies considerably among individuals and at different times in the same individual. It is influenced by many factors—age, sex, physical exercise, food, smoking, drugs, and changes in posture. Emotional excitement particularly may send your blood pressure up, whereas sleep sends it down. Repeated blood pressure recordings often give lower levels overall than just a single casual recording. And so it is important to remember that your doctor cannot really tell whether your blood pressure is slightly or moderately higher than "normal" from a single blood pressure reading. Nor can he tell you whether it is "high" without considering your age, weight, sex, nationality, family history, and so on. An individual is considered to have a raised blood pressure (hypertension) only if the pressure is consistently raised in the absence of any factors which may cause a temporary increase during the recording. There are two groups of hypertension. The first is very common, and because we do not know what causes it we call it "essential" or "idiopathic" hypertension. The other group, called secondary hypertension, is caused by a known disorder such as kidney disease, adrenal disorders, toxemia of pregnancy, narrowing of the main artery from the heart or of an artery supplying a kidney, and certain disorders of the nervous system.

The blood pressure recording consists of two readings. The upper reading is the pressure at the point where the contractions (systole) of the heart force the pulse wave of blood through the artery from which the pressure is being recorded (this is usually the artery at the front of the elbow). This is called the systolic blood pressure. The second reading is the pressure recorded between the pulse waves when the heart is relaxed and filling with blood (diastole), ready for the next pumping action. This is called the diastolic blood pressure. The readings are recorded as the systolic over the diastolic pressures—e.g., 120/80—and the units are in millimeters—e.g., 120/80 mm.

Systolic blood pressure may be raised independently by emotion, fever, pregnancy, and old age when the arteries harden and narrow. An increased systolic blood pressure is considered to be of less importance than an increased diastolic blood pressure, because the latter appears to be more related to resistance to the flow of blood caused by constriction of the peripheral arteries.

High blood pressure is significant because there is an increased predisposition to illness and death among people with this condition. It has been found to be more common among patients with coronary artery disease. There appears also to be a connection between high blood pressure and disease of the blood vessels; for example, of blood vessels supplying the brain, which may produce an increased risk of a stroke. Sustained high blood pressure may also be associated with heart failure and kidney damage (which in turn causes an increase in pressure, since damaged kidneys sometimes produce a chemical which increases the blood pressure). High blood pressure may also damage blood vessels in the eye.

We know very little about what causes essential hypertension. Blood pressure increases with age. In early life the pressure is higher in men than in women, but from middle age (around forty-five years) the pressure becomes higher in women than in men. Men are much more likely than women to develop complications such as coronary artery disease, and in men the higher the pressure the higher is the risk of premature death. Hereditary, dietary, environmental, psychological, and racial factors have all been considered in attempts to account for the development of essential hypertension. Raised blood pressure is also considered (by some) to be related to obesity, so that reduction in weight may help, although differences in thickness of the arm (at the point where the cuff is applied when measuring the blood pressure) may also alter the recordings.

There are differences of opinion over exactly what constitutes a raised blood pressure as well as differences of opinion over how and when to treat the condition. The situation is made even more confusing by the different types of drugs available, many of which produce serious adverse effects. Unfortunately, the diagnosis of "high blood pressure" and its treatment has and is often used when no such diagnosis is necessary and no drug treatment needed. It is a common myth among patients, particularly elderly women, that a high blood pressure is responsible for numerous minor symptoms such as flushing of the face, dizziness, headache, and so on.

Drugs used to treat high blood pressure are complex chemicals with many actions and effects upon the body. Used appropriately, they prolong life, but when wrongly used or when given in wrong dosage, they may be dangerous as well as useless.

The aim of using drugs is to try to limit or reverse the damage which occurs in blood vessels of patients with raised blood pressure. The procedure involves lowering the blood pressure with drugs to a level just above the accepted "normal," achieving this state with a minimum of tolerable adverse effects. Such adverse effects include faint feelings on standing up after sitting or lying down, failure to ejaculate in men, diarrhea, pain in the cheeks, mood changes, blurred vision, drowsiness, stuffy nose, and changes in sexual desires.

With appropriate drug treatment, patients with severe blood pressure now have a far better chance of living much longer than they did ten years ago. Many symptoms disappear, and the risk of heart failure, angina, and stroke may be impressively reduced. The effects of high blood pressure upon the arteries of the eyes may also be decreased. The drug treatment of moderately high blood pressure also produces much benefit. In patients of early middle and middle age, life can be prolonged by the treatment of mildly or moderately high blood pressure. These patients may have a raised blood pressure recording even though they may be without any of the complications caused by raised blood pressure. Appropriate treatment delays the appearance of these and prolongs life. Because of greater risks, men need treatment more than women.

There are several groups of drugs which may be used to reduce blood pressure:

ADRENERGIC-NERVE BLOCKING DRUGS block those nerves which supply arteries and which are normally responsible for maintaining the resistance to the flow of blood by causing constriction. Guanethidine is the main drug used in this group. It is taken by mouth, but its absorption from the gut (and therefore its effective dose) varies among individuals. Tolerance to it is not common. It is cumulative and has a long duration of action. A person taking guanethidine may suffer a fall in blood pressure upon standing up (postural hypotension). This produces faintness.

METHYLDOPA interferes with the production and action of chemicals in the body which act on blood vessels to raise the blood pressure. It has a complex action on the nervous system. It is slow to work, and its effects continue for several days after it has been stopped. It is much less apt to produce postural hypotension (an abrupt fall in blood pressure when you stand up) than guanethidine and related drugs and is very widely used.

RAUWOLFIA ALKALOIDS AND RELATED COMPOUNDS have been used for centuries as sedatives. They deplete the tissues, brain, and nerve endings of stored chemicals which act on blood vessels to raise the blood pressure. They thus cause a fall in blood pressure but also affect mood. The principal drug used in this group is reserpine.

When reserpine is given by mouth its onset of action is slow. Effects appear in three to six days and continue for many days after the drug has been stopped. It may cause severe, possibly suicidal, mental depression. Injections of reserpine may cause postural hypotension. Adverse effects produced by reserpine and related drugs are usually dose-related and disappear when the dose is reduced or stopped. They should be used with caution in patients with psychological disorders, particularly persons who are anxious or depressed. They should also be used with caution in patients with impaired heart or lung function, in debilitated or elderly patients, and in patients with peptic ulcers or ulcerative colitis.

GANGLION BLOCKING DRUGS block nervous impulses in nerves supplying internal organs and tissues not under voluntary control. They affect blood vessels and reduce the blood pressure, but they also produce numerous adverse effects because of their other actions. These adverse effects are so severe that the drugs are now scarcely used at all except in emergencies. The principal drug in the group is trimethaphan.

ALPHA-RECEPTOR BLOCKING DRUGS act on nerve receptors in artery walls. They block the effects of stimulation of the nerves which cause blood vessels to contract, resulting in dilation of the vessels, a fall in resistance, and a fall in blood pressure.

One alpha-receptor blocking drug—phenoxybenzamine—is long-acting and is used to treat a rare disorder of the adrenal glands (pheochromocytoma) which causes sudden and severe increases in blood pressure. Phenoxybenzamine and related drugs are of no use in treating patients with "ordinary" high blood pressure, but it has been shown that phenoxybenzamine may be of use in helping patients who have developed a resistance to drugs like guanethidine. In these patients the combination of a receptor blocker and a nerve blocker may possibly be of use. Tolazoline and phentolamine also have alpha-receptor blocking properties.

BETA-RECEPTOR BLOCKING DRUGS are discussed on p. 101, under the drug treatment of angina. They are increasingly being used to lower mild blood pressure, particularly in younger patients. Unlike most drugs that treat blood pressure, they also reduce the lying-down blood pressure.

THIAZIDE DIURETICS (see p. 104) reduce body fluids and have a lowering effect on the blood pressure, an effect which possibly is in part due to their direct dilating effect upon the peripheral blood vessels. Diazoxide, when given by injection, produces a rapid fall in blood pressure. As noted on p. 105, there is a danger of potassium loss associated with the use of diuretics.

OTHER DRUGS. Clonidine acts on the central nervous system to reduce blood pressure, slow the heart rate, and produce a sedative effect. It is less likely than guanethidine and similar drugs to cause a drop in blood pressure when the patient stands up. When use of clonidine is to be discontinued, this must be done *gradually* to prevent sudden and dangerous increases in blood pressure.

Hydralazine is used to treat patients with high blood pressure, because it dilates arterioles all over the body. To be effective it must be given in large doses, which produces severe adverse effects. Prolonged high dosage may produce a disorder resembling acute rheumatoid arthritis with skin rashes. Hydralazine should be used with caution in patients with coronary artery disease.

Nitroprusside, a vasodilator given only by intravenous injection, has recently become a drug of choice for quickly and reliably reducing life-threatening high blood pressure.

### Choice of Drugs for Blood Pressure

Because there are many drugs available and many different ways of combining one drug with another, treatments vary widely. The drug and dosage regimen should be tailored to the individual. The mainstay of therapy is often a diuretic, and many of the other classes of drugs for high blood pressure cause the body to retain sodium and water, necessitating the concurrent use of a diuretic.

A thiazide diuretic is usually the first drug of choice in moderately raised blood pressure. In cases in which blood pressure is moderate to severe, it may be combined with propranolol or methyldopa. However, fixed-dose combination products are not recommended, because the dose of each constituent drug must be varied to meet the individual patient's needs.

For moderately to severely raised blood pressure, methyldopa may be tried on its own and is well tolerated by some patients. Others may prefer propranolol. Guanethidine is an alternative because it may be taken only once a day, but some may not tolerate the diarrhea and postural hypotension that it sometimes produces. In difficult cases, hydralazine may be added to a diuretic and propranolol.

For mild to moderate blood pressure, reserpine combined with a long-acting diuretic such as chlorthalidone may be useful. However, the risk of depression limits its use, and it should not be used with elderly patients or persons with a history of depressive episodes. Beta-receptor blocking drugs (see p. 101) are also becoming popular.

# THE RELIEF OF PAIN

We all experience pain at some time or another, and each of us varies in the amount of pain we can tolerate. Severe, continuous, or unusual pain must be explained and relieved. If we have sprained an ankle, we can understand the cause of the pain and it is reasonable to take a pain reliever. But all too often we take pain relievers for unexplained pain, particularly headaches, without attempting to identify the cause. Pain is only a symptom. Therefore, you should always try to determine its cause. If you have toothache, do not just take pain relievers—go to your dentist. If you get recurrent headaches, try to figure out what brings them on—noise, smoking, worry, something in your diet, and so on. Very often pain produces fear and anxiety: somebody with chest pain may think that he has a bad heart and somebody with headache may worry about a brain tumor. If you have a pain that is continuous or unusual for you or if you find yourself becoming anxious about a pain, you have sufficient reason to consult your doctor. We are not all stoics, and continuous pain can make most people depressed and irritable. By far the most common pains are headaches and those from muscles and joints, such as are caused by rheumatic and arthritic disorders. Drugs to relieve this sort of pain are among the most frequently used of all drugs.

Nerve endings highly sensitive to pain are widely distributed throughout various tissues of the body. Their response to pressure or stretching produces the sensation of pain. Nerve endings are also very sensitive to chemical stimulation (for example, a burn with no tissue injury). The area of pain can usually be identified: in the skin or subcutaneous tissue, in muscles or joints, in an internal organ such as the heart or lungs, gall bladder, stomach, or bowels. The relief of these pains does not necessarily require pain-relieving drugs. Cold water applied to a skin burn may relieve the pain, heat or massage may relieve muscle pain, and an alkali mixture may relieve the pain of a peptic ulcer. It must be obvious, therefore, that the *best* way to treat pain is to attempt to relieve the underlying cause. Where the cause of the pain cannot be removed, then pain relievers should be used.

There are two main types of pain-relieving drugs: those that work at the site of the pain and those that work on the brain. For example, a local anesthetic injected into a nerve in your finger will "freeze" that finger and cut off the transmission of painful stimuli through the nerve to the brain. A general anesthetic, on the other hand, reduces your brain function so that you are unaware of the pain. Those pain relievers that work at the site of pain block painful impulses; those that work on the brain both interfere with perception of pain (probably by the thalamus) and alter the appreciation of pain by the brain centers. There are thus two nonspecific approaches to the relief of pain which may be used in combination.

Drugs which depress the central nervous system are often called narcotics. The term is also used to include general anesthetics, hypnotics, and opiates. Others use the term "narcotic" when talking about derivatives of the opium plant. "Opiates" or "opioids" refer to any naturally occurring or synthetic drug that has morphinelike actions. Many consider the term "narcotic" to be equivalent to "addiction-producing," and legally narcotics can cover all sorts of drugs, including cocaine. When discussing pain relievers (analgesics) it is usual to talk about narcotic analgesics (those analgesics of natural or synthetic origin with actions like morphine) and nonnarcotic analgesics (such as aspirin). Narcotic analgesics act principally on the brain and may produce physical drug dependence; nonnarcotic analgesics act principally at the site of the pain. The former are used frequently and effectively to relieve pain from internal organs, and the latter are used to relieve skin, muscle, joint, bone, or tooth pains.

Numerous psychological factors make us feel pain more at one time than at another. We feel pain much more if we are tense, anxious, worried, or depressed, and of course the reverse applies too. Therefore, testing done on animals or on human volunteers under laboratory conditions may not give a true indication of a drug's effectiveness in real patients. The marked individual variations in response to drugs are further influenced by weight, sex, physical or psychological disorders, time of treatment, and place of treatment. Also, about one in three patients can get relief of pain from placebo pills or injections—though with repeated doses the placebo effect soon wears off.

## MORPHINE AND NARCOTIC PAIN RELIEVERS

Opium has been used since prehistoric times. It is obtained from the seed pods of the opium poppy and contains a variety of drugs called opium alkaloids. The most widely used of these is morphine. Opium also contains codeine, used to relieve pain, as a cough suppressant, and to relieve diarrhea; papaverine, used to relieve spasms in involuntary muscles (e.g., in bronchospasm and intestinal colic); and noscapine, used as a cough suppressant.

In addition to opium and its alkaloids there are many synthetic narcotic pain relievers. These include heroin (not legal in the United States), meperidine, anileridine, hydromorphone, oxycodone, propoxyphene (dextropropoxyphene), dihydrocodeine, levorphanol, methadone, and pentazocine.

MORPHINE produces its main effects upon the brain and the bowel. In the brain it brings relief of pain, suppression of the cough center and stimulation of the vomiting center, drowsiness, and a relaxed mood. Sleep may occur. Sometimes it produces the opposite effect, causing mild anxiety and fear. Mental clouding with inability to concentrate may occur. It also causes constriction of the pupils and sweating. With increased doses these effects increase and the patient may develop nausea, vomit, and suffer depression of respiration (the latter is a major adverse effect of morphinelike drugs).

Morphine is therefore dangerous to patients with chest disorders such as asthma and to patients with heart failure due to chronic bronchitis and other chest diseases. It may also be harmful to patients after operations. Not only does it discourage deep breathing, it also suppresses cough, with the result that the patient may get a collapsed lung through accumulation of bronchial secretions. Also, morphine-induced vomiting can be harmful in patients recovering from stomach operations, or those who have just had a coronary thrombosis or a cataract operation. For this reason it is sometimes given in combination with an antivomiting drug such as demenhydrinate or promethazine. It is often used to treat pain caused by a coronary thrombosis.

Morphine also acts on the muscles of the gut, causing constipation, and should preferably not be given for gut pain. (Meperidine is more suitable, but still may produce a degree of constipation.) It causes a rise in pressure in the gall bladder and should not be used for gall-bladder pain, which it may make worse. In patients who have had their gall bladder removed, morphine can cause quite severe pain resembling a coronary thrombosis. It may cause a fall in blood pressure and dilatation of the blood vessels in the skin (probably by releasing histamine). It should, therefore, be used with caution in patients who are shocked through loss of blood. Rarely, patients may develop delirium and insomnia. Increased pain sensitivity may remain after the effects of the drug have worn off.

Tolerance and drug dependence develop with morphine. Physical dependence can occur within twenty-four hours if morphine is given every four hours. When it is stopped after even a short period of use, patients may experience such mild withdrawal symptoms as sweating, nausea, weakness, headache, and restlessness.

MEPERIDINE is a synthetic pain reliever with effects similar to morphine but a lesser tendency to cause constipation. It does not constrict the pupils, but like morphine it may cause nausea and vomiting, particularly in children. Meperidine is used to relieve moderate to severe pain. It is more powerful than codeine but less so than morphine.

METHADONE is a synthetic drug with actions identical to those of morphine. It is effective for the relief of moderate to severe pain. It has an extended duration of action in narcotic-dependent individuals and is used to treat heroin addicts (see pp. 31–2). Vomiting is as common as with morphine, but sedation is less. It is effective when taken by mouth and is also used to suppress cough. Because of its long-lasting effects it should not be used in childbirth; it can depress the respiration of the newborn baby.

### Effects of Moderate to Severe Pain Relievers
The narcotics used to relieve moderate to severe pain differ from one another markedly in structure, yet all have similar actions and effects. Their adverse effects are similar too—nausea, vomiting, drowsiness, dizziness, constipation, and respiratory depression. In pain-relieving doses there is not much difference in the incidence of these adverse effects. They do differ, however, in their onset and duration of action,

in whether they are effective by mouth, and in the way that individuals respond to them. They all cause tolerance and physical dependence and are potential drugs of abuse. They increase the effects of alcohol and other depressant drugs, and they should not be taken by patients who drive motor vehicles or operate machinery.

## Mild to Moderate Pain Relievers

CODEINE (methylmorphine) is obtained from opium and is present in numerous preparations. It produces less mood change and is not as effective as morphine in relieving pain. It is more effective by mouth than by injection and is used to relieve mild to moderate pain (often in combination with aspirin, acetaminophen, or some other pain reliever). It is also used in cough medicines and diarrhea mixtures.

DIHYDROCODEINE relieves mild to moderate pain, suppresses cough, and is effective by mouth. It produces adverse effects like those of morphine but of a generally less severe character. It may produce dependence of the morphine type and should not be given to patients with impaired liver function or asthma and other respiratory disorders.

PROPOXYPHENE has effects and uses similar to those of codeine. It is slightly less effective and is usually given in combination with other pain relievers by mouth.

## Narcotic Antagonists

In 1953 a morphine antagonist—nalorphine—was found to bring on acute withdrawal-like effects in patients who had been on morphine or heroin for brief periods. In addition, it was found to have good pain-relieving properties. However, it was unsuitable for use because it affected mood adversely and produced vivid daydreams, hallucinations, difficulty in focusing the eyes, sweating, nausea, and feelings of being drunk.

The most impressive effects of nalorphine were its abilities to prevent or abolish many of the actions of morphine and to precipitate withdrawal symptoms in patients who were physically dependent upon morphine or related narcotics. Naloxone, a related antagonist with no respiration-depressing effect of its own, is now the preferred treatment for depression of respiration caused by narcotic overdose.

The discovery of these drugs led to research for pain relievers with less risk of dependence than morphine. One of these, pentazocine, was introduced in 1967. It is an antagonist with pain-relieving properties between those of codeine and morphine.

Unlike aspirin and related drugs, pentazocine has no anti-inflammatory properties, and it does not reduce a high temperature. It is more effective when given by injection than by mouth. It is mildly sedative and produces less respiratory depression than morphine. The incidence of nausea and vomiting is about the same as with morphine and is especially likely in patients who are not confined to bed. The drug rarely causes constipation. In high doses it may cause a rise in blood pressure and heart rate. Cases of physical drug dependence of the morphine type have been reported in patients taking pentazocine by injection over a long term.

### The Choice of Narcotic Pain Relievers

These are all potential drugs of dependence, and most of them are subject to regulations concerning dangerous drugs. They should be used with caution. Morphine is the narcotic analgesic of choice for severe pain, but the other drugs give your doctor the chance to vary effects and adverse effects according to your individual needs. These include pain-relieving properties, dependence and abuse potential, effects on the brain and mood, individual sensitivities, and whether the drug works effectively by mouth. Pentazocine may be a useful alternative to morphine in treating the pain of coronary thrombosis; morphine may cause the blood pressure to fall. For moderate pain, oral codeine, oxycodone, propoxyphene, and dihydrocodeine are useful. Their effectiveness can often be enhanced by the addition of nonnarcotic pain relievers such as acetaminophen or aspirin.

### ASPIRIN, NONNARCOTIC PAIN RELIEVERS, AND DRUGS USED TO TREAT RHEUMATISM AND ARTHRITIS

These are all mild pain relievers. Some of them also bring down temperature, and some have anti-inflammatory properties. According to their effects they may be used to relieve pain, to treat rheumatism and arthritis, and to treat gout. Many authorities claim that there is little to choose among drugs in the various groups except for differences in adverse effects.

The anti-inflammatory effects of the nonnarcotic pain relievers are often difficult to separate from their pain-relieving effects. However, aspirin has been shown to antagonize many substances involved in the process of inflammation. Aspirin, salicylates, indomethacin, and some of the newer drugs have also been shown to inhibit the production of substances called prostaglandins, which are involved in the production of inflammation and perhaps pain.

### Salicylates

ASPIRIN is one of the most widely used drugs. It relieves mild pain, particularly in toothache or headache and pains in muscles, ligaments, and joints. Its long-term use does not lead to tolerance or physical dependence. It brings down the temperature and relieves inflammation. It stimulates respiration, causes a fall in blood sugar, and if taken regularly it reduces certain blood fat levels. Aspirin in high doses makes the kidneys pass out urates (see Drugs Used to Treat Gout, p. 124), but in low doses it can cause retention. It antagonizes all drugs which cause a fall in blood uric acid levels. It is therefore of no use in treating gout. Aspirin alters the blood salts (acid/base balance) and interferes with some of the processes involved in blood clotting. It also causes water retention when given in high doses, and speeds up the body's metabolic rate.

Aspirin in mild overdosage may produce "salicylism"—deafness, noises in the ears, nausea, and dull headache. These are related to dose and disappear if the drug is stopped. It is irritant and can cause pain in the stomach with nausea and vomiting, and may interfere with the process by which the cells lining the stomach are shed. It is considered by many to produce superficial ulcers in the stomach, which may bleed and lead to iron deficiency anemia. This may occur without indigestion symptoms and seems to be independent of when the aspirin is taken (before or after meals) or the type of aspirin preparation. This may be a real danger in elderly patients on poor diets low in iron, in women with heavy menstrual periods, and in debilitated patients.

Aspirin should not be taken on an empty stomach. It should be taken preferably in a soluble form with plenty of fluids. If you have peptic ulcers, a hiatus hernia, or a bleeding disorder you should *not* take aspirin. It is considered to be a causative factor in many patients admitted to a hospital with bleeding from the stomach or duodenum, especially when taken after alcohol. For long-term use a specially coated aspirin (called enteric-coated) is available; it does not dissolve until it enters the small intestine. However, it takes up to six hours to work.

Aspirin is excreted mainly by the kidneys, and a dose every four to six hours is sufficient to maintain effective blood levels. It dissolves in the stomach faster and is absorbed more quickly if it is taken with a large amount of warm water or an alkali mixture (the basis of some commercial preparations containing sodium bicarbonate which fizz in water).

Aspirin is a very useful drug, but it is used so indiscriminately that it is not surprising that adverse effects occur. You should be aware of the danger of aspirin use in babies, elderly and debilitated patients, and persons with impaired function of their kidneys, liver, or blood. It should not be given to patients with heart disease except in special conditions, because it increases the work of the heart. Children with fever should be given no more than the recommended dose, and then only if they are able to drink more than their normal amounts of fluids. It should not be used in feverish children who are dehydrated due to vomiting, diarrhea, or lack of fluid intake, and it should never be taken by anyone who has abdominal pain, or is nauseated or vomiting.

Aspirin overdose can be serious, especially in children—always take the patient to the nearest hospital. Remember: aspirin is present in hundreds of compound preparations; always read the contents and note that aspirin may be called acetylsalicylic acid.

SALICYLAMIDE has effects and uses like aspirin but is not as effective.

## Aniline Derivatives

PHENACETIN has been frequently used as a mild pain reliever and antipyretic. It does not possess anti-inflammatory or antirheumatic properties. After absorption it is rapidly converted into acetaminophen, which provides its pain-relieving properties. Because there is now much circumstantial evidence that phenacetin may cause kidney damage, its use is no longer recommended, although it is still found in numerous pain-reliever preparations.

ACETAMINOPHEN is an effective mild pain reliever and antipyretic. It is a suitable alternative for patients sensitive to aspirin. It has no anti-inflammatory or antirheumatic properties. Overdose is dangerous because it may cause liver and kidney damage. Acetaminophen should not be used indiscriminately simply because it produces less stomach upset than aspirin. *Acetanilid* is a more toxic form of phenacetin and should not be used at all.

Poisoning with phenacetin, acetaminophen, or particularly acetanilid may cause blueness of the lips and skin (cyanosis). The blue color is due to a decrease in the oxygen-carrying power of the red blood cells. Sometimes the red blood cells can be destroyed. Anemia may result from the use of any of these three drugs, and this may be associated with kidney failure. In severe poisoning, circulatory collapse may occur.

Mixtures of phenacetin with aspirin, caffeine, and/or codeine have been widely available in various combinations and doses. Those containing phenacetin are considered by some authorities to cause kidney damage with prolonged daily use, and are best avoided. Other mixtures containing aspirin, acetaminophen, codeine, and caffeine should be used with caution. Avoid prolonged regular daily use.

## Pyrazolone Derivatives

PHENYLBUTAZONE is related to phenazone and aminopyrine and was introduced in 1947 for the treatment of rheumatoid disorders. It should *not* be used to bring down fever, and its pain-relieving properties are inferior to aspirin for nonrheumatic disorders. It possesses anti-inflammatory properties, increases the excretion of uric acid by the kidneys (see Drugs Used to Treat Gout, p. 124), causes retention of salt and a reduction in urine volume, reduces the uptake of iodine by the thyroid gland, and may occasionally cause goiter or underworking of the thyroid gland.

Phenylbutazone is well absorbed from the gut. It becomes bound to plasma proteins, competes with other drugs, and affects enzymes in the liver which help in drug breakdown. For these reasons it can cause many drug interactions.

Phenylbutazone should not be used by patients with peptic ulcers, high blood pressure, impaired heart, kidney, or liver function, or a previous history of a peptic ulcer or drug allergy. If you are on this drug you are advised to restrict your salt intake, never to take the drug on an empty stomach, and to stop it if you get any ankle swelling, indigestion, sore throat (which may be an early sign of a blood disorder), or skin rash. Some experts consider that its use should be restricted to short-term courses of one or two weeks at a time.

OXYPHENBUTAZONE is a derivative of phenylbutazone and has similar actions, effects, and adverse effects. The same warnings apply.

### Indomethacin
This drug produces effects similar to those of aspirin. It relieves pain, reduces inflammation, and brings down temperature. Read about its adverse effects in Part III. It may produce peptic ulceration with bleeding, and so the same sort of decisions that apply to the use of aspirin also apply to indomethacin.

### Ibuprofen
The same warnings as those described under indomethacin apply to this drug. It is really a matter of balancing desired effects with adverse effects, particularly stomach ulceration and bleeding, which may be less of a problem from this drug than with aspirin, phenylbutazone, oxyphenbutazone, and indomethacin.

### Mefenamic Acid
This drug has effects similar to those of aspirin but is said to produce less irritation and bleeding in the stomach. It is also less effective than aspirin, and can produce serious adverse effects. Its use should not extend beyond seven days, and it should not be given to children, or to women of childbearing age.

### Corticosteroids and Corticotropins
Corticosteroids (e.g., prednisone, prednisolone) and corticotropins (e.g., ACTH) reduce inflammation. They are discussed beginning on p.

160. They are not curative, and joint destruction may progress even though the symptoms are relieved. They should be used only as reserve drugs when other treatments fail to produce relief. Preferably they should be used for no more than one or two months at a time, although some doctors continue treatment indefinitely because when the drugs are reduced and stopped, symptoms flare up and make life for the patient intolerable again. Very important precautions should be applied to the use of these drugs. Look them up in Part III.

## Gold
Gold is often most effective in active, progressive rheumatoid arthritis. It is usually given by deep intramuscular injection at weekly intervals. The total course should not exceed 1,000 mg. It should be given with caution to pregnant women, to elderly and debilitated patients, and to those with high blood pressure. Frequent blood tests are necessary.

## Chloroquine and Hydroxychloroquine
These antimalarial drugs are sometimes used in high doses to treat rheumatoid arthritis. Prolonged use of high doses may lead to the development of corneal opacities, causing misty vision, and irreversible damage to the retina of the eye, resulting in blindness. Patients on these drugs should have periodic eye examinations, although symptoms may come on long after the drug has been stopped. These drugs should never be given to pregnant women because they cause damage to the unborn baby's sight and hearing.

## Penicillamine
This drug aids the elimination of toxic metals from the body. It is used in lead poisoning and to treat certain disorders of copper metabolism. Occasionally it is used as a reserve drug in the treatment of severe rheumatoid arthritis that has not responded to other treatments.

## Choice of Mild Pain Relievers
For mild pain, aspirin is the drug of choice. A soluble aspirin is probably better than plain aspirin. Some people may prefer buffered aspirin (i.e., aspirin mixed with an antacid). Gastric upset and bleeding may be lessened by using enteric-coated tablets of aspirin, but these are of use only if you are on long-term treatment, as for rheumatoid arthritis.

Acetaminophen is an effective alternative, particularly if you cannot take aspirin. Preparations containing codeine and aspirin or codeine and acetaminophen in suitable doses are very useful, but don't forget that codeine may constipate.

Numerous preparations prescribed by doctors contain aspirin or acetaminophen combined with a narcotic pain reliever (e.g., propoxyphene). These are useful for relieving moderate pain, but because they contain narcotics they should be used with caution over prolonged periods.

## Choice of Drugs in the Treatment of Rheumatic and Arthritic Disorders

I have used the vague terms "rheumatic" and "arthritic" to cover a multitude of disorders ranging from a "rheumatic" condition causing mild pain and swelling in one joint to the serious disease called rheumatoid arthritis, which may affect one or many joints and be associated with other disorders of the arteries and various internal organs. Therefore treatment will of course vary, and reserve drugs such as corticosteroids, gold, and chloroquine will be used only in serious cases and under specialist care.

Of the commonly used antirheumatic drugs—aspirin, phenylbutazone, indomethacin, ibuprofen, and related drugs and mefenamic acid, the choice is a matter of balancing adverse effects of stomach irritation and bleeding with the beneficial effects. Other adverse effects such as salt retention, bone marrow damage, and potential risks of interaction with other drugs should be considered. And so the selection of the most appropriate drug will require skill and patience depending on the severity of the disorder being treated. As a patient, you should be aware of these problems.

Aspirin is the drug of first choice. But for rheumatic disorders it must be given in high doses. If aspirin does not work, phenylbutazone or indomethacin may be tried. The latter may also be tried as a suppository. Ibuprofen or related drugs are alternatives.

Depending on the severity of your symptoms a moderate pain reliever may have to be used in addition (particularly at night), for example, dihydrocodeine, pentazocine, or dextropropoxyphene. Codeine compounds with aspirin or acetaminophen are alternative mild pain relievers.

Corticosteroids such as prednisone and prednisolone by mouth and adrenocorticotropin (ACTH) by injection are reserve drugs if other treatments fail to produce relief. Local injections of hydrocortisone into a joint may help but have been criticized by some experts, as has the use of gold, chloroquine, and penicillamine.

### Osteoarthritis

Aspirin, phenylbutazone, indomethacin, ibuprofen, and related drugs may relieve some pain and stiffness in osteoarthritis. Acetaminophen and codeine compounds relieve mild pain but do not help the inflammation. Phenylbutazone and indomethacin are said to be superior to aspirin in the treatment of ankylosing spondylitis.

# DRUGS USED
# TO TREAT GOUT

Gout is a relatively uncommon disease, rare in women. It causes recurrent attacks of acute pain and swelling, at first affecting one joint (usually the big toe) and later many joints. It is a hereditary disease, and usually comes on after the age of forty. It is more common in temperate climates and sometimes diet may bring on an acute attack. The effects of gout are caused by an increased production of uric acid and uric acid salts (urates), which are deposited in the tissues around joints and in the kidneys.

Drugs are used to relieve pain and inflammation in an acute attack of gout. They are also used to avoid attacks by increasing the elimination of urates by the kidneys or by blocking the production of uric acid.

## Acute Attacks of Gout

Colchicine (obtained from the autumn crocus) relieves the pain and inflammation of gout within a few hours. It is absorbed from the gut and broken down in the liver. Some is excreted unchanged in the bile and goes back into the gut, causing abdominal pain, vomiting, and diarrhea. As well as being used to treat an acute attack of gout, it is also useful in preventing attacks.

Other drugs for treating acute attacks of gout include phenylbutazone and indomethacin (see section on antirheumatic drugs, p. 123). If these fail, corticosteroids or adrenocorticotropin (ACTH) may be used.

## Recurrent Gout

By reducing the reabsorption of urates from the urine by the kidneys, probenecid promotes their excretion. It has no pain-relieving properties and is of no use in an acute attack of gout. It may even *set off* an acute attack of gout in the first few weeks of treatment, so the patient must be warned. Sulfinpyrazone is related to phenylbutazone but causes excretion of urates. It is more effective than probenecid but more toxic, and, again, it may also trigger an acute attack of gout in the first few weeks of treatment. Its adverse effects are similar to phenylbutazone and it has more adverse effects than probenecid.

Allopurinol affects uric acid production and reduces the concentration of uric acid in the blood. Acute attacks of gout may be triggered in the early stages of treatment, but after a few weeks or months acute attacks stop and deposits of uric acid salts in cartilage get smaller. (These deposits are often visible in the cartilage of the earlobes and are known as *tophi*.) It may prevent kidney damage in gout and also stops the formation of uric acid stones in the kidneys. Allopurinol is therefore useful for treating gout in patients with kidney disorders, whereas other antigout drugs may not be effective or may not be advisable to use. It also prevents a rise in blood uric acid levels in patients with gout being treated for heart failure with thiazide diuretics, since these can cause a rise in blood uric acid.

## Choice of Drugs in Gout

Colchicine, phenylbutazone, indomethacin, and some of the newer antirheumatic drugs are all alternative drugs of choice, depending upon how the patient responds. Colchicine may cause troublesome diarrhea in some people. Indomethacin acts quickly and is very useful because it can be given as a suppository, thus avoiding stomach upsets. Allopurinol is the drug of choice for long-term prevention, but probenecid may have to be added or used as an alternative. Allopurinol is the drug of choice for patients with kidney disorders or uric acid stones. It is also the drug of choice in patients being treated with thiazide diuretics.

# DRUGS USED
# TO TREAT MIGRAINE

It is often difficult to differentiate between migraine and ordinary headache. Some doctors label any one-sided headache as migraine, particularly if it is accompanied by nausea and vomiting. Others look for all the classic symptoms of migraine: one-sided headache associated with nausea and vomiting and preceded by visual symptoms (e.g., flashing lights), speech disturbances, or disturbances of sensation (e.g., pins and needles in a foot or hand).

Migraine is uncommon under the age of five years, and then its incidence increases until middle age. In old age, the incidence declines. It is more common in women than in men, and it may be associated with menstruation. There are many myths about migraine sufferers; for example, that they are more tense, neurotic, or obsessional than nonsufferers. There is no evidence that this is true. Nor is there evidence to suggest that they are more likely to be professional people, that they are more intelligent, that they suffer more from high blood pressure or visual disturbances, or that they are more involved in work which involves close vision. Nor is there any convincing evidence that migraine runs in families.

Many statements about migraine sufferers are made by doctors who only see a small self-selected group—those who have decided to consult a doctor. These patients cannot be assumed to be representative of migraine sufferers in general.

An attack of migraine is associated with changes in the caliber of the blood vessels supplying the head and brain. It is thought that these changes occur in response to certain chemicals produced by the body and by some chemicals which are present in various foods such as cheese. Underlying constitutional factors which may be biochemical possibly cause a predisposition to develop migraine in response to external factors.

Factors which may trigger a migraine attack include:

PSYCHOLOGICAL: anxiety, tension, worry, emotion, depression, shock, excitement.

PHYSICAL: overexertion, lifting, straining, bending.

EXTERNAL FACTORS: sunlight, weather, traveling, change of routine, staying in bed, watching television, noise, smells, smoking, drugs.

DIETARY: irregular meals, fasting, such foods as cheese, onion, cucumber, bananas, chocolate, fried foods, pastry, cured meats (hot dogs, ham, bacon), alcohol.

The most important part of treatment is to try to prevent an attack, and this means attempting to identify trigger factors. If you develop migraine, always go through a check list of possible trigger factors. The solution may be something simple like not eating cheese or cured meats containing sodium nitrates or nitrites. Or it may be very difficult, like trying not to get tense or anxious and learning to relax. It may take time and patience, but it will be worth it. Some migraine clinics teach relaxation and other useful methods of preventing an attack, but on the whole the vast majority of sufferers manage without such help. Many learn how to cope with an attack, but they should also realize that it is worth trying to prevent attacks in the first place.

The usefulness of drugs in treating migraine is really very limited. Some drugs may reduce the number of attacks in some people but not in others; they may also reduce some symptoms of an attack in some patients but not in others. The use of drugs is aimed principally at reducing the dilation of blood vessels in the head, which is thought to be responsible for migraine at least in some people.

Ergotamine is the main drug used by doctors to treat an acute attack. It may be dissolved in the mouth (sublingual), inhaled through the mouth, taken as tablets or capsules, suppositories, or injections. The sooner it is taken in an attack the better, and the quicker it gets to work the better. Injections work faster than suppositories, which in turn work faster than tablets by mouth. Caffeine, which appears to enhance the effectiveness of ergotamine in the treatment of migraine, is often added to the tablet and capsule preparations.

Ergotamine should not be used to prevent attacks but only in the treatment of acute attacks. Whatever the preparation or route of administration there is a maximum safe dose which should be strictly observed—always read the instructions carefully.

Dihydroergotamine produces less vomiting, and there is less risk of circulatory disorders than with ergotamine (see Part III). It works best by injection.

Sedatives, tranquilizers, or mixtures of ergotamine with sedatives and/or atropinelike drugs are frequently prescribed but have never been subjected to satisfactory testing.

Methysergide is an effective drug in *preventing* attacks, but it is not known how it works, and it causes frequent and sometimes very serious adverse effects. It should not be given to pregnant women or to patients with impaired function of their kidneys or liver, high blood pressure, circulatory disorders, or peptic ulcers. It is of no value during an acute attack. "Rebound" headaches may occur upon withdrawal of the drug.

Drugs to prevent attacks should be used only when all trigger factors have been examined and eliminated and when the attacks are interfering with the individual's ability to cope with his everyday existence.

Ergotamine remains the drug of choice in acute attacks if you do not respond to ordinary pain relievers.

# ANTIHISTAMINE DRUGS

### Allergy

To defend itself against infecting organisms, the body produces antibodies that combine with protein in the invaders to neutralize any effects which they may have upon the body. By means of this defense mechanism the body develops resistance or immunity. Such immunity often gives protection against reinfection by the same organism (for example, you never get chicken pox twice). An antibody is a protein (globulin) which reacts only with the protein of the infecting organism (usually called an antigen) responsible for its formation. There is no cross-antibody formation to other antigens (cross-immunity), between measles and polio, for example. Sometimes renewed exposure to an infection produces a different or altered response. This is called allergy. It results because the body has been sensitized to that organism. In some people this type of reaction occurs not only to infecting organisms but also to drugs, house dust, pollens, certain foods—all sorts of things. These are usually grouped under the general term "allergens." The reason why some people become sensitized and not others is not understood. We are all, for example, exposed to pollen spores, and yet some of us will develop hay fever and others will not. Nor is the nature of allergic reactions fully understood; it may be a fault in the immunity mechanisms, resulting in faulty antibody production, or an inherited defect in the tissues concerned.

The allergic reaction consists mainly of the local release, or release into the bloodstream, of a chemical called histamine and several other chemicals. A single allergen may cause reactions at several sites; thus a patient sensitive to a certain food may develop stomach symptoms, a rash, and wheezing. Allergens may affect the body through the skin (e.g., contact dermatitis from detergents), in food (e.g., allergy to strawberries), by inhalation (e.g., hay fever and asthma due to grass pollens), and by injections (e.g., insect bites and allergy to antitetanus serum). The resulting reactions may appear as skin rashes; as swelling of the eyelids, face, lips, and throat; as abdominal symptoms (vomiting, diarrhea, and colic); or (commonly) as hay fever (itching eyes, running nose, and sore throat) or as wheezing (asthma). Allergic reactions may be sudden and transient (for instance, sneezing) or last for years (for instance, eczema). They may be trivial, or so serious as to cause sudden death from what is called anaphylactic shock—collapse of the circulation, fall in blood pressure, and acute asthma. This usually occurs in patients given an injection which contains a protein to which they have already been made sensitive by a previous injection (e.g., antitetanus serum or bee stings). It is extremely rare.

Histamine, a principal chemical involved in allergic reactions, is present in most tissues of the body and is released when cells are injured. It causes the small blood vessels of the body (capillaries) to open up, particularly those in the skin, which becomes hot and red. It also makes the vessels more permeable so that plasma flows from inside the blood vessels out into the surrounding tissues to produce swelling. When histamine is injected into the human skin it produces what is called a triple response (a hive): first, a localized red spot which extends within a few seconds, reaches a maximum in about a minute, and then becomes bluish; second, a bright red "flame" that spreads out from this spot; third, local swelling that forms a weal, often associated with itching and pain. Histamine also causes the blood vessels in the brain to dilate, producing migraine-type headache. It causes a fall in blood pressure and may increase the heart rate. Large doses may produce shock. It stimulates the muscles of the small bronchial tubes to constrict, resulting in asthma, and it stimulates the production of acid in the stomach. Histamine is released in anaphylactic shock, allergy, and injury. Its concentration is particularly high in the skin, the stomach lining, and the lungs.

The release of histamine does not account for all allergic reactions, and it is obvious that what was thought to be a straightforward antigen-antibody reaction is in fact more complex. A whole spectrum of allergic responses, both direct and indirect, accounts for the lack of effect of antihistamine drugs in some cases: in fact the drugs may themselves sometimes produce an allergic response.

Any chemical that causes tissue damage will cause the release of histamine, but some drugs may do this with little sign of tissue damage —for example, certain household detergents. The allergic effects produced by drugs may vary from an itchy skin rash to death from anaphylactic shock. In addition to drugs, any physical process—e.g., sunburn, cold, light, or friction—may cause the release of histamine. The juice of the stinging nettle contains histamine which produces a skin rash called urticaria (nettle rash). This sort of rash may also appear in patients with psychological disorders; in fact most allergic disorders may be aggravated by emotional disturbances.

## Antihistamines
The antihistamine drugs counteract in varying degrees most, but not all, of the effects produced by histamine. They may also reduce the intensity of allergic and anaphylactic reactions. They act not by preventing the release of histamine but by occupying its sites of action. They block its action on the muscles of the gut and bronchial tubes, they reduce the weal produced by histamine, and they reduce hay fever symptoms, itching skin rashes, and swelling. They have no effect on stomach secretions (with the exception of a new drug, cimetidine —see p. 79).

In addition to their actions in blocking the effects of histamine the antihistamines produce other effects, particularly on the brain. In some patients they may cause stimulation. But their usual effect is to depress the brain, which causes drowsiness and sleep; in overdose they may lead to excitation and convulsions. They are used, often in combination with a sleeping drug, to produce sleep. Another use of their depressing effect on the brain is their ability to reduce motion sickness. Some, but not all, antihistamines have this property, and those that do may also be used to prevent nausea and vomiting during pregnancy and symptoms produced by disorders of the organ of balance (e.g., dizziness or vertigo).

In effective dosage all antihistamines produce adverse effects, but these vary from individual to individual and from drug to drug. The commonest is drowsiness; others include dizziness, noises in the ears, incoordination, fatigue, blurred vision, double vision, changes of mood, nervousness, delusions, hallucinations, insomnia and tremors, loss of appetite, nausea, vomiting, diarrhea or constipation, dryness of the mouth, cough, frequency and difficulty in passing urine, palpitations, headache, tightness in the chest, tingling, heaviness and weakness of the hands. You may even become allergic to an antihistamine, particularly if it is applied to the skin. Very rarely, antihistamines may cause serious blood disorders.

## Use of Antihistamines

There are numerous antihistamines to choose from, and bearing in mind the individual variations in response, it is often a matter of trial and error before you find one that will relieve your particular allergic symptoms and produce a minimum of adverse effects.

• Antihistamines are useful in relieving the symptoms of seasonal hay fever (pollinosis), but do nothing to cure the basic condition in sensitive individuals.

• They are virtually useless in treating asthma, including allergic asthma, and may make an attack worse by drying up the bronchial secretions.

• They may relieve allergic swelling of the face but are of little value if the swelling affects the throat and threatens life. Furthermore, they are of little value in anaphylactic reactions.

• Some patients who suffer from perennial nasal congestion, running nose, and sneezing (vasomotor rhinitis) respond to antihistamines. Antihistamines are of very doubtful and unproven value in cough medicines; in fact they may have undesirable effects because they dry the lining of the nose and respiratory tract, thus impairing natural defense systems. Even so, cough mixtures containing antihistamines are among the most frequently taken drugs. And apart from providing some relief from a running nose, they are of no benefit in treating the common cold.

• Some skin rashes, such as allergic nettle rash, respond well to antihistamines. Longstanding rashes are little affected. Antihistamines may be used to relieve itching. However, although they produce their best effect when applied to the skin, there is a serious danger of producing allergic dermatitis to antihistamine preparations. Given by mouth or injection they relieve the itching and swelling produced by insect bites.

• They are of use in relieving the rash in serum sickness (an allergic reaction following the injection of a serum), but they do not relieve fever and joint pains very much.

• They are of benefit in treating blood transfusion reactions.

• They are of no value in treating allergic reactions affecting the stomach or gut—nausea, vomiting, diarrhea.

• Many drug reactions respond well to antihistamines—but do not forget to stop the drug that caused the reaction.

• Some antihistamines are effective in preventing motion sickness.

• Some are useful sedatives.

## Warnings

You must by now realize that antihistamine drugs are complex chemicals which have many actions in the body and produce numerous effects, including adverse effects ranging from loss of appetite to serious blood disorders. They increase the effects produced by alcohol and sedative drugs and interfere with mental function. Overdose with antihistamines is serious and difficult to treat. Even though they are available over the counter from pharmacists, you must bear these dangers in mind.

Antihistamines may produce alarming reactions in some children (stimulation, fever, and convulsions), and reports have associated high dosages of chlorcyclizine, cyclizine, and meclizine with abnormalities in newborn babies. These reports have not been fully confirmed.

Because of the variations in response among individuals taking antihistamines, it is often necessary to try different ones. If a drug does not relieve your symptoms within about three days it is unlikely to do so at all. If it produces drowsiness take it at bedtime. Always take antihistamines with food because they irritate the stomach. If you are just starting a course, try taking the first dose on Friday—then you have the weekend to overcome adverse effects. Avoid prolonged-release preparations until you know the nature and intensity of the adverse effects caused by the antihistamine drug in question. Prolonged-release preparations are most useful taken at bedtime in order to reduce early morning symptoms.

### Desensitization

Hay fever, urticaria, allergic asthma, contact dermatitis, and other allergic disorders are often due to oversensitivity to such things as certain foods, pollen, fur, feathers, dust, hair, mites, and cosmetics. Contact dermatitis of the skin may occur through contact with drugs (e.g., streptomycin), metals (e.g., nickel), plants, paint, resins, and cosmetics. Most people get to know what they are sensitive to and can avoid that substance in the future. In some cases it is not possible to identify or to avoid a particular substance. Therefore, skin tests to certain allergens may be carried out, although the results of these tests are often difficult to assess. If you are found to be sensitive to an inhaled allergen such as grass pollen, then you may be desensitized by having a series of injections of the allergen under the skin at intervals, using gradually increasing strengths. These courses are usually given in winter and may have to be repeated for several years, with varying success. There are several preparations of allergens on the market. Some contain a mixture of commonly occurring allergens (e.g., grass pollens), while others are prepared individually for each person's requirements after skin tests. Desensitization is of little use in skin allergies and drug reactions.

*Note:* For the use of cromolyn sodium in the treatment of allergic asthma and hay fever, see p. 141 and read about it in Part III of this book.

# DRUGS USED
# TO TREAT COMMON COLDS

There is no such thing as a cold cure. Apart from a possibility that high doses of vitamin C may shorten the duration or decrease the intensity of the symptoms of a common cold in *some* individuals, there is no drug on the market which prevents colds or reduces their duration. Because there is no cure, there are numerous remedies.

The common cold produces swelling and inflammation of the lining membrane of the nose, resulting in blockage and a runny nose. This may be accompanied by a sore throat, cough, headache, aching back or limbs, and a mild fever. In an attempt to relieve these symptoms, drug companies produce nose drops, inhalants, sprays, aerosols, ointments, tablets, powders, capsules, and mixtures, in all shapes, colors,

and sizes. Treatment is aimed at two target groups of symptoms—
aches, pains, and fever; and blocked and runny nose.

### Relief of Aches, Pains, and Fever

Pain relievers such as aspirin or acetaminophen will relieve your aches
and pains and will bring down your temperature. They must be taken
according to the instructions on the package and with plenty of fluids
(on dangers of aspirin and acetaminophen, particularly in babies and
infants, see pp. 119 and 120, and Part III). They will have no effect
upon the duration or outcome of the cold, and they may be harmful
in some people who are encouraged to do physical work when they
should be resting or taking it easy.

There are hundreds of pain-relieving preparations on the market,
and yet the choice boils down to two drugs—aspirin or acetaminophen. Remember to take aspirin with water or with food or milk to
minimize stomach irritation. If you have a peptic ulcer or history of a
peptic ulcer, if you get indigestion or have any stomach upset, do not
take aspirin. Acetaminophen is a suitable alternative. *There is no point in
spending money on any preparations because they fizz or taste fruity.* Furthermore,
many proprietary remedies contain drugs which expose you to the
risk of several adverse effects. They are often expensive and best
avoided.

### Nasal Decongestants

These are usually applied locally in the nose by nasal spray or drops,
but there is increasing pressure from advertising to take such drugs by
mouth. The majority of decongestant drugs belong to a group known
as sympathomimetic drugs (see pp. 139, 148). When applied locally to
the surface of the nose or throat they produce constriction of small
blood vessels, returning nasal passages toward normal. Long-acting
members of this group are used to relieve runny nose and nasal congestion. They all share one disadvantage: their use may be followed by
an *increase* in nasal congestion ("rebound" or "aftercongestion"), particularly when used for extended periods of time. Some irritate the
lining of the nose and sting when applied. Their effectiveness decreases
with repeated use, and some experts believe that they actually prolong
a cold and that their use may not be without complications.

The use of these drugs in nasal drops or sprays should be avoided
in infants and young children. Two of them—naphazoline and tetrahydrozoline—may cause unconsciousness and a significant fall in
body temperature in infants.

The blood vessels supplying the lining membranes of the nose have
not been shown to be more sensitive to these drugs than any other

vessels in the body. The use of doses by mouth which relieve nasal congestion will therefore produce constriction of blood vessels elsewhere in the body and so increase the blood pressure. This may be dangerous in patients who suffer from angina, coronary thrombosis, high blood pressure, diabetes, or overworking of the thyroid glands, and in patients who are receiving monoamine oxidase antidepressant drugs. Adverse effects include giddiness, headache, nausea, vomiting, sweating, thirst, palpitations, difficulty in passing urine, weakness, trembling, anxiety, restlessness, and insomnia. Some individuals may be very sensitive to them, while others may be able to tolerate high doses.

Other drugs used to decrease nasal congestion include belladonna alkaloids and antihistamines.

The belladonna alkaloids (see atropine, p. 146) reduce secretions in the upper and lower respiratory tract. They are a common constituent of proprietary cold remedies, usually in such small doses as to be totally ineffective. But, of course, if they were given in effective doses by mouth they would produce very unpleasant adverse effects.

Antihistamines are present in numerous common cold remedies, and yet there is no evidence that they are of the slightest value. They are not the sort of drugs which should be taken casually—for example, they influence brain function, causing drowsiness, and may interfere with ability to drive a motor vehicle. Their effects are increased by alcohol. They do tend to "dry up" the respiratory tract. However, this reduces natural barriers to bacteria, and in the presence of infection this effect is considered to be harmful by some experts.

### Treating the Common Cold
Drink plenty of fluids and take some rest in the acute phase of a cold. Alcohol has no beneficial effect on the cold but may help you to rest. Antiseptic gargles, mouth washes, and throat lozenges have no effect on the cold virus.

Aspirin or acetaminophen in appropriate dosage and with appropriate precautions are the only drugs worth taking by mouth, and even these drugs will relieve only pain and fever. For social emergencies (for example, an unavoidable party), a nasal spray may be used, but not repeatedly.

This may seem hard advice. But to take a proprietary cold remedy which contains a decongestant, pain reliever, stimulant (e.g., caffeine), and antihistamine is somewhat like taking a sledge hammer to crack a nut, except that the nut is virtually uncrackable! No drug has a single effect, and to take several drugs with many diverse effects and adverse effects in order to dry up a few square centimeters of the lining membrane of the nose is quite irrational. One last warning: Taking a decongestant drug by mouth can very easily be toxic if you use a decongestant nose spray or drops at the same time. If you have to use a local application in a social emergency, stay with a nose spray that is mixed with water, not oil. Oil may be inhaled into the lungs and cause inflammation or even pneumonia.

# DRUGS USED
# TO TREAT COUGHS

Coughs frequently serve a useful purpose—to get rid of an inhaled foreign body or to cough up sputum. These coughs are said to be productive. A cough which is simply dry and irritating is said to be unproductive. As with cold remedies, the marketing of cough medicines is a lucrative business, and so the market is flooded with preparations. Many of these are mixtures containing such small doses of individual drugs as to render them pharmacologically ineffective. But, of course, a large proportion of us respond to inert mixtures—we *think* they do us good, and thus to a degree they do.

The purpose of cough medicines is to give comfort to those people with a productive cough and to help them cough up their sputum. For those people with a dry, irritating, unproductive cough, the aim is to suppress it. Therefore, two main groups of drugs are used to treat cough: expectorants and cough suppressants. Expectorants liquefy the sputum, so that it is easier to cough up. Cough suppressants work locally at the site of the irritation in the throat, or they act on the cough center in the brain, reducing the desire to cough. Some cough mixtures contain drugs which act on the conscious part of the brain, producing sedation and making one less aware of throat irritation.

### Cough Expectorants
A wide variety of drugs are used in order to help expectoration, but there are two main groups: those that stimulate coughing and those that "thin" the sputum (mucolytic drugs).

Stimulant expectorants act by irritating the lining of the stomach. This stimulates the nerves supplying the glands in the bronchi. The result is supposed to be an increased production of secretions, thus making the sputum more "watery" and easy to cough up. However, the dose required to do this would, in fact, with most of these drugs, produce stomach pains and vomiting. Stimulant expectorants include ammonium chloride, acetates, bicarbonates, potassium iodide, sodium citrate, glyceryl guaiacolate, ipecac, squill, creosote, eucalyptus, and menthol. They are present in many cough medicines, and from the point of view of effectiveness you may as well choose them by taste or color.

The stickiness of sputum depends on the amount of water it contains, which in turn depends upon the general degree of hydration of the body. Patients with chronic bronchitis and other chest disorders which produce dry sticky sputum may well benefit from increasing their fluid intake. Inhalation of water or steam may also be very useful, and it does not really matter whether these are made to smell pleasant by the addition of menthol, eucalyptus, or benzoin.

Chymotrypsin and other enzymes (e.g., pancreatic dornase, streptokinase-streptodornase) have been shown to "digest" sputum in the laboratory, but their effect on sputum in the bronchial tubes has been variable. Cysteine compounds (e.g., acetylcysteine) are available for inhalation or instillation. These may liquefy sputum production so much that it becomes necessary to clean the airway with a suction device. They also may cause fever. They should be used with caution in elderly patients with severe breathing difficulties. They may produce spasm of the bronchi, nausea, vomiting, stomatitis, and runny nose. Some patients have coughed up blood. Acetylcysteine may actually produce asthmalike attacks in certain individuals, and difficulties in breathing in some infants and children.

Mucolytic drugs liquefy sputum production, but this may in no way be related to improvement in the breathing capacity of the patient. The reduction in stickiness of sputum may, however, be helpful and of some use in some patients with bronchitis, asthma, and other serious respiratory diseases.

## Cough Suppressants (Antitussives)

The most important cough suppressant in people who smoke is to stop smoking. For coughs caused by irritation or inflammation in the throat above the larynx (voice box), hundreds of different makes of throat candies, tablets, lozenges, and cough drops are available. Many contain antiseptics (such as creosote, thymol, benzoin, cetylpyridinium, domiphen) in doses which are totally useless. (However, were the doses effective, they could be harmful.)

Most cough drops contain demulcents—soothing substances which act on the surface of the throat—such as honey, licorice, and glycerin. Such preparations also contain pleasant-smelling and -tasting substances like peppermint, eucalyptus, cinnamon, lemon, clove, and aniseed. Others contain menthol, camphor, or chloroform. The main effect of these preparations is that their smell or taste may help you feel better. They may increase the production of saliva, which is soothing and helps to wash the inflamed surfaces of the throat. Some preparations contain a topical anesthetic (e.g., benzocaine), which may reduce the pain of inflammation. Many cough medicines contain the same ingredients in liquid form—irrational, since they are swallowed, go directly into the stomach, and have only a fraction of a second to work locally on the throat. There is no evidence that any of these cough preparations are any more effective than sucking ordinary candy or chewing gum.

For nonproductive irritating coughs caused by inflammation below the larynx, steam inhalations may be very useful and can be made to smell pleasant by adding such substances as menthol.

The main drugs used to suppress cough may be divided into two groups, narcotic and nonnarcotic.

Narcotic cough suppressants include hydrocodone, oxycodone, and hydromorphone. These are discussed in the section on narcotic pain relievers, p. 115. In addition to suppressing the cough reflex, they also tend to dry up and thicken bronchial secretions. They are drugs of dependence and should not be used routinely. Codeine is also discussed under narcotic pain relievers. It is present in many cough medicines, usually in noneffective doses. In appropriate dosage it is an effective cough suppressant but may cause constipation.

Nonnarcotic cough suppressants include dextromethorphan (present in many cough mixtures), levopropoxyphene, and noscapine.

## Cough Mixtures

There are numerous mixtures on the market, some containing up to ten drugs. Some are useless, some are harmful, many are expensive, some are addictive, and it is difficult to find out what some of them contain, because the labels are not informative. Some mixtures sold over the counter or prescribed by doctors contain mixtures of an expectorant and a suppressant, which seems contradictory: the suppressant dries and thickens the bronchial secretions and blocks the reflex which clears them from the bronchial tubes, whereas the expectorant liquefies and increases the secretions.

In addition to expectorants, demulcents, and suppressants, many cough medicines contain antihistamines. Yet there is no support at all for the popular belief that antihistamines are of use in treating cough. They also tend to dry up and thicken bronchial secretions. They may produce sedation, which could help at night, but they should not be used casually.

### Drugs of Choice in Treating Cough

For a dry throaty cough (i.e., one caused by inflammation or irritation above the larynx) anything that may be sucked or chewed will help. There is little point in taking special cough lozenges or mixtures. If the cough is very irritating it is better to take a dose of a cough suppressant along with something to suck or chew.

For a cough in the chest (below the larynx) which is irritating and nonproductive, a straight cough suppressant is best—e.g., codeine, dextromethorphan, or noscapine. Dextromethorphan may be less sedating than codeine and is safer in cases of accidental poisoning, particularly with children. For the ordinary dry cough associated with a common cold only three or four doses at appropriate intervals will be required. If you find yourself having to take a cough suppressant for more than a few days, see your doctor. Also see your doctor if the cough does not clear up after one or two weeks, if your sputum turns yellow or green (you may need an antibiotic), if there is blood in your sputum, if your cough is associated with chest pain and/or fever, or if it is associated with breathlessness.

Steam inhalations are of benefit to both dry throaty coughs and nonproductive chest coughs.

A productive cough may be helped by a warm drink or steam inhalations. A simple expectorant mixture (such as a sodium chloride compound) may help, but these mixtures may produce stomach pains and upsets if taken over prolonged periods. If you have the bad habit of taking cough medicines every day and suffer from indigestion, it might be the cough medicine that is causing it. *Any patient with a cough should stop smoking.* Patients with chronic cough from, say, bronchitis may be helped by bronchodilator drugs (see below), but the repeated daily use of any medicine should be avoided unless recommended by a physician.

# DRUGS USED TO TREAT BRONCHIAL ASTHMA

### Bronchodilators

Drugs which open up the airways are called bronchodilators. They act by dilating (opening up) the bronchial tubes. They are used to reverse or decrease obstruction to the flow of air to the lungs caused by narrowing of these tubes. This occurs in bronchial asthma when narrowing of the airways is produced by spasm of the muscles. This spasm (bronchospasm) is often associated with swelling of the lining surfaces and an increased production of secretions.

Narrowing of the airways may also occur in chronic chest disorders such as emphysema and bronchitis. In these disorders the small bronchial tubes are scarred, distorted, and narrowed by repeated infections. In addition, repeated infections affect the secretory glands in the walls of the bronchial tubes and in the lining membranes. These increase in size and produce more secretions (sputum) resulting in a chronic productive cough (a cough which produces sputum). Also, in such chronic disorders as emphysema the lung tissues lose their normal elasticity, and this causes many small bronchial tubes to close up when the person breathes out. Thus the two types of obstruction to the airways produced by asthma and chronic bronchitis differ; the extent to which they can be treated by drugs also differs. Much more benefit from bronchodilator drugs may obviously be obtained when the airways are obstructed due to spasm, as in asthma, than when it is due to scarring, as in chronic bronchitis or emphysema. Machines which measure the volume of air breathed out by an individual in a given time show this clearly.

There are two main groups of bronchodilator drugs: sympathomimetic compounds (epinephrinelike drugs) and theophylline compounds.

SYMPATHOMIMETIC DRUGS

These drugs, as their name implies, mimic the effects of stimulating the sympathetic division of the autonomic nervous system (see p. 148). They include chemicals which are produced in the body; e.g., epinephrine and norepinephrine (which is the main chemical messenger at nerve endings of the sympathetic nervous system). Numerous synthetic chemicals also mimic stimulation of the sympathetic nervous system—e.g., isoproterenol, ephedrine, and amphetamines. Drugs which have sympathomimetic effects may act directly on the site of nerve endings (e.g., epinephrine, norepinephrine, isoproterenol); indirectly by causing a release of the chemical messenger at the nerve endings (e.g., amphetamine); or by both direct and indirect actions (e.g., ephedrine). This is a very simple description of what really is a most complex physiochemical process. It is made more complicated by factors that influence stores of norepinephrine in the body, causing sympathomimetic drugs to act differently if given for short or prolonged periods of time.

The sites of action of the nerve endings are called receptor sites, and these are widely distributed throughout various tissues of the body.

Three types of receptors have been recognized: alpha receptors, beta-1 receptors, and beta-2 receptors (see p. 148).

Drugs which stimulate beta receptors are used in treating obstruction to the airways because they relax bronchial muscles. However, most sympathomimetic bronchodilator drugs act on both beta-1 and beta-2 receptors so that in addition to relieving bronchospasm they also produce unwanted effects upon the heart and circulation and may produce serious disorders of heart rate and rhythm.

Over the last decade there has been an increasing tendency to give drugs such as isoproterenol by inhalation, often as pressurized aerosols. This is not without danger. There is now convincing evidence that the increased deaths from asthma among young people in Great Britain in recent years has been directly related to the use of aerosols containing high doses of isoproterenol.

Selective beta-2 receptor stimulants are available which dilate bronchial muscles but produce fewer effects upon the heart. These appear to be safer than the isoproterenol-like drugs, are longer-acting, and may also be given by mouth or by inhalation. They include salbutamol, terbutaline, metaproterenol, and isoetharine.

Sympathomimetic drugs used to treat asthma and nasal congestion include: epinephrine (in numerous inhalers); ephedrine (in numerous preparations); isoetharine (in bronchodilator inhalants); isoproterenol (in numerous preparations); metaproterenol; pseudoephedrine (in numerous preparations); salbutamol; terbutaline.

To understand the effects, adverse effects, and use of these drugs it is best to know two or three drugs well. Look up ephedrine, isoproterenol, and salbutamol in Part III.

### THEOPHYLLINE COMPOUNDS

Theophylline and related compounds relax bronchial muscles, stimulate the respiratory center in the brain, and increase coronary artery blood flow to heart muscles. They may be given by injection, by mouth, or as suppositories. Their effectiveness depends upon the amount of theophylline which enters the bloodstream. Suppositories are useful at night.

Theophylline is a xanthine present in small amounts in tea. However, more soluble derivatives such as aminophylline are used. But because aminophylline is an irritant, various preparations containing it are available, aimed at producing less irritation when the drug is taken by mouth. A different theophylline preparation, oxtriphylline (choline theophyllinate), may be less irritating to the stomach. Generally, various preparations are less irritating because they contain less theophylline—but they are therefore less effective.

## Choice of Bronchodilator Drugs

Because of the risks produced by isoproterenol, either salbutamol or metaproterenol by mouth is probably the drug of choice to control recurrent attacks of asthma. In patients with damaged bronchial tubes due to chronic bronchitis it is better to have special breathing measurements carried out and the most appropriate drug (if any) selected in the light of these tests. Ephedrine is a useful alternative.

To stop an acute attack, an aerosol containing salbutamol or terbutaline is possibly the safest preparation. In emergencies epinephrine or aminophylline by injection may be used, alone or in combination with salbutamol. Severe attacks may require corticosteroid drugs (see p. 160), and so may incapacitating asthma which fails to respond to any other available drug or combination of drugs.

## Allergic Asthma

The drug called cromolyn sodium (sodium cromoglycate) acts on the lining surfaces of the airways to interfere with the allergic reaction in patients who develop allergic asthma. The allergic effects (spasm of the bronchial muscles and swelling of the lining membrane) are stopped or reduced if the drug is present on the airway surfaces at the time when the allergic reaction begins; it is not effective if taken after the reaction has started. It is, therefore, of use in preventing asthma and rhinitis (inflammation of the nasal passages) due to allergy. It is taken by inhalation and may cause bronchospasm and slight irritation of the throat, especially if used during or after a respiratory infection. It may produce contact dermatitis in people who handle it. It should not be used during pregnancy. The drug is available as a dry powder in a gelatin capsule. A special inhaler punctures the capsule and allows the powder to be delivered into the lungs. A small dose of salbutamol or metaproterenol may be added to cut down bronchospasm, which can occur in some patients on inhalation of a dry powder. Cromolyn sodium is not effective in all cases, and it is very expensive.

## Corticosteroids

These are discussed beginning on p. 159. They are used in the treatment of a number of allergic or infectious respiratory disorders, the most important of which is asthma.

Corticosteroids may be used to treat asthma of varying degrees of severity. The most serious form of asthma attack is called status asthmaticus. In an emergency such as this, the use of corticosteroids by injection into a vein can be lifesaving, although their maximum effects may not occur until one to four hours after the injection. For this reason additional treatment, such as the intravenous injection of aminophylline, is often required to obtain some immediate relief for the patient.

Severe attacks of asthma may be helped by the use of oral corticosteroids (e.g., prednisone or prednisolone), starting with a high dose and slowly reducing the daily dose over a six-day period. Some patients will benefit by intermittent courses when necessary, but a few will need a maintenance daily dose of prednisone with increased dosage during an acute attack. However, a maintenance daily dose of above 10 mg. of prednisone (or equivalent dosage for other oral corticosteroids) may produce serious adverse effects. In particular, the body's own production of corticosteroids is suppressed, bringing added associated dangers from injury, infections, and surgery. In order to minimize these adverse effects, whenever possible, corticosteroids should be given on alternate days in the morning.

An alternative to oral corticosteroids may be injections of adrenocorticotropin hormone (ACTH), which stimulates the body's adrenal glands to produce corticosteroids. This is not without danger —see adverse effects of corticotropin in Part III. Long-lasting depot injections of a corticosteroid are also used.

The recent development of a beclamethasone *inhalation* preparation offers a substantial improvement in the therapy of steroid-dependent asthmatics by allowing a reduction or discontinuation of oral steroid therapy, thereby substantially reducing adverse effects. See beclamethasone in Part III.

Corticosteroids are also used to treat certain rare chest diseases, such as sarcoidosis and fibrosing alveolitis. Their use in pulmonary tuberculosis is now restricted to those patients with fluid in their pleural cavity (pleural effusion). Corticosteroids may cause old tuberculosis to flare up. Therefore, patients with a previous history of tuberculosis should have their chest X-rayed at intervals and be under the care of a chest physician if they are taking corticosteroids.

# DRUGS USED
# TO TREAT EPILEPSY

Epilepsy is characterized by an abnormal and excessive stimulation of the nerve cells in the brain. This results in a fit which may also be called a convulsion or seizure. The excessive stimulation taking place in the brain may be measured by an electroencephalograph. Epileptic attacks can occur when the brain is "irritated" by an infection (e.g., meningitis, encephalitis), by a head injury, by a tumor, by a stroke (a thrombosis or hemorrhage into the brain), or by some drugs. The most common type of epilepsy occurs without any recognized abnormality and is therefore called idiopathic epilepsy.

Idiopathic epilepsy includes two main types: grand mal (major epilepsy) and petit mal (minor epilepsy). Grand mal epilepsy is preceded by a warning sensation or aura (e.g., flashing lights, a smell, taste, or noise), which is followed by a sudden loss of consciousness, then an attack of rigidity and breath holding, followed by twitching that may last for a minute or two. The person may urinate and foam at the mouth. The attacks may be followed by coma, sleep, confusion, or headache. Petit mal attacks are transient attacks of impaired consciousness which may last only a fraction of a second. There are of course many degrees of severity of grand mal and petit mal epilepsy. Automatism may follow both types. This is a state in which the patient carries out his normal routine without knowing that he has done so.

There are other types of epilepsy which may be localized to certain parts of the brain—focal or local epilepsy. These start with spasm of one group of muscles and then spread (e.g., from the fingers to the arm) without the patient losing consciousness. Other local epilepsy attacks may produce sudden changes in mood. Psychomotor epilepsy, for example, is confined to the temporal lobes of the brain.

In general, the idiopathic epilepsies—grand mal and petit mal—are controlled more easily by drugs than epilepsy secondary to brain irritation caused by injury or disease. Any general depressant of the nervous system will decrease or abolish an epileptic fit, but the ones used to treat epilepsy have been selected because they reduce excessive stimulation in the brain without depressing such vital centers as the respiratory center, or without sending the patient to sleep. Bromide was the first effective antiepileptic drug (or anticonvulsant), but it is now obsolete. Phenobarbital has been used since the 1910s and phenytoin (diphenylhydantoin) was discovered in the 1930s. Since then numerous anticonvulsant drugs have been introduced.

The selection of the most appropriate drug and dosage regimen is critical to the individual being treated. It may take several months to achieve control on a particular drug regimen. The dose must be increased slowly, and the drugs must be taken strictly as directed. All adverse effects should be recorded.

Most patients with epilepsy receive great relief from anticonvulsant drugs, and some are able to stop taking the drugs after two or three years. This, of course, depends upon many factors such as age of onset, type of attack, frequency of attack, and so on. A few children may prove very difficult to treat. Also, be aware of factors which can trigger an attack—fever, stress, and infection.

## Anticonvulsant Drugs
These include barbiturates, such as phenobarbital; barbiturate-related drugs, such as primidone; hydantoins, such as ethotoin, mephenytoin, and phenytoin (diphenylhydantoin); oxazolidines, such as paramethadione and trimethadione; succinimides, such as ethosuximide, methsuximide, and phensuximide; phenylacetylurea derivatives, such as phenacemide; and other drugs, such as carbamazepine, diazepam, and ACTH. In emergencies, diazepam, phenytoin, or paraldehyde is given by injection.

## The Choice of Anticonvulsants
For grand mal epilepsy and focal epilepsies, phenobarbital, phenytoin, and primidone are often the most effective drugs. They are long-acting, but they cause changes in the liver which affect their rate of breakdown, and therefore their dose must be carefully adjusted according to individual needs. Phenobarbital or phenytoin is the drug of first choice (being cheaper and relatively less toxic), then primidone, and then phenobarbital combined with phenytoin. Genetic and other factors affect the way that the liver deals with phenytoin, so effective blood levels may vary considerably. Also, other anticonvulsant drugs such as diazepam may cause high blood levels of phenytoin. If phenobarbital and phenytoin together fail to control fits, then primidone may be substituted for the phenobarbital, even though primidone is a barbiturate derivative which is partially converted to phenobarbital in the body. It is really a matter of testing the various drugs and combinations of drugs until the attacks are controlled. This requires patience. For example, phenobarbital may actually cause increased activity and aggression in some children. Thus it can be seen how difficult it sometimes is to arrive at the most appropriate treatment.

For petit mal epilepsy (which occurs more commonly in children) ethosuximide appears to be the drug of choice and trimethadione may be useful. Phenobarbital may make the attacks worse. Other drugs such as acetazolamide (see under Diuretics, p. 106) and paramethadione may be effective. Diazepam appears to be the drug of choice for epilepsy characterized by twitching of a limb (myoclonus) and infantile spasms, with ACTH as an alternative.

Primidone or phenytoin should be tried in patients suffering from psychomotor epilepsy which seems to be aggravated by phenobarbital.

For status epilepticus (a succession of fits without the patient regaining consciousness), diazepam by intravenous injection is now regarded as the drug of choice, but paraldehyde, phenytoin, and phenobarbital may also be used.

Treatment in epilepsy should aim at keeping the individual free from fits for two to three years, at which time the drug should be slowly tapered off and stopped. Sudden withdrawal may cause status epilepticus.

# DRUGS WHICH ACT ON THE AUTONOMIC NERVOUS SYSTEM

The autonomic nervous system, as the name implies, is not under direct voluntary control. It supplies internal organs—the stomach, intestine, bronchi, heart, blood vessels, bladder—as well as the eyes and sweat glands. It therefore controls all sorts of functions, from breathing to sexual activity, from sweating to digestion. It consists of two divisions, sympathetic and parasympathetic. These divisions oppose each other, but a careful balance is maintained by special centers in the brain.

Impulses from the brain and spinal cord join the autonomic network of nerves along nerve fibers which run into ganglia (rather like electrical switch boxes). The impulses are transmitted at these junctions by chemical transmitters. The nerve fibers running *to* the junctions are called *pre*ganglionic nerve fibers, and they all use the same chemical transmitter—acetylcholine. This transmitter works for only a very short time, because once it is liberated at nerve junctions to act as a chemical transmitter another chemical starts to break it down. The latter chemical is an enzyme called cholinesterase. Nerve fibers running *from* the nerve junctions (ganglia) are called *post*ganglionic nerves.

Parasympathetic postganglionic nerves also use acetylcholine as a chemical transmitter; they are therefore known as cholinergic nerves. The sympathetic postganglionic nerve fibers, which use epinephrine and norepinephrine as chemical transmitters, are known as adrenergic nerves.

## Drugs Which Act on the Parasympathetic Nervous System

Drugs which act like acetylcholine are called cholinergic drugs; they may also be called parasympathomimetic because they mimic the actions of the parasympathetic nervous system.

Stimulation of the parasympathetic division produces stimulation of secretory glands—salivary, tear, bronchial, and sweat. It slows the heart rate, constricts the bronchi, produces increased movement of the gut, contracts the bladder, and constricts the pupil. It stimulates nerve endings in voluntary muscles, stimulates and then depresses the brain, and dilates blood vessels.

CHOLINERGIC DRUGS

There are three groups of cholinergic drugs:

CHOLINE ESTERS: carbachol, methacholine, bethanechol. These act at all sites like acetylcholine.

ALKALOIDS: pilocarpine, muscarine. These act selectively on those nerve endings which respond to acetylcholine.

CHOLINESTERASE INHIBITORS OR ANTICHOLINESTERASE DRUGS: physostigmine and neostigmine. These inactivate the enzyme (cholinesterase) which is responsible for breaking down acetylcholine, allowing acetylcholine to go on working.

Not all effects occur with each cholinergic drug. Also, the intensity of effect varies. Methacholine may be used to slow down fast heart rates, and carbachol may be used to stimulate bowel and bladder function after surgical operations. They both have to be given by injection under the skin. Bethanechol is related and may be given by mouth. Pilocarpine is used to constrict the pupil and decrease the pressure inside the eye in patients with glaucoma. The anticholinesterase drug physostigmine is used to stimulate the bowel and bladder after surgery, in the treatment of myasthenia gravis (a disease caused by defective transmission of impulses by acetylcholine, and characterized by severe muscle weakness and fatigue), and as an antidote to neuromuscular blocking drugs. Many related drugs are also "used" as nerve gases, and some are pesticides.

## Drugs Which Oppose Parasympathetic Activity

These may be called acetylcholine antagonists or parasympatholytics. They prevent acetylcholine from acting as a transmitter. There are three groups anticholinergic drugs, which act principally at parasympathetic nerve endings, ganglionic blocking drugs, which act on ganglia; neuromuscular blocking drugs, which act on nerve endings in voluntary muscles.

ANTICHOLINERGIC DRUGS

Typical of these drugs is atropine, and they are therefore often referred to as atropinelike drugs. Atropine is an alkaloid from the plant *Atropa belladonna*. It competes for the same chemical receptors as acetylcholine, thus blocking its effects. It produces dry mouth and a reduction in all secretions except milk, effects opposite to that of stimulation of the parasympathetic division. In the stomach it reduces the amount of acid produced. Sweating is inhibited, and bronchial secretions are reduced. It causes a relaxation of muscles in the bowel, bronchi, and bladder and is used to relieve muscle spasm in these organs (e.g., intestinal colic, bronchospasm). It dilates the pupils and increases the pressure inside the eyes. It increases heart rate, stimulates the brain, reduces motion sickness, and decreases the tremor and rigidity of Parkinsonism. Higher doses of atropine produce a rapid heart rate, dry mouth, blurred vision, dilated pupils, and restlessness. In overdose, atropine produces excitement, hallucinations, delirium, mania, and coma.

Other atropinelike drugs are: scopolamine, which depresses the brain and is used preoperatively and in motion sickness; homatropine, used to dilate the pupils; scopolamine butylbromide, which relaxes involuntary muscles and is used to relieve colic; cyclopentolate, used as eye drops to dilate the pupils; and propantheline, one of many anticholinergic drugs used on their own or in combination with alkalis or sedatives in the treatment of peptic ulcers. Many anticholinergic drugs have been used to treat Parkinsonism.

The principal uses of anticholinergic drugs therefore includes their use in Parkinsonism, for motion sickness, as sedatives, to dilate the pupils, to dilate the bronchi and reduce bronchial secretions, to reduce acid production by the stomach in the treatment of peptic ulcers, to relieve spasm of the gut, to treat colic, and to reduce sweating.

GANGLION BLOCKING DRUGS

These have been used in the past to treat raised blood pressure. They lower blood pressure by blocking the nerves which normally keep blood vessels constricted, therefore producing a fall in peripheral resistance. They include mecamylamine, pentolinium, and trimethaphan. Because they are not selective and block ganglia in both parasympathetic and sympathetic divisions, they produce numerous adverse effects—particularly constipation. They are seldom used now.

NEUROMUSCULAR BLOCKING DRUGS

When an impulse passes down a nerve to a voluntary muscle it causes the release of acetylcholine at the nerve ending. The acetylcholine acts as a chemical transmitter, stimulating the muscle to contract. Neuromuscular blocking drugs interfere with this chemical transmission. Curare, used on poisoned arrows by natives in South America, is the most famous example of this group of drugs. There are two main ways in which neuromuscular blocking drugs work. Tubocurarine, gallamine, and pancuronium compete with acetylcholine and block the impulse being transmitted to the receptor organ in the muscles. They cause a flaccid paralysis of voluntary muscles. Drugs such as succinylcholine (suxamethonium) mimic the action of acetylcholine. At first they cause the muscles to contract, but this effect wears off quickly, leaving the muscle no longer receptive to stimulation by acetylcholine. They are said to work by depolarization because they block the complex physiochemical process called polarization. Thus neuromuscular blocking drugs work in two ways—by competition and by depolarization. They are used to provide muscular relaxation during surgery and also during electroshock therapy.

## Drugs Which Act on the Sympathetic Nervous System

Those drugs that imitate the effects of stimulation of the sympathetic division are called sympathomimetic drugs. Those that oppose its effects are called sympatholytic.

SYMPATHOMIMETIC DRUGS

This group of drugs includes epinephrine, the main hormone produced by the medulla of the adrenal glands, and norepinephrine, the main chemical transmitter at postganglionic sympathetic nerve endings. These are called adrenergic drugs, while those that oppose their action are called adrenolytic or sympatholytic.

Norepinephrine is produced and stored at adrenergic nerve endings. It can be liberated from these stores by stimulating the nerve, or by drugs such as amphetamines, ephedrine, reserpine, and guanethidine. Sympathomimetic drugs (or adrenergic drugs) may act directly on the receptors at the nerve endings of the sympathetic nervous system (epinephrine, norepinephrine, and isoproterenol); indirectly, by stimulating the liberation of norepinephrine from the stores at the nerve endings (amphetamines work this way) or by both indirect and direct actions (as with ephedrine and metaraminol).

Sympathomimetic drugs act on the adrenergic receptor sites found widely distributed throughout the body. These receptors are classified simply into alpha and beta-1 and beta-2 receptors. Stimulation of alpha receptors produces what are called alpha effects—constriction of the blood vessels in the skin and gut, a rise in blood pressure, and dilation of the pupils. Beta-1 receptors are principally located in the heart; stimulation produces an increase of heart rate and increased output of blood from the heart. Stimulation of beta-2 receptors produces relaxation of bronchial muscles, relaxation of the uterus, and dilation of blood vessels, chiefly in muscles. Stimulation of both alpha and beta receptors in the gut produces relaxation. Alpha and beta stimulation also produces a raised blood sugar and a raised level of blood fatty acids. The mobilization of sugar from the liver is an alpha effect, and that from the voluntary muscles is a beta effect. Epinephrine produces both alpha and beta effects, norepinephrine produces chiefly alpha effects, and isoproterenol produces beta-1 and beta-2 effects.

Sympathomimetic drugs are principally used as nasal decongestants (read the section Drugs Used to Treat Common Colds, p. 132); to treat bronchospasm (read the section Drugs Used to Treat Bronchial Asthma, p. 138); and to treat low blood pressure: Because they constrict blood vessels in the skin they increase resistance and raise the blood pressure. They may be used in severe states of low blood pressure caused by coronary thrombosis, anesthetics, or drug overdose. They are not as popular as they once were.

SYMPATHOLYTIC DRUGS

These drugs oppose sympathetic activity by:

1. Blocking transmission of nerve impulses along postganglionic sympathetic nerves (adrenergic nerves) or their nerve endings. They are called adrenergic neurone blocking drugs and include guanethedine. These drugs are discussed in the section Drugs Used to Treat Raised Blood Pressure (p. 108).

2. Blocking the alpha receptors. These are called alpha-receptor blocking drugs and include phentolamine, phenoxybenzamine, and tolazoline. The principal effect of these drugs is to produce dilatation of the blood vessels in the skin. They are discussed under the section Drugs Used to Treat Disorders of Circulation (p. 94).

3. Blocking the beta receptors. These are called beta-receptor blocking drugs. They are used to treat angina, disorders of heart rhythm, and raised blood pressure. They are discussed primarily under Drugs Used to Treat Angina (see p. 101).

# DRUGS USED
# TO TREAT PARKINSONISM

Parkinsonism is a disorder of the nervous system in which voluntary movement is disturbed, involuntary movements occur, and the tone of muscles is altered. Voluntary movements become slow and trembly (tremor), and muscles become stiff (rigidity). The group of signs and symptoms produced are usually referred to as Parkinson's disease or simply Parkinsonism. There are several causes and many different groups and degrees of involuntary movements and muscle rigidities. These days one frequent cause is the use of drugs from the major tranquilizer group.

There is no drug available which *cures* Parkinsonism, but if the most appropriate drugs are used, many patients may benefit. The centers in the brain which control movement balance their control through two physiochemical processes. The chemical transmitters are acetylcholine and dopamine (a precursor of norepinephrine and a chemical transmitter itself). They are thought to function in the brain as do the two opposing chemical transmitters in the peripheral autonomic nervous system—acetylcholine and epinephrine. These two processes in the brain are often referred to as the cholinergic system and the dopaminergic system respectively. In Parkinsonism the dopaminergic system appears to be defective, so that the control mechanisms of movement become unbalanced and the cholinergic system dominates the control. Chemical suppression of this dominance may, therefore, be possible by the use of drugs which block or interfere with the action of acetylcholine (for example, anticholinergic drugs). Alternatively, drugs which increase the effect of the dopaminergic system will have beneficial effects (e.g., levodopa or amantadine).

The main aim of treatment in Parkinsonism is to try to ease both the difficulty in starting movements and the slowness of movement (hypokinesia) and to reduce tremor and muscle rigidity.

For over a century Parkinsonism has been treated with anticholinergic drugs. Atropine was the first to be used, and since then many atropinelike drugs have been used. Antihistamines such as promethazine and diphenhydramine have also been used, but these may have helped because they produce mild atropinelike effects (see the section Antihistamine Drugs, p. 127). Many other drugs have been claimed to be of benefit in treating patients suffering from Parkinsonism, but the two real advances in recent years have been the respective discoveries of the effects of levodopa and amantadine.

## Anticholinergic Drugs

A wide choice of anticholinergic drugs is available for the treatment of Parkinsonism. These include trihexyphenidyl, benztropine, cycrimine, procyclidine, and biperiden. Orphenadrine and chlorphenoxamine are antihistamines, and ethopropazine is a phenothiazine, but all are used here for their anticholinergic properties.

The anticholinergic drugs are discussed in more detail on p. 146. Their beneficial effects in Parkinsonism are very limited. Muscle rigidity and tremors may be helped, but hypokinesia (slowness of movements), one of the most disturbing effects of Parkinsonism, is unaffected by them.

The adverse effects produced by these drugs are the result of their blocking actions on the parasympathetic division of the autonomic nervous system. The different drugs available may produce some or all of the effects in varying intensities according to dosage. They should be used with caution in patients with enlarged prostate glands or heart disorders. They should not be used in patients with closed-angle glaucoma or in patients who are receiving monoamine oxidase inhibitors or have received them in the previous ten days. Their effects may be increased by other drugs such as major tranquilizers and antihistamines. Trihexyphenidyl may produce confusion and hallucinations. These drugs should be slowly reduced before stopping, since sudden withdrawal may produce severe rigidity and tremor.

## Levodopa

Levodopa is the chemical forerunner of dopamine. Although levodopa is quickly converted to dopamine in the body, enough of it enters the brain to be effective if it is given in high dosage. The worst features of Parkinsonism—difficulty in starting movement and slowness of movement—improve during treatment with levodopa. This is often impressive, resulting in improvement in walking, eating, and talking. The rigidity is also helped, and other effects of Parkinsonism—difficulty in balancing, drooling, and involuntary eye movements—may also improve slowly.

Levodopa may produce many adverse effects related to dosage. In particular, abnormal involuntary movements (dyskinesia) of the tongue, lips, face, and limbs may occur, as well as tremors and rapid breathing. There are many precautions associated with its use.

Pyridoxine (vitamin $B_6$) in small doses blocks the effects of levodopa. Since this vitamin may be present in vitamin preparations, patients taking levodopa should check with their pharmacist or doctor to see whether or not such preparations may be taken.

## Amantadine

Amantadine is thought to work by acting on nerve endings to produce the release of dopamine. In some patients it may be beneficial to all three main factors of Parkinsonism—hypokinesia, rigidity, and tremor—but less so than with levodopa. It is sometimes used in combination with levodopa, particularly in patients who are unable to tolerate full therapeutic doses of levodopa. Its true value in the treatment of Parkinsonism requires more study.

### Choice of Drug

All patients with Parkinsonism should be offered levodopa, but its use requires careful control and close cooperation between patient and doctor. The dose must be built up slowly, and repeated blood tests should be carried out at intervals to check for damage to white blood cells, to test for anemia, and to test liver function. An electric tracing of the heart rhythms should be made before starting treatment and at regular intervals. It may take several months to reach the most appropriate dose. Amantadine is an alternative. The anticholinergic drugs are of more use for patients suffering from drug-induced Parkinsonism, but they may help patients who have not responded to levodopa or amantadine. They may also be given to patients who are already taking and responding favorably to levodopa, because they help to reduce the nausea and vomiting which are common side effects.

A major problem with levodopa is that it is rapidly metabolized in the body into dopamine. Dopamine cannot cross the blood-brain barrier, whereas levodopa can. Given in high dosage, sufficient levodopa enters the brain before it is converted into dopamine. However, levodopa adverse effects are dose-related. A drug called carbidopa blocks levodopa metabolism in the body by inhibiting the enzyme dopa-decarboxylase, but it does not enter the brain. It cannot therefore interfere with the conversion of levodopa to dopamine in the brain. When carbidopa is given along with levodopa, the metabolism of levodopa outside the brain is blocked and the blood level of levodopa increases, with a corresponding decrease in stomach irritation. An effective treatment, therefore, is to give a dose of levodopa and carbidopa together. The addition of carbidopa reduces the dose of levodopa required. Fixed-dose combination products are available, and their use seems promising. In giving carbidopa and levodopa separately there is a risk that too high a dose of levodopa may be given. Also, the fixed-dose preparation ensures that the patient takes the appropriate amount of each.

# IRON

Iron is necessary for the manufacture of blood. A deficiency in iron leads to anemia. There are many other causes of anemia, but an iron deficiency is by far the commonest cause and the easiest to treat. Iron-deficiency anemia is common in women, infants, and elderly people. It may result from a diet lacking iron-rich foods—liver, meat, eggs, whole-meal cereals, oatmeal, peas, beans, and lentils. Such faulty feeding is likely to occur with babies and infants and with the elderly who live alone. Blood loss during menstruation (particularly at the menopause, when menstruation may be heavy and frequent), from a peptic ulcer, from the stomach due to the regular consumption of aspirin and other antirheumatic drugs, and during childbirth may produce iron deficiency anemia. Worm infections of the gut can cause iron deficiency, as can disorders of the stomach (e.g., surgical removal of part of the stomach in the treatment of duodenal ulcer) and intestine (e.g., ulcerative colitis). Thus treatment of iron-deficiency anemia will require special attention to its cause, as well as the giving of iron.

The symptoms produced by anemia may be produced by many disorders—some physical, some psychological, some mild and some serious. If you develop such symptoms as tiredness, breathlessness, and weakness and feel that you are anemic, consult your doctor, who may arrange for a blood test. If you look pale, then similarly consult your doctor and ask for a blood test.

Unfortunately doctors and patients use iron preparations quite indiscriminately as pick-me-ups. It should be obvious that iron will do no good for someone who is not suffering from iron deficiency. On the other hand, there is no substitute for it in cases where it is needed.

Iron is essential for the formation of the pigment called hemoglobin in red blood cells. These cells are responsible for carrying oxygen to the tissues from the lungs and carbon dioxide from the tissues back to the lungs. Two-thirds of the body's iron is present in the hemoglobin. The rest is stored in the bone marrow, spleen, and muscles. Absorption of iron from food takes place principally through the duodenum and the upper part of the small intestine. Its absorption is helped by acid from the stomach, and it is more easily absorbed in the inorganic ferrous state. Only a small proportion of iron in food is absorbed, but even so the iron content of the average diet in the Western world is sufficient for our needs. Obviously, a woman will usually need more if she is pregnant, breast feeding, or having heavy menstrual periods. The mechanisms for controlling the body's iron content exercise a careful control over the absorption of iron from the gut: if we are iron-deficient, absorption is increased. If we are not, then absorption is decreased. Vitamin C in appropriate doses increases absorption of iron, as does succinic acid. Because of menstruation, women need to absorb about twice as much iron as men each day.

Iron-deficiency anemia responds well to iron treatment, but as stated earlier the underlying cause must be diagnosed and treated. This must of course include attention to diet. In order to produce a suitable response in cases of iron deficiency, it is necessary to take a large amount of iron each day—about 200 mg. A good response will increase the hemoglobin level (which is an indication of the degree of anemia) by about 1 percent per day. However, in order to ensure a satisfactory level and to replenish the body's stores, treatment should continue for at least three to six months. It is no use trying to deal with iron-deficiency anemia by taking the tablets for only a few weeks.

Iron may be given by mouth or by injection into a vein or muscle. By mouth, it may irritate the stomach and gut to produce nausea, vomiting, diarrhea or constipation, and abdominal pains. Stools become black and tarry in consistency.

There are numerous oral iron preparations on the market; the cheapest effective preparations are ferrous sulfate, ferrous gluconate, ferrous succinate, ferrous fumarate. Stomach upset or diarrhea may be avoided by taking the drug with meals (although absorption is not as good as before meals) and by starting on a small daily dose—one tablet daily —and then increasing the daily dose up to two or three tablets over a period of one to two weeks. Combination with a sufficient amount of vitamin C increases absorption, and therefore the dose of iron may be reduced, in hopes of reducing stomach upsets. If you still have problems taking iron, then more expensive preparations in a slow-release form may be of use, although some such preparations may release insufficient quantities of iron. Many of these have the added advantage of requiring only one dose daily.

Injections of iron may be necessary if iron cannot be absorbed from the gut and in certain emergencies such as severe anemia in late pregnancy. Response to injected iron takes about fourteen days, and both the dose and the interval between doses should be calculated on the basis of the patient's hemoglobin level and body weight. However, it is important to remember that the speed of response to injected iron is no faster than to oral iron.

Iron sorbitex is a citric acid complex which is given by deep intramuscular injections. Injections can be painful, cause staining of the skin at the site, and produce headache, blurred vision, painful muscles, disorientation, flushing, nausea and vomiting, a metallic taste in the mouth, or loss of taste. Some of it is excreted by the kidneys, turning the urine black. Intramuscular iron sorbitex injections should not be given to patients with kidney disorders or infections.

Iron-dextran solution is widely used. It is absorbed more slowly from deep intramuscular injections and it may leave a residue. Repeated use of deep injections of iron-dextran solutions has been shown to produce sarcoma (a type of cancer) at the injection sites in rats, but no such change has been shown in human beings. Injections of iron-dextran solution may cause pain and staining of the skin at the site of the injection, necessitating a special injection technique. After deep intramuscular injections, fever and rapid beating of the heart may occur, as well as allergic reactions. Infusion into a vein may cause venous thrombosis, fever, and rapid beating of the heart. Allergic reactions to intravenous infusion occasionally cause death. Iron-dextran solution should not be given to patients who have severe liver damage or depressed blood production in the bone marrow. It should be given with utmost caution to anyone who has previously suffered from any drug reaction, and the patient should be kept under close observation for at least one hour after intravenous infusion. Local inflammatory reactions are much less frequent with intravenous administration than with intramuscular administration. However, shock and adverse effects on the heart, though still rare, are more common.

Finally, iron itself is a drug which may produce adverse effects. Overdose can cause liver and kidney damage, collapse, and death. Iron preparations, like any drug, must be kept out of the reach of children.

# VITAMINS

Vitamins are substances which are essential for the maintenance of normal body function, but they are not manufactured by the body. We therefore have to rely upon an outside source—and this, in a healthy individual, is a normal well-balanced diet.

When vitamins are not taken as part of the diet but in highly concentrated forms, they must be regarded as drugs. As such, they may produce adverse drug effects. Those that are soluble in water (the B vitamins and vitamin C), if taken in excess of the body's requirements, are quickly excreted. They thus do little harm, but their use is often unnecessary and wasteful. However, the fat-soluble vitamins (A, D, K, and E), if taken in excess of daily requirement, become stored in the body fat, where they may reach toxic concentrations.

Vitamins may be used to treat recognized disorders produced by vitamin deficiencies. In these cases doctors often use incredibly high doses. They are also administered to *prevent* the development of vitamin-deficiency disorders, as supplements to the individual's diet. Much confusion over dosage has therefore arisen between the doses used to treat established vitamin-deficiency disorders and the doses used in supplementary treatment. Supplementary dosage need only be at the level of recommended daily intake, and there is no merit in taking in more than this. Unfortunately, many over-the-counter preparations contain vitamins, and these are the subject of intense advertising and sales promotion. The thoroughly misleading message being given by the manufacturers is that if 100 units of a vitamin does you good then 1,000 units will do you even better. The promotion also quite wrongly implies that extra vitamins give you vitality and zest— that you don't really "live" until you take added vitamins.

Most people who take supplementary vitamins could afford a well-balanced diet and don't need them. Still, if they think vitamins will make them feel better, then vitamins probably will, but they ought to know the hazards of overdosage and they should not try to push these drugs onto everybody else.

Doctors are equally guilty in their indiscriminate use of vitamins. Yet many patients who may benefit from them (for example, the elderly person living alone) never receive vitamins, whereas they are frequently prescribed as "tonics" for the well-nourished. Supplementary vitamins may be of great value to those people whose diet is inadequate—those who are poor, isolated, elderly, or debilitated; those who are faddy about their food; those on certain diets, such as weight-control diets; and alcoholics and others who take in too little food. Similarly, some disorders of the stomach and gut may produce inadequate vitamin intake, and people with such disorders will require supplementary vitamins. Pregnant women and women who are breast feeding need supplementary vitamins, and they may be required by babies and by children at puberty, during debilitating illness, and in certain glandular disorders. But, of course, they are no substitute for a good nutritious diet. After all, vitamins are only a small part of food. There is no evidence that minor deficiencies of vitamins cause debility or increased risk of getting colds and other infections.

Since deficiency of a single vitamin is rarely encountered, it is best to supplement with several vitamins in doses not larger than the recommended daily requirements contained in a "normal" diet.

## Vitamin A
Carotene (pre-vitamin A) and vitamin A are present in dairy produce (milk, eggs, butter, cheese), in green vegetables and carrots, in liver and fish liver oils. Margarine has added vitamin A. Deficiency causes defective vision in dim light and thickening and hardening of the skin (metaplasia and hyperkeratosis). Such thickening also affects the cornea of the eyes. Vitamin A is fat-soluble, and if large amounts are taken the result is such adverse effects as loss of appetite, itching, skin disorders, loss of weight, enlargement of the liver and spleen, debility, and painful swellings of bone and joints.

### Vitamin B Complex

It includes vitamin $B_1$ (thiamine), vitamin $B_2$ (riboflavin), vitamin $B_6$ (pyridoxine), niacin (nicotinic acid—an alternative form is niacinamide —nicotinic acid amide, nicotinamide), folic acid (pteroylglutamic acid), and vitamin $B_{12}$ (cyanocobalamin).

#### VITAMIN $B_1$ (thiamine)

Vitamin $B_1$ is present in wheat germ, eggs, liver, peas, beans, and vegetables. Deficiency causes inflammation of nerves (peripheral neuritis), heart failure, edema, nausea, and vomiting. This group of disorders is known as beriberi. Vitamin $B_1$ deficiency may also damage the brain (Wernicke's encephalopathy) and cause mental confusion (Korsakoff's syndrome).

#### VITAMIN $B_2$ (RIBOFLAVIN)

Vitamin $B_2$ is present in yeast, milk, liver, and green vegetables. Deficiency produces sore lips (angular stomatitis), ulcers of the mouth, a sore magenta-colored tongue, skin rashes (seborrheic dermatitis), and blood vessels on the cornea of the eye (vascularization of the cornea).

#### VITAMIN $B_6$ (PYRIDOXINE)

Vitamin $B_6$ is present in liver, yeasts, and cereals. Deficiency may produce anemia.

#### NIACIN

Niacin (which is converted into niacinamide in the body) is present in liver, yeast, milk, vegetables, and unpolished rice. Deficiency produces pellagra, a disease affecting the mouth, stomach, and gut that results in sore tongue, stomatitis, gastritis, and diarrhea. Deficiency also affects the brain, causing dementia, and skin, producing dermatitis.

#### FOLIC ACID (PTEROYLGLUTAMIC ACID)

Folic acid is present in green vegetables, yeast, and liver. It is necessary for cell division and for the normal production of red blood cells. Symptoms of folic acid deficiency include sore tongue, anemia, diarrhea, and loss of weight. Folic acid deficiency may occur in patients with certain disorders of their stomach and bowels which interfere with absorption (e.g., sprue, coeliac disease, after gastrectomy), after prolonged use of large doses of pyrimethamine (used to prevent malaria), and in patients with epilepsy treated with anticonvulsant drugs (particularly primidone and phenytoin but also phenobarbital). In this last disorder, folic acid deficiency can lead to mental deterioration, which can be prevented by giving folic acid and vitamin $B_{12}$. Folic acid deficiency may also occur in pregnancy, and it is now often given routinely along with iron during the prenatal period.

VITAMIN B$_{12}$ (CYANOCOBALAMIN)

Vitamin B$_{12}$ is present in meat, milk, and eggs. To be absorbed into the bloodstream it has to combine with a substance secreted by the stomach known as the intrinsic factor, after which it is absorbed through the small intestine. Vitamin B$_{12}$ is stored in the liver. Its main action is upon blood formation by the bone marrow. Deficiency produces a special type of anemia called pernicious anemia. Such an anemia may also follow the surgical removal of large parts of the stomach and may occur in disorders of the small intestine. Only rarely is it caused by dietary deficiency of vitamin B$_{12}$, in strict vegetarians or in those living in the tropics.

## Vitamin C (Ascorbic Acid)

Vitamin C is present in citrus fruits, rose hips, and green vegetables. Cooking reduces the vitamin C content of food. Deficiency causes scurvy, a disease characterized by anemia, hemorrhage into the skin and gums, bruising, and bone pains. In children, vitamin C deficiency may delay bone growth. It is claimed by some that large daily doses of vitamin C (1,000 mg.) reduce the chances of getting the common cold, and/or reduce the severity of a cold.

## Vitamin D

Vitamin D is present in dairy produce and fish oils. It is also produced by the body after exposure of the skin to sunshine. The average diet of babies and some children may not provide sufficient vitamin D, particularly if they are not exposed to sufficient sunshine. Vitamin D deficiency produces rickets in children by interfering with calcium absorption, and osteomalacia (bone softening) in adults. Excessive dosage produces a rise in blood calcium which causes debility, drowsiness, nausea, abdominal pains, thirst, constipation, loss of appetite, deposits of calcium in various tissues and organs, kidney damage, and kidney stones.

## Vitamin K

Vitamin K$_1$ is present in greens and vegetables, and vitamin K$_2$ is produced by bacteria in the gut. Vitamin K is necessary for the production of various blood-clotting factors by the liver. Vitamin K$_1$ is fat-soluble and requires bile salts for its absorption from the gut. Deficiency causes a reduction in blood clotting factors, resulting in bleeding and delayed blood clotting. It may be caused by disorders of the gut which interfere with its absorption, obstruction to the production of bile (obstructive jaundice), and by some drugs (e.g., sulfonamides and tetracyclines) which affect the bacteria in the gut that produce vitamin $K_2$.

## Vitamin E
Vitamin E is present in the oil from soybeans, wheat germ, rice germ, cotton seed, maize, and such greens as lettuce leaves. Opinion on the importance of vitamin E is divided. In animals deficiency of vitamin E has been claimed to produce numerous effects on the reproduction system, muscular system, heart and circulation, and blood. Because deficiency in rats was found to produce adverse changes in early pregnancy in females and wasting of the testes in males, it quickly became known as the "antisterility vitamin" and was once widely promoted for its alleged enhancement of virility. But there is no unequivocal evidence to suggest that its use is of any benefit. In fact, because of its effects upon certain fats in the body, some experts consider that it may even cause premature aging.

## Recommended Daily Requirements
Tables of recommended daily vitamin requirements are easily found in books on nutrition, human biology, medicine, and so on. However, they specifically refer to diet and indicate that your *food* should contain the stated amounts. Unfortunately, but quite purposefully, the manufacturers of vitamin preparations give the impression that these amounts are to be *added* to your normal diet. They even sell products which have no food value but which are "enriched" with vitamins. Do not be misled: vitamins may be required to *supplement* an inadequate diet but never to *complement* a sensible diet. High-dose vitamin preparations should be avoided particularly.

# CORTICOSTEROIDS

The metabolic functions of the body are under the control of several glands whose internal secretions (or hormones) are released into the bloodstream. These glands include the master gland, called the pituitary, the thyroid and parathyroid glands, the pancreas, the adrenal glands, and the sex organs. The effect of the hormones released by these various glands is to stimulate particular body processes.

Under the direction of the brain, the front part (anterior lobe) of the pituitary gland exercises control over the thyroid gland, part of the adrenal glands, and the sex glands. It produces stimulating hormones which cause these organs (often known as target glands) to produce in turn their own secretions of hormones. In addition, there is a feedback mechanism, so that the production of a stimulating hormone by the pituitary is itself controlled by the circulating level of hormone from the target gland. For example, if the level of adrenal hormones increases in the blood, the adrenal-stimulating hormone decreases and vice versa. Thus the adrenal glands may be encouraged to secrete by giving the patient a stimulating hormone obtained from the pituitary glands of slaughtered animals. Furthermore, the effects of the adrenal glands may be "mimicked" by giving adrenal cortex extract or synthetic adrenal hormones, which can also decrease the production of the adrenal-stimulating hormone by the pituitary.

There are two adrenal glands. They lie above the upper ends of each kidney. Each consists of a center (medulla) which produces epinephrine and norepinephrine (see p. 148) and an outer layer known as the *cortex*. Over thirty hormones have been isolated from the adrenal cortex, the two most important ones being hydrocortisone and aldosterone. The adrenals (and from now on this term will be used instead of saying adrenal cortex) produce three groups of hormones (known as adrenocortical hormones), which may be categorized according to their main function: *glucocorticoids*, which act on sugar, protein, and calcium metabolism; *mineralocorticoids*, which act on salt and water metabolism; and *sex hormones*. Except for aldosterone, their production is under control of adrenocorticotropic hormone from the pituitary gland, a substance generally referred to as corticotropin or ACTH. There is an overlap of actions and effects produced by these hormones, again excepting aldosterone.

The glucocorticoids reduce inflammatory, allergic, and rheumatic reactions. They are, therefore, often referred to as anti-inflammatory hormones, as corticosteroids, or simply as steroids (since they belong to a chemical group known as steroids). They may also affect salt metabolism. Aldosterone controls retention of sodium and excretion of potassium by the kidneys; see p. 107 in the section Diuretics.

The sex hormones produced by the adrenals (in addition to those produced by the sex organs) include male sex hormones (androgens) and female sex hormones (estrogens). Their balance affects the degree of femininity and masculinity of the body. See the immediately following sections: Male Sex Hormones, Anabolic Steroids, and Female Sex Hormones.

## CORTICOSTEROIDS

Corticosteroids are important drugs that have become widely used. Their anti-inflammatory usefulness, however, may be in some cases limited by their metabolic effects. A huge number of synthetic preparations, related to hydrocortisone and producing similar effects, and also known as corticosteroids, have been manufactured in hopes of separating the two main effects: the anti-inflammatory, antiallergic, and antirheumatic effects from their metabolic effects on sugar, salts, and water. Modifications of the basic cortisone structure have led to drugs possessing greatly enhanced anti-inflammatory properties, particularly when applied to the skin. Available preparations include hydrocortisone, desoxycorticosterone, fludrocortisone, prednisolone, prednisone, dexamethasone, methylprednisolone, triamcinolone, and betamethasone to name a few. Adrenocorticotropin (ACTH) increases the production of adrenocortical steroids by the adrenal glands and may also be used.

To produce desired anti-inflammatory and other effects, however, corticosteroids have to be given in doses far in excess of the body's needs. This greatly increases the risk of adverse effects. In these doses their effects on metabolism are complex: for example, hydrocortisone affects salt and water balance, producing salt and water retention and potassium loss; sugar and carbohydrate metabolism is affected, producing a raised blood sugar and sugar in the urine (glycosuria); protein metabolism is affected, producing weakening of the bones (osteoporosis), retarded bone growth in children, wasting of the skin with appearance of stripes (striae), and delayed wound healing; fat metabolism is affected, resulting in fat being laid down on the face (moon face), shoulders (buffalo hump), and abdomen; calcium metabolism is affected, producing increased calcium excretion in the urine and the risk of kidney stones; and uric acid excretion is increased. In addition, hydrocortisone's ability to reduce the inflammatory response may sometimes be harmful. It can mask symptoms and signs of infections, such as tuberculosis. It also reduces the allergic response, interferes with the processes which produce immunity, and decreases the ability of the white blood cells to fight infection. It may cause mood changes, and it suppresses the complex nervous and hormonal response to stress, which may result in collapse and death.

The various corticosteroids used to treat inflammatory, allergic, and rheumatic disorders produce the same effects as hydrocortisone, but to very different degrees, so that their net effect may vary quite markedly. It all depends upon their chemical structure and dosage. The general term "corticosteroid" is convenient, but it is really so broad as to rob it of much of its meaning, particularly since it is usually applied to those chemical variations which have been developed specifically for their anti-inflammatory effects.

Hydrocortisone is the most commonly used corticosteroid by injection, and prednisone is the most popular preparation by mouth. Injections of hydrocortisone are used in such emergencies as severe asthma attacks. Short-term tapered courses of prednisone are given by mouth in the treatment of bronchial asthma, allergies, and other disorders. Long-term daily maintenance doses of prednisone are used in such disorders as asthma, rheumatic disorders, skin diseases, and blood disorders.

### Dangers Connected with the Use of Corticosteroids

In the individual with normally functioning adrenal glands the production of corticosteroid hormones is increased by the stress of, for example, injury, surgery, and infections. This problem of increased need during stress is exaggerated in patients who use corticosteroids in doses in excess of normal "replacement" therapy. The amount of circulating corticosteroids in the blood suppresses the production of ACTH by the pituitary gland, leading to "disuse" changes in the adrenal glands. If these drugs have been used for more than a few weeks in high doses the body may fail to react in the normal way to stress. The patient may collapse and even die. For this reason the daily dose should be increased threefold or fourfold during such episodes, and corticosteroid drugs should never be stopped suddenly. They should be tapered off very slowly over many weeks (depending, of course, on how long the patient has been on them). These dangers mean that every patient on corticosteroids should carry a warning card. If he has received them for one month or more in any two-year period he should *continue* to carry a steroid warning card; collapse can occur during a surgical operation up to two years after stopping the drugs.

In order to minimize most of the above adverse effects of corticosteroids, the shorter-acting preparations (e.g., prednisone) should whenever possible be administered on alternate days in the morning. This is possible in the case of a great many diseases normally treated with corticosteroids.

### Adrenocorticotropic Hormone (ACTH or Corticotropin)

This very complex chemical was first isolated in pure form from the pituitary glands of slaughtered animals in the 1940s, and first synthesized twenty years later. The synthetic preparations are less likely to cause allergic reactions because they are not contaminated with animal protein. ACTH stimulates the adrenals to produce corticosteroids (the most important of which is hydrocortisone) and to a lesser extent male sex hormones (androgens).

The principal effects produced by ACTH are those produced by corticosteroids. Therefore, it should not be used, although it often is, with the idea that it will produce selective anti-inflammatory effects.

It will *always* produce disturbances of salt and water balance. ACTH is inactive when given by mouth and has to be given by injection. When given by intravenous injection it produces rapid effects which quickly wear off. Its effects may be prolonged by giving the injection under the skin or into a muscle, but even then they last only about six hours. Long-acting ACTH preparations are also available. They contain gelatin, which delays the release of ACTH so that its effects may last for twenty-four to seventy-two hours, or zinc hydroxide, which makes the injection effective for about forty-eight hours. With the exception of adrenal deficiency disorders such as Addison's disease, and overactivity disorders of the adrenals, ACTH is used only to treat disorders which also respond to corticosteroids. Because it does not produce disuse changes in the adrenals, it is easier to withdraw ACTH than corticosteroids, and therefore it may be of use in short-term therapy. However, over the long term it is not as useful (because it is not as selective) as oral anti-inflammatory corticosteroids, and as it has to be given by injection is less convenient. It may produce the adverse effects described under corticosteroids; in particular, diabetes may be made worse and insulin dosage may have to be increased. High blood pressure and acne occur more frequently, but stomach troubles occur less frequently. It may produce allergic reactions and increase skin pigmentation. Long-term use may cause the adrenal glands to undergo changes of "overuse" and the pituitary changes of "underuse"—it should always be slowly withdrawn if it has been administered on a long-term basis.

# MALE SEX HORMONES

The development and maintenance of reproductive organs are under the control of chemicals known as steroid hormones. These hormones are produced by the male and female sex organs, the adrenal glands, and the placenta (afterbirth). The hormones concerned with the development and maintenance of the male reproductive system are called androgens. Several androgens are produced by the testes and adrenal glands. The most powerful of these is known as testosterone.

The pituitary gland produces a hormone called gonadotropin which stimulates the testes to make male sex hormones. At puberty the hormones are made in sufficient amounts to produce physical changes in males. The larynx enlarges and the voice gets deeper, the genitals get bigger, and hair begins to appear in various parts of the body. Male hormones are responsible for the growth and development of the testicles to produce sperm. At puberty there is a spurt in growth and a buildup of body protein; muscles develop and bones grow. The latter effects may be separated from the effects upon the sex organs; because they are related to protein buildup, they are called anabolic effects. Male sex hormones, therefore, have two principal effects: androgenic (affecting the development and maintenance of reproductive organs and function) and anabolic (affecting growth, muscle bulk, and protein buildup).

Those male sex hormones which produce predominantly androgenic effects will also produce some anabolic effects, and those which have principally anabolic effects will also produce some androgenic effects. Testosterone is the natural androgenic hormone produced by the testes, but several synthetic preparations are available. Similarly, much attention has been directed to manufacturing synthetic anabolic steroids. Those with marked androgenic properties and also some anabolic properties include mesterolone, fluoxymesterone, methyltestosterone, and testosterone.

Male sex hormones with mainly anabolic properties and relatively weak androgenic effects are discussed in the following section, Anabolic Steroids.

Androgenic male sex hormones are used principally to treat disorders caused by failure of the testes to produce these hormones. This failure may be primary, due to lack of development or underdevelopment of the testes, or secondary, due to failure of the pituitary gland to produce sufficient gonadotropin. In cases of underdevelopment, or if used in adolescent males, the androgenic hormones encourage development of the secondary sexual characteristics. They can stimulate growth, but because they also close off the growing ends of the long bones in the body, they may stunt growth. In small doses they stimulate the production of sperm. In high doses, however, they suppress the production of gonadotropin by the pituitary, thus reducing sperm production. Androgenic hormones are also used to shrink enlarged breasts in males.

Male sex hormones are of no use in treating male sterility unless it is due to underdevelopment of the testes. Nor are they of use in treating impotence, unless this too is due to testicular failure, which is rare compared with the number of patients suffering from impotence. Male sex hormones were previously used to treat women with abnormal menstruation, painful periods, and suppressed milk production after childbirth. They may be used to treat certain patients with breast cancer. Small doses combined with female sex hormones (estrogens) have been used to treat menopausal symptoms.

They all may be taken by mouth. Testosterone may also be given by injection. The adverse effects produced by testosterone and other androgens may be related to their dual androgenic and anabolic effects. These include increase in skeletal weight, salt and water retention, edema, increase in the number of blood vessels in the skin, increased blood calcium levels, and increased bone growth. In women they may affect gonadotropin production by the pituitary and lead to suppression of the ovaries and menstruation. Large and continued doses cause masculinization in women—deep voice, male pattern of baldness, hairiness, shrinking of the breasts, and enlargement of the clitoris with an increase in sexual drive. Androgenic steroids should not be given to patients with cancer of the prostate gland, and they should not be used in pregnancy because the unborn baby may be affected. They should be used with caution by patients who would be adversely affected by salt and water retention (e.g., those with heart failure, impaired kidney function, or epilepsy). Phenobarbital may reduce the effects of testosterone by increasing its breakdown in the liver. Dose-related jaundice may occur with methyltestosterone. Isolated cases of cancer of the liver have been reported in association with the use of certain anabolic and androgenic steroids for prolonged periods.

# ANABOLIC STEROIDS

We have seen in the preceding section that male sex hormones may produce two main effects—androgenic and anabolic. Many anabolic compounds have been developed and vigorously marketed as body builders. These products have been widely promoted for the treatment of disorders involving an increased breakdown of body protein—for instance, after major surgery or a severe accident, and for treating patients with longstanding debilitating diseases. Administering an anabolic steroid may seem reasonable in these disorders, but it is much more important to ensure that the patient takes a nourishing diet, high in protein, so that the body's own mechanisms control the required buildup. The value of these drugs has not been proved. They are of value in suppression of lactation and in certain types of breast cancer in women. They are not to be used in *men* with breast cancer.

The anabolic steroids which are available are all derivatives of testosterone. They include dromostanolone, ethylestrenol, methandrostenolone, oxandrolone, nandrolone, oxymetholone, and stanozolol.

All anabolic steroids produce adverse effects similar to those produced by testosterone (see preceding section, Male Sex Hormones). They may be given by mouth or injection. Those taken by mouth may cause jaundice when used over a prolonged period of time. They should not be given to patients with impaired liver function, and they may increase the effects of some anticoagulant drugs. The main adverse effects of anabolic steroids are fluid retention and masculinization. They should not be used in pregnant patients or in those suffering from cancer of the prostate gland.

There are few if any reasons for using anabolic steroids for medical disorders. Yet while doctors have slowly moved along their typical path of enthusiastic and widespread use followed by more cautious assessment, these drugs have become increasingly employed for nonmedical purposes in sports—a practice which needs careful investigation because of their potential for toxicity and the effects of drug-induced body building upon competitive sports.

# FEMALE SEX HORMONES

The newborn baby girl's ovaries contain thousands of eggs or ova. Each ovum is in a little fluid-filled sac called a follicle. Before puberty many of these follicles enlarge but then shrink. After puberty only a few hundred of the thousands will grow and produce ova which are discharged from the ovaries each month during the reproductive phase of a woman's life.

## Puberty
At puberty the ovaries begin to undergo cyclical changes under stimulation from hormones produced by the pituitary gland. The uterus and vagina enlarge, the breasts develop, fat is laid down in certain areas, giving the characteristic female figure, and hair starts to grow under the arms and on the pubes.

## Menstruation
The anterior pituitary gland produces two gonadotropic hormones (hormones which affect the growth of the ovaries). One, the follicle-stimulating hormone (FSH), stimulates the development of follicles around the ova in the ovaries. This makes the follicles grow, and as one of them starts to grow more than the others it begins producing its own female sex hormones, called estrogens. These estrogens then start to work on the lining of the uterus, making it grow thicker. As the blood

concentration of estrogens increases, the pituitary's production of FSH decreases. The other gonadotropic hormone is called luteinizing hormone (LH). It acts on the follicle, making it rupture and release the ovum, a process known as ovulation. LH also ensures the continuing development of the follicle after it has released the ovum and converts it into a yellowish body (corpus luteum). This body produces a different female sex hormone called progesterone, which belongs to the group of female sex hormones known as progestins. Progestins also act on the lining of the uterus, making it ready to receive a fertilized ovum.

The first changes in the uterus when its lining thickens under the influence of estrogens is called the proliferative phase, or phase of growth. The subsequent phase, after ovulation, when progesterone makes it undergo special changes in preparation for receiving a fertilized egg, is called the secretory phase. This term derives from the fact that cells develop which will secrete nutritious fluids if conception occurs and the fertilized egg settles on the lining of the uterus. By taking a scraping from the lining of the uterus, doctors are able to tell whether or not the lining has undergone both changes—proliferative and secretory—and thus determine that the patient has ovulated. They are also able to see whether estrogens and progesterone have been made in sufficient quantities to produce the changes.

Progesterone inhibits the production of LH by the pituitary, whereas estrogen stimulates it. There is plainly a delicate balance between FSH and LH production by the pituitary gland, and the production of estrogens and progesterone by the developing follicle and the corpus luteum respectively.

Before puberty, the production of FSH and LH by the pituitary is not enough to stimulate the development of a follicle around an ovum, and only small quantities of estrogens and progesterone are produced by the ovaries. Two or three years before the development of menstruation, puberty changes are already taking place. This is thought to be due to the growth and development of the pituitary gland and also part of the brain known as the hypothalamus, which exerts control over nervous and hormonal activity in the body. As the pituitary gland develops, it starts to increase its production of FSH and LH. These get to work on the ovaries and cause groups of follicles to develop. As the follicles grow they start to produce more and more estrogens. The estrogens work on various tissues in the body, producing the secondary sexual characteristics, and in addition the lining of the uterus starts to thicken.

After the first menstrual period, the pituitary and hypothalamus continue to develop. At times they produce too little gonadotropic hormone to affect the production of estrogen by the ovaries. Thus the lining of the uterus fails to thicken, and a young girl may go several months with irregular periods or none at all. As the pituitary settles down, the periods will become more regular and menstrual periods will start to occur approximately every 28 days.

During these first few months, ovulation does not usually occur because the pituitary does not produce sufficient LH hormone. But as the cycles without ovulation (usually known as anovulatory cycles) continue, more and more estrogens are produced by the follicles, and LH production increases, causing ovulation—the release of the ovum.

If the ovum is not fertilized, LH production falls and the corpus luteum shrinks, resulting in a decreasing production of progesterone and estrogens. As the level drops, the blood vessels supplying the lining of the uterus close off, the lining disintegrates, and menstrual bleeding starts. As the result of the decline in progesterone production by the shrinking corpus luteum, the pituitary responds by producing more LH. Also, in response to decreased production of estrogens, the pituitary starts to produce more FSH and the cycle starts all over again. The increasing production of FSH and LH goes to work on the ovaries, a new group of follicles begin to develop, and the whole sequence of changes is repeated.

### Pregnancy

If the ovum is fertilized, it burrows into the lining of the uterus and becomes anchored. It develops a surrounding layer of cells (the trophoblast) which multiply and eventually form the placenta (the afterbirth). At this early stage the trophoblast cells surrounding the developing fertilized ovum (now called an embryo) start to produce chorionic gonadotropic hormone. (It is called "chorionic" because it is produced by the cells which go to form part of the placenta called the chorion and "gonadotropic" because it works on the gonads—or ovaries.) Chorionic gonadotropin, like LH, works on the corpus luteum in the ovary and maintains its development. This results in an increased production of progesterone by the corpus luteum despite the fall-off in LH production by the pituitary.

Under stimulation from progesterone, the lining of the uterus continues to provide nutrition for the developing embryo until the placenta is developed. The placenta then takes over essential duties—supplying nutrients, carrying away unwanted products, and supplying oxygen and other gases to the developing baby. In addition, the placenta (which links the baby's blood supply directly to the mother's) continues to produce chorionic gonadotropin but also starts to produce its own estrogens and progesterone.

This delicate and complex balance of hormones ensures that the pregnancy becomes established. After about 12 weeks the chorionic gonadotropin production by the placenta starts to fall off; at 16 to 18 weeks the corpus luteum shrinks, and production reaches a low level which lasts throughout the pregnancy. At the same time production of estrogens and progesterone by the placenta continues to increase throughout the pregnancy, falling abruptly after delivery. The fall in estrogens then stimulates the pituitary to produce FSH. Gradually a group of follicles start to develop in an ovary, and the menstrual cycle is set in motion again. The high estrogen and progesterone levels during pregnancy are responsible for breast development. Some chorionic gonadotropic hormone is excreted in the urine and provides a positive test for pregnancy early in the term.

After childbirth, the sucking of the baby at the breast stimulates production of a milk-producing hormone (prolactin) by the pituitary gland. This stimulates further milk production to ensure that supply meets demand. At the same time prolactin serves a useful purpose by stopping the production of FSH by the pituitary and thus preventing the development of follicles in the ovaries. This prevents the breast-feeding mother from menstruating—though not necessarily from conceiving again—for several months after delivery, depending, of course, on how long she breast-feeds.

## Menopause

As the ovaries get older, the follicles start responding less and less to FSH. This results in a decreased production of estrogens and for a time an increased production of FSH. Also LH production falls and ovulation fails to occur during some cycles. As ovarian function continues to decline, ovulation stops altogether. Estrogen and progesterone production falls off completely, and eventually menstrual periods stop. The rise in FSH production may affect other pituitary hormone production, causing various menopausal changes. These include increase in weight, hot flushes, bone changes, and psychological symptoms. The lack of estrogens produces shrinking of the secondary sex organs —the breasts become smaller, the vulva and vagina undergo changes, and the ovaries and uterus shrink.

From this brief description of the hormonal control of puberty, menstruation, pregnancy, and the menopause it can be seen that there are two groups of hormones which control numerous functions in the female body: estrogens and progestins. Many synthetic preparations of these hormones are available, and they are used for a wide variety of disorders.

## Estrogens

The main sources of estrogens are the ovaries and the placenta. Estrogens are also produced in smaller amounts by the adrenal glands and by the testes in the male. More than twenty different estrogens have been isolated from the urine of pregnant women. The three main estrogens produced by the ovaries and placenta are called estrone, estradiol, and estriol. The first two may be converted into each other by an enzyme present in many tissues of the female body. They exert a major effect upon the lining of the uterus. Estriol is produced in large quantities by the placenta during pregnancy. It has a marked effect upon the neck of the uterus (cervix) and upon the vagina.

Preparations available for use include naturally occurring estrogens such as estradiol and estrogens obtained from the urine of mares. Estrogens are steroid chemicals, and there are numerous synthetic steroid estrogens available which resemble estradiol in structure. These are broken down more slowly in the body than naturally occurring estrogens, and thus their effects in the body last for a longer time. The two main synthetic estrogens, ethinylestradiol and mestranol, are present in many female hormone preparations, particularly oral contraceptive drugs. Other chemicals are available which, although not steroids, have estrogenic effects. The main one in this group is diethylstilbestrol (stilbestrol).

The various estrogen preparations available include benzestrol, chlorotrianisene, dienestrol, ethinylestradiol, hexestrol, mestranol, methallenestril, estradiol, diethylstilbestrol, conjugated estrogens, and esterified estrogens.

Many preparations of female sex hormones contain both estrogens and progestins. They are marketed in a profusion of doses, sizes, and shapes for a multiplicity of symptoms and disorders. Yet the majority contain the same drugs. Diethylstilbestrol is the cheapest estrogen available. Ethinylestradiol is the strongest and is present in many combination products; so too is mestranol. These last three are long-acting and may be taken once daily. Conjugated estrogens are less effective and may require several daily doses when high dosage is required.

Estrogens are used as replacement treatment in patients who have deficient estrogen production due to underdevelopment of the ovaries, a cause of delayed puberty and absence of periods (primary amenorrhea), to treat menstrual irregularities (e.g., dysmenorrhea), to suppress milk production after childbirth, to treat menopausal symptoms, to treat cancer of the prostate gland, to minimize softening of bones (osteoporosis) in postmenopausal women, to treat subfertility, to treat cancers of the breast and uterus in selected cases, to delay menstruation, to treat premenstrual tension, and in oral contraceptive preparations. They have been used to treat habitual abortion and senile vaginitis and other disorders such as acne.

Adverse effects from estrogens include nausea and vomiting (which are directly related to dose), tenderness and enlargement of the breasts, headache, dizziness, fluid and salt retention, irregular vaginal bleeding, and enlargement of breasts in men. The estrogens in oral contraceptive preparations may be responsible for changes in blood clotting, leading in rare cases to the risk of venous thrombosis and strokes. Also, the use of high doses of estrogens to stop milk production just after childbirth may be associated with an increased risk of thrombosis. Diethylstilbestrol has been linked with the production of cancer of the vagina in young teenagers whose mothers had taken the drug in early pregnancy.

Estrogens should not be used if there is a family or personal history of cancer of the breast, uterus, or genital tract. They should not be used if there is a history of thrombosis, and they should not be used postoperatively. They should be used with caution in patients who are obese or have varicose veins or diabetes. They should preferably not be used to stop milk production just after childbirth.

## Estrogen Replacement Therapy

The term "menopause" refers to the cessation of the menstrual periods, and "climacteric" generally describes the longer-term effects produced when ovarian function gradually ceases, but the whole process is usually referred to as "the menopause."

Menopause can be very distressing both physically and mentally, and estrogen replacement can be very helpful to some women. However, authoritative medical opinion considers that estrogens should be used in patients with menopausal symptoms only in minimal effective dosage and that treatment (cycles of three weeks treated, one week untreated) should be intermittent and tapered off as soon as possible except in special cases. The aim should be to allow the body to adjust to the decreasing production of estrogens. High and continued dosage will prevent this natural process. Others argue for the benefits of long-term use, but we need much more information before such a recommendation can be considered.

## Progestins

Progesterone is responsible for the secretory changes in the lining of the uterus during the last two weeks of the menstrual cycle following ovulation. It is also necessary for maintaining pregnancy. In addition, it has many other effects. It plays an important role in the development of the placenta, and it stops movements of the uterine muscle. It stops ovulation during pregnancy and plays a part in further breast development. It is produced by the corpus luteum and acts only on tissues which have been previously subjected to the actions of estrogens. Progesterone increases the use of energy by the body, causing the body temperature to rise at ovulation and stay up until menstruation (that is, during the secretory phase). This characteristic makes it possible to discover easily whether ovulation is occurring. It is an indicator of the time of ovulation, when pregnancy is more likely to take place. Progesterone also affects salt excretion by the kidneys.

Progesterone is rapidly broken down in the liver to pregnanediol. It is, therefore, inactive by mouth and has to be given by intramuscular injection or by implanting a pellet under the skin. It is insoluble and cannot be injected into a vein.

Synthetic progestins which may be taken by mouth have been developed. The first to be developed, ethisterone, has both estrogenic and androgenic (male sex hormone) properties in addition to its progesteronelike actions. Chemically, ethisterone is related to the male sex hormone testosterone, and it is from this basic structure that most of the progestins have been developed.

Female sex hormones with predominantly progestational effects include chlormadinone, dimethisterone, dydrogesterone, hydroxyprogesterone, medroxyprogesterone, megestrol, norethynodrel, norgestrel, and progesterone. Sex hormones with estrogenic and progestational properties and also some androgenic properties include ethisterone, ethynodiol, ethylestrenol, and norethindrone.

Progestins are used in oral contraceptive preparations. They are also used, combined with estrogens, to control heavy and irregular periods. Painful periods may be reduced by stopping ovulation with an oral contraceptive agent which contains a progestin. They may also be helped by a progestin called dydrogesterone, which does not stop ovulation and has no estrogenic and androgenic properties. Similarly, such a nonestrogenic progestin may be of use in treating such premenstrual symptoms as tension, headaches, breast fullness, and the pain which comes on during the week preceding a period. Progestins were previously used without much success to treat threatened miscarriage (abortion) and in recurrent miscarriages (habitual abortion). Similarly, they have been used with unproven results in treating premature labor.

Progestins have few adverse effects: they may produce greasy hair, acne, breast tenderness, and depression of mood before a period. Those used in oral contraceptives may also cause increase of appetite and weight, cramps in the legs and abdomen, changes in libido (sex drive), fluid retention, white vaginal discharge, reduced menstrual loss, dry vagina, and bleeding between periods (breakthrough bleeding).

Progestins with some androgenic properties should be avoided during pregnancy (they may cause masculinization of an unborn baby girl) and should not be used by patients who have had jaundice or other liver diseases. They should be used with caution in patients with impaired kidney function or Addison's disease.

Estrogen and progestin combination products are widely prescribed. Their most common use is as oral contraceptives. Combination products were frequently used to diagnose pregnancy before the rapid urine test became standard practice among most doctors and pharmacists. Many authorities now oppose their use for diagnosing pregnancy, and the long-term risks to the developing baby have never been assessed.

# ORAL CONTRACEPTIVE DRUGS

To understand the use of oral contraceptives, you must understand the hormonal control of the menstrual cycle, and in particular the parts played by the female sex hormones, estrogen and progestin (see preceding section, Female Sex Hormones).

There are three types of oral contraceptives: combined estrogen/progestin preparations (the "pill"), sequential preparations containing estrogens and progestins, and progestin-only preparations.

The progestins used in oral contraceptives belong to two groups. One group consists of drugs, chemically related to the male sex hormone testosterone, that are to some degree estrogenic, androgenic, and anabolic as well as progestinic in their action—norethindrone and ethynodiol. The other group is more closely related to the naturally occurring progesterone and includes megestrol. Progestins have varying effects in preventing ovulation by blocking the production of LH (see pp. 166–7).

The estrogens used in oral contraceptives are ethinylestradiol and mestranol. Mestranol is converted into ethinylestradiol in the body, so any discussion of estrogens in oral contraceptives usually concerns ethinylestradiol. Estrogens stop the production of FSH; thus the follicle does not develop and ovulation is prevented. However—and this is very important—the production of FSH is related to the circulating level of estrogen, and therefore a small dose of estrogen may actually lead to *increased* FSH production and *stimulation* of the follicle-producing ovulation. Equally important, a medium dose of estrogen may merely delay ovulation. But, as we shall see later, the principal risk of the pill is probably related to its estrogen content, so the smallest effective dose should be used. In some women, this may not be enough to prevent ovulation. The safest dose now seems to be 0.05 mg. (50 micrograms) or less of ethinylestradiol or mestranol. The name of the estrogen and progestin in your pills will be entered in small type on the packet. Be sure to check.

In the most common versions of the pill, the dose of estrogen is usually 0.05 mg. Some contain as little as 0.01 mg., and some are still available which contain doses as high as 0.075 mg. and 0.1 mg. The dose of progestins also varies, but there is a much wider margin of contraceptive safety here, and since progestins also prevent ovulation, affect the lining of the uterus, and alter the stickiness of the mucus in the cervical canal (all useful ways to prevent conception), they introduce a large additional safety factor. For example, the dose of the frequently used progestin norethindrone varies from 0.5 mg. to 10 mg. in various oral contraceptive preparations. The higher-dose progestin pills may be useful if you get breakthrough bleeding (bleeding between periods) on a small-dose progestin pill.

Low-dose estrogen and low-dose progestin pills may cause some women to miss a period, followed by breakthrough bleeding. Ovulation may also occur in these cases. Therefore, there is a risk of pregnancy if you are on a pill which gives you breakthrough bleeding. Check with your doctor; you should perhaps switch to a pill with a higher progestin content. High-dose progestin combination pills also give a wider margin of safety if you happen to forget to take one.

SEQUENTIAL PREPARATIONS of estrogens and progestins are presented in such a way that you take an estrogen-only pill on the first 15 days and then a combined estrogen and progestin pill daily for the next 5 or 7 days. The latter combination pills have less effect upon the lining of the uterus, and sequential preparations rely largely on the first 15 days of estrogen to prevent ovulation. Remember, however, that estrogens prepare the lining of the uterus to receive the ovum, and also stimulate mucus production in the cervical canal (the entrance to the uterus). There is, therefore, a risk of pregnancy with sequential preparations. They may also cause loss of periods followed by breakthrough bleeding. What is more, they rely upon a higher dose of estrogen than do most combination pills. Because of these risks there really is no point in taking a sequential preparation.

PROGESTIN-ONLY oral contraceptives are started on the first day of the cycle and then taken every day, all through the cycle, without missing a day. They may be used before menstrual periods start after childbirth, provided you are not breast-feeding the baby. Progestin makes the mucus in the cervical canal sticky, thus preventing sperm from entering the uterus. There is, therefore, a much greater risk of pregnancy if you forget to take one of these pills on a day you have sexual intercourse. They may produce heavy and irregular periods and breakthrough bleeding. And they are not foolproof—with progestin-only pills there is a risk of pregnancy even if you do take one every day. However, they produce fewer adverse effects than the combination preparations because of the absence of estrogens. For patients who cannot tolerate combination pills, the progestin-only pill is an alternative. It is also of use in patients due to have a surgical operation, since estrogens should not be taken at these times. But remember, there *is* a risk of pregnancy.

The use of diethylstilbestrol, known as the morning-after contraceptive pill, has been associated with serious risks (p. 171).

## How to Take the Pill

For convenience the term "the pill" is used here (and generally) to refer to the most commonly used oral contraceptive, the estrogen-progestin combination taken daily. The first course is started on the fifth day of the menstrual period. Take the day that the period started as the first day and count forward five days. Whether the period lasts two or three days or six or seven days, you must start your very first course of an oral contraceptive on the fifth day after the onset of the period. You then take a pill daily for 20, 21, or 22 days or for whatever number of days it states in the instructions on the packet. The different number of days recommended for different preparations does not really matter; what does matter is that you take yours daily for the recommended number of days. The number of days is adjusted so that you have a menstrual cycle of 28 days, because this is what most women are used to and perhaps feel happier with. When you have finished the first month's course of 21 days or whatever it is, you will get a period in three to four days. You then start the next course according to the instructions. For ease, many preparations contain 21 pills in a package so that in a 28-day cycle you take the pill for three weeks and stop it for one week. The packages are push-out types, and the days of the week are often marked so that it is easy for you to remember when you stopped and need to restart. If you lack a good memory, there are preparations available which contain seven dummy tablets (a recent preparation contains seven iron tablets). The dummy tablets are a different color from the contraceptive pills, but all you have to do, having started the first course, is to take one pill every day without stopping.

Because intercourse is more common at night, a lot of women take the pill before going to bed. This is fine, but it does not really matter what time of day you take it so long as you take it every day (that is, every 24 hours), preferably at the same time. Avoid any risk of getting pregnant (by using additional contraceptive techniques) during the first two weeks of your first month on the pill—in subsequent months you will be safe. Also, when changing from one contraceptive preparation to another, particularly from a high-dose to a low-dose estrogen preparation, do not run the risk of getting pregnant during the first two weeks (some say four weeks) on the new pill. If you forget to take the pill *one* day, take it as soon as you remember (certainly within twelve hours of the right time), and then take the day's pill at your usual time. If you forget to take the pill for *two* days (36 hours or more) ovulation may occur. Read your instructions carefully and follow them. Some may say to take a double dose for the next two days and then carry on with your normal routine while others say carry on as normal but do not run the risk of getting pregnant. If you miss *three* days, stop, wait seven days (during which time you should have a period), and start a new course—but avoid the risk of getting pregnant for the first two weeks. If you think you may have become pregnant during the days when you forgot to take the pill, or if you are scared or worried about being pregnant, then stop the pill. If you have a "normal" period then start the new course, *but* if you are at all suspicious and particularly if your period is scanty or does not start, do *not* start a new month's course. *Wait* until *40* days from the first day of your previous period and get a urine pregnancy test done. (You may get a false negative if the test is done before this time. You must also advise your doctor or pharmacist of any other drugs you are taking, as some may interfere with the test.) If the urine test is negative, avoid getting pregnant and start your next course on the fifth day of your next period. Avoid the risk of getting pregnant in the first two weeks on the pill because this will be the same as starting a new course.

Remember, if you have an episode of diarrhea or vomiting while on the pill, this may interfere with its absorption. Take extra precautions for the rest of that month.

While on the pill, if you do not have a period, proceed as usual to take the next month's pills on schedule. If you miss two periods, stop the pill and have a urine pregnancy test done. If you have been on the pill for some time and then get breakthrough bleeding between periods, stop the pill and consult your doctor.

### Adverse Effects from the Pill
(Combined Estrogen-Progestin Preparations)
The commonly used estrogens in the pill are mestranol and ethinyl estradiol, and the commonly used progestins include norethindrone,

norgestrel, megestrol, norethynodrel, dimethisterone, and ethynodiol.

The preceding section, Female Sex Hormones, explains the adverse effects produced by estrogens. These adverse effects are related to dose and may therefore occur to a varying degree in different individuals. Patients on the pill *may* experience them. In addition, they may also experience adverse reactions to progestins, which when used with estrogens may cause depressed mood, increased appetite, cramps in the legs and abdomen, changes in libido, fluid retention, white vaginal discharge, reduced menstrual loss, dry vagina, and increased weight.

These are the dose-related adverse effects of progestins and estrogens taken together. In addition, there are other adverse effects produced by such combinations. In some individuals, they may affect the circulation, producing headaches, migraine, flushing, dizziness, changes in blood pressure, swelling of the ankles, and thrombophlebitis. These tend to occur with higher-dose estrogen and medium-dose progestin preparations. Blood clotting may be affected by high synthetic estrogen preparations which may predispose to thrombosis.

The progestin in the pill may cause a depressed mood in some individuals. However, it is not the progestin alone that produces this unpleasant effect, but the combination with estrogen. Norethindrone particularly seems to be related to depression of mood, so check which pill you are on if you feel depressed. There is a suggestion that vitamin $B_6$ (pyridoxine) may help to control depression from this source.

The greatest—though rare—risk from the pill is the possibility of a thrombus in a vein, part of which could break off and reach the lungs and so cause death. This process is called thromboembolism, and the most dangerous thrombosis usually occurs in the deep veins of the legs or pelvis. It may also occur in the vessels supplying the brain (cerebral thrombosis), producing a stroke.

This remote possibility of thrombosis is not related to how long you have been on the pill. The risk is thought to be roughly proportional to the amount of synthetic estrogen in a preparation. There is no obvious difference between mestranol and ethinylestradiol. The safety level for estrogen appears to be about 0.05 mg., and, as stated above, the majority of pills do not now go above this level.

There has been no proved association between taking the pill and developing a *coronary* thrombosis. Of course, there may be an added danger of this in high-risk patients—those with raised blood pressure and a heavy smoking habit, or those with high blood fat levels and a family history of a parent or brother or sister dying from a coronary thrombosis under the age of sixty.

Oral combined contraceptive pills have many effects upon the body's metabolism; over fifty have been recorded. For example, blood sugar and fat levels may be raised, and liver function tests, blood clotting factors, and thyroid function tests all altered. They may predispose to infections of the cervix particularly by thrush (candida) and cause loss of periods in someone who has previously had irregular or scanty periods. Itching vagina (pruritus vulvae) may be produced by the pill. Vaginal discharge and pruritus vulvae is even more likely to occur if you are given a tetracycline or other such "broad-spectrum" antibiotic for some other infection, such as bronchitis. Itching of the skin may occur, and some women get brownish spots on the face (chloasma—often seen in pregnancy). A blistering skin rash (porphyria) on exposure to sun may rarely occur, and some women lose hair for a few months after stopping the pill.

After stopping the pill, some women fail to have a period. This is more common in women who had late puberty and previously irregular periods. It is caused by failure of the pituitary to recover from its suppression due to the high blood levels of estrogens and progestins while on the pill. The hypothalamus may also not recover full function. The lining of the uterus in these women may not respond to estrogens produced by their own ovaries because they have been under daily influence for many months from the estrogen and progestin in the pill they have been taking. If no period occurs for four to six months, clomiphene may be given, which stimulates ovulation. But loss of periods does not appear to be harmful, and if a woman does not want to get pregnant there is no need to give a drug. Remember also that after being on the pill it may take some women a few months to get pregnant, but this is not related to the length of time that the pill was taken.

Studies involving the long-term risk of cancer of the breasts, uterus, cervix, or vagina are conflicting, and as yet there is no clear evidence to indicate such risks. Problems in studying such effects include the often prolonged delay between administration of the estrogen and subsequent development of cancer, and the complicating socioeconomic factors known to influence the incidence of such cancers. Women taking oral contraceptives should have regular medical examinations.

## Precautions

• To reduce the risk of thrombosis, it is better to use a pill that contains 0.05 mg. of estrogen or less.

• To reduce the risk of depression it is better to use a lower-dose progestin pill.

• It is best not to use the pill if you have a high blood fat level.

• You should not take the pill if you have had a previous deep-vein thrombosis or embolism. Previous superficial thrombophlebitis is not a reason for not taking the pill, but requires regular medical supervision.

• Do not take the pill within one month after childbirth or within one month of a surgical operation.

• Do not take the pill if you have had an attack of jaundice or severe itching of the skin during pregnancy.

• Do not take the pill if you have or have had a cancer of a breast.

• Do not take the pill if you have an acute or severe longstanding liver disorder.

• Do not take the pill if you have attacks of severe migraine (that is, migraine associated with pins and needles in hands and feet). An increase in the frequency or severity of headaches requires a medical examination.

• If you are at the menopause (and being on the pill will not affect your symptoms), stop the pill for two or three months to see if a period comes on. If it does, go back to the pill for two to three months. If you do not have a period, then stop the pill but take alternative contraceptive precautions as long as you have reason to believe you might become pregnant.

• If you have a family history of diabetes, then you should be cautious. Still, having diabetes does not prevent your using the pill, although it may increase your insulin requirements.

• If you are due to have thyroid tests, stop the pill for two months beforehand—it interferes with tests for thyroid functions.

• Do not take other drugs which may affect liver function—for example, chlorpromazine.

• Be cautious when using corticosteroids such as prednisone; they may elevate your blood pressure.

• Remember the effectiveness of the pill may be affected by other drugs, such as phenobarbital, which affect estrogen breakdown in the liver. Varicose veins are not considered to be a reason for not taking the pill, but check carefully with your doctor. Piles (hemorrhoids) are not a reason for not taking the pill. If you have a raised blood pressure, your doctor should keep you under regular observation. The same goes if you have epilepsy, otosclerosis (a type of progressive deafness), multiple sclerosis, porphyria, or any disease which is likely to get worse during pregnancy.

• It may be best not to take the pill if you have had previous episodes of severe mental depression, but discuss this with your doctor.

• Remember that you can get depressed if you change from a high-dose to a low-dose estrogen pill.

• Read the instructions in this book and also on the packet insert about breakthrough bleeding, spotting, and scanty or absent periods.

• Read in this book and also on the packet insert about what to do if you forget to take a pill.

• Check in this book and also on the packet insert about when to avoid the risk of getting pregnant.

• If you got brown pigmentation on your face (chloasma) in pregnancy, then be careful about exposure to the sun while on the pill.

• Young girls (under 15 years of age) should not go on the pill until their periods have started and are occurring regularly.

• Young girls on the pill for more than nine months should stop their pill for one month and have their daily temperatures checked to see if they are ovulating (see pp. 171–2). If they are, then they can continue taking the pill. If they are not ovulating, they should not be on the pill. They should be referred to a gynecologist.

## When to Stop the Pill Immediately

• If you get pregnant.
• If your blood pressure rises.
• Four weeks before a surgical operation or when confined to bed after an accident or an illness.
• If you get jaundice.
• At the first signs of a thrombosis.
• If you get migraine and have never previously had an attack.
• If you have had migraine before and develop a very severe attack.
• Any severe or unusual headaches.
• Any disturbance of vision.

## Changes in Menstruation

"Spotting," a very slight show of blood between periods, is usually of no significance. Continue with the pill, since it usually clears up. If it recurs the next month, consult your doctor.

"Breakthrough bleeding," bleeding between periods like a small period, may be stopped by taking two pills a day for two or three days and then going back on the normal course. Alternatively, you may go on with the course and see how things are with the next month's course. If it recurs consult your doctor. Another way is to stop the pill for seven days and then restart another course. Whichever you choose, if breakthrough bleeding occurs two months running you must see your doctor and have a gynecological examination, which will usually include a cervical smear test. Such an examination is also necessary if spotting or breakthrough bleeding occurs for the first time after prolonged use of the pill or if it recurs at irregular intervals.

Decreased menstrual flow is nothing to worry about.

## The Choice of Pill

Progestins act on the uterus, which has been subjected to the effects of estrogens. Various preparations may therefore be compared as to how long they can delay a period when given in equally effective doses. In this way estrogens may also be compared, and from such studies we have learned that ethinylestradiol is about twenty times more potent than the naturally occurring estradiol. It is about twice as potent as mestranol. Similarly, the progestins can be ranked in order of potency (from strongest to weakest)—norgestrel, ethynodiol, norethindrone, megestrol.

In the body, the ratio of estrogens to progestins is delicately balanced to produce optimum chances of getting pregnant. Some women may produce too much estrogen and therefore have heavy, frequent periods, whereas others may produce too much progestin and suffer from scanty and irregular periods. Neither of these groups of women produce the ideal balance of hormones to encourage conception, and they may therefore be subfertile. It follows, therefore, that if an estrogen is given to some women it may produce heavier periods, whereas progestins may produce scanty periods or even absent periods if given in sufficient dosage. When the drugs are stopped, withdrawal bleeding will occur. Effects produced by estrogens can be balanced by adding progestins. As the doses of progestins increase, the risk of pregnancy decreases. Unfortunately, adverse effects start to increase, too. High doses of estrogens will produce the adverse effects mentioned earlier; so too will increasing dosage of progestins. Thus there is a spectrum of effects and adverse effects produced by the various combination estrogen/progestin pills. The choice of pill should be based upon the regularity and heaviness of your periods, and according to the drugs' potential for producing adverse effects in *you*. Reread this section and the preceding section, Female Sex Hormones, and make a note of the important facts which apply to *you*. For example, consider whether you previously had scanty periods or heavy periods, whether you are overweight and smoke, whether you have abnormal blood pressure or have had a previous thrombosis, whether you have previously had some episodes of depressed mood, what adverse effects you have felt on certain contraceptive preparations, and so on. You may be on the pill for many years, so it is most important for you and your doctor to choose the pill which suits *you*.

# DRUGS USED
# TO TREAT DIABETES

Diabetes is the term used to refer to diabetes mellitus, a disorder characterized by a deficiency or diminished effectiveness of insulin. Insulin, a hormone produced by the pancreas, is responsible for lowering the blood sugar level by encouraging the tissues to burn up sugar to produce energy. Insulin is also responsible for converting glucose into a substance called glycogen for storage in muscles and the liver for future use, and for the formation of fat for storage. It also influences protein buildup.

There are many factors which contribute to these processes; but, very simply, diabetes may be regarded as a disorder which results in too little insulin production by the pancreas for the body's requirements or the failure of the insulin produced to be effective in carrying out the necessary processes—or both. In diabetes, glucose removal from the blood is reduced and the release of glucose into the blood by the liver is increased. Glucose is overproduced and underused, resulting in a high blood sugar level, a condition called hyperglycemia. Diabetes may be caused by a disorder of the pancreas, resulting in its failure to produce insulin; by the presence of body chemicals which block the effects of insulin; or by increased production of glucose by the liver. Epinephrine, for example, increases the breakdown of liver glycogen and pushes up the blood sugar levels.

High blood sugar levels may cause sugar to appear in the urine because the kidneys cannot cope with the high concentrations; through osmosis this results in an increased volume of urine, leading to salt and water loss and thirst. Because the diabetic patient is unable to use the glucose in the blood, his body fat is mobilized and used for energy. This causes an increased amount of fat breakdown products to accumulate in the blood, producing what is called ketosis and an alteration in the acidity of the blood. Such chemical changes can cause coma and death if untreated. In addition, protein is also broken down, which produces wasting of muscles and loss of weight.

Many things influence the development and progress of diabetes—hereditary factors, age, sex, weight, infections, stress, and physical disorders. There are many stages of the disease, ranging from a slight depression in insulin effectiveness to a total lack of insulin production.

It can develop rapidly in children (juvenile diabetes) or slowly with advancing age (maturity-onset diabetes). Its treatment is difficult but rewarding and should always be in the hands of experts. Successful treatment of diabetes should be a joint effort between doctor and patient. Such successful treatment demonstrates how important it is for the patient to know what is wrong with him, to know about the drugs he is taking, to know the effects and adverse effects of these drugs, to know when to adjust the dosage, and to know what other drugs to take and not to take.

There are two main approaches to the drug treatment of diabetes: one is insulin by injection; the other is blood-sugar-lowering drugs taken by mouth, called oral antidiabetic drugs or oral hypoglycemic drugs (*hypo*glycemia meaning low blood sugar).

## Insulin

Insulin is a hormone produced and stored by the beta cells of the pancreas. As a drug, its principal source is from slaughtered animals. It has been synthesized, but this process is as yet too expensive for general use. Pork and beef insulins are the ones used routinely. The choice is not critical, except that some patients may in rare cases become allergic to one type. Insulin must be given by injection because it is inactivated when given by mouth. An enzyme called insulinase found mainly in the liver is responsible for its breakdown in the body.

Insulin production by the pancreas is principally regulated by the blood sugar level, but many other factors may also affect its production and breakdown. For example, many diabetic patients require doses of insulin far in excess of "normal" output in order to control their symptoms. It has been suggested that insulin antagonists may account for this by interfering with its effects.

Insulin is used to treat diabetes in young patients and in diabetes developing in older individuals in whom no improvement has been obtained in response to diet control (restricted sugars and carbohydrates). Insulin is also necessary during pregnancy and in elderly patients (who normally do well on diet and oral antidiabetic drugs) when they have a severe infection or are undergoing surgery. At these times —during infections, injury, or surgery—the body normally requires more insulin.

Initial treatment with insulin should always be carried out in a hospital, where repeated estimations of blood sugar level may be made. Where appropriate, patients are shown how to give themselves their own injections of insulin. They should be allowed to experience the effects of an underdose and an overdose, and know how to correct these. The process of finding the correct dose is known as stabilization:

it is most important and should not be hurried. The patient is ready for discharge when the most appropriate dosage regimen of insulin has been worked out in order to control his symptoms, blood sugar levels, and the amount of sugar in his urine. But he should not be discharged until he understands his diet, how (if necessary) to give himself his injection, test his urine for sugar, and know when and how to increase the dose as required.

The choice of insulin preparation will depend on many factors and in particular is related to the duration of action of the various preparations available.

Injected insulin is rapidly inactivated by the liver. Therefore, much work has gone into making insulin injections long-acting by ensuring their slow absorption into the bloodstream from the injection sites.

To reduce the possibility of allergic reactions to the pancreatic tissue in some patients, small quantities of zinc have been added to insulin mixtures, producing a clear solution of insulin that causes fewer allergic reactions and gives a more uniform effect. Such preparations of beef or pork insulins (termed soluble insulin, ordinary insulin, regular insulin, or unmodified insulin) are available as injections.

However, soluble insulin is acidic, and a neutral solution is more easily absorbed into the bloodstream. Neutral insulin is such a preparation; it acts more rapidly than soluble insulin and has a more prolonged effect. Biphasic insulin is a mixture of beef insulin and a neutralized solution of pork insulin.

By altering the acidity and the amount of zinc added to the suspensions, much more zinc can be combined with the insulin, producing large particles. These act after injection as a depot to produce a slow release of insulin. Such preparations are called insulin zinc suspensions or lente insulins (*lente* meaning "slow"). They include insulin zinc suspension (IZS, insulin lente); insulin semilente amorphous (amorphous IZS, insulin semilente); and insulin zinc suspension crystalline (crystalline IZS, insulin ultralente).

Another method of making insulin last longer is to add protamine (a protein obtained from fish sperm) to a suspension of insulin. The protamine and insulin form a complex which is much less soluble than the insulin suspension alone, and from which insulin is slowly released after injection. The duration of action of this complex may be further prolonged by adding zinc to form protamine zinc insulin. Its use is complicated by the danger that if the blood sugar is controlled through the daytime it may fall hazardously low during the night and early morning. Attempts to balance this effect led to the combined use of protamine zinc insulin and soluble insulin in one injection. The combined effects provide sufficient cover during the day, without too high a dose of protamine zinc insulin continuing to work through the night.

Such a combination is still needed by some severe diabetics, but its use has now been generally replaced by the lente insulins. Some patients may be allergic to protamine, and an alternative protein preparation, globin zinc suspension, is available. There is also a preparation containing less protamine and zinc called isophane insulin. It lasts for a relatively long time.

However, the most significant advance in insulin preparation has been made in the past few years. By means of chromographical separation techniques, it has been possible to remove pancreatic impurities from the insulin, thus reducing both the risk of allergic reactions and the risk of antibody formation which greatly reduced the effectiveness of the insulin. Preparations so refined are available in the modern form of fast-acting soluble insulin, intermediate-acting like the semilente insulins, and a long-acting preparation like the lente insulins. With these new preparations it is possible to provide a 24-hour cover tailored to the individual's needs with the important advantage of reduced allergic effects.

The commonest adverse effect of insulin treatment is hypoglycemia, or low blood sugar. This happens when the patient receives too much insulin, which may occasionally occur if he misses a meal or eats a diet lacking sufficient carbohydrates. The early symptoms are weakness, giddiness, pallor, sweating, increased production of saliva, a sinking feeling in the stomach, palpitations, irritability, and trembling. If these are not immediately relieved by taking a glucose sweet or sugar the patient may develop changes in mood, be unable to concentrate, lack judgment, and lose self-control. Loss of memory, paralysis, double vision, pins and needles in the hands and feet, unconsciousness, convulsions, and death may occur. Every diabetic patient should be allowed to experience the early warning effects of hypoglycemia and then be taught the correct treatment to prevent an attack. If the patient is unable to understand these effects and instructions, the nearest relative or friend should be instructed.

Other adverse effects from insulin include allergic reactions—skin rashes, itching, and swelling of the face and throat. These may sometimes be controlled by changing the preparation; for example, one patient may be allergic to beef insulin but not to pork insulin or vice versa. Nettle rash and other local reactions may occur at the site of injections, resulting in wasting of the fatty tissue under the skin. The incidence of these local reactions is said to be declining with the development of more highly purified insulins. Alternatively, fatty swellings (lipomata) may occur, but rarely.

In rare cases an immune reaction to insulin may occur, resulting in a dramatic increase in the amount of insulin required. The insulin becomes "neutralized" and less effective. This reaction is more common with beef insulin than with pork insulin. Certain glandular disorders—e.g., underworking of the pituitary gland or adrenal gland—may increase sensitivity to insulin, resulting in low blood sugar levels. Oral contraceptive agents and thiazide diuretics may make diabetics worse by reducing the effects of insulin, so that more insulin is required.

If you are on insulin you should carry a warning card saying that you are a diabetic and giving the name and dose of the insulin preparation you are taking. The card should state that if you are found behaving strangely you should be given sugar by mouth.

## Oral Antidiabetic Drugs

Oral antidiabetic (or hypoglycemic) drugs are drugs which may be taken by mouth to produce a reduction in the blood sugar level. There are two main groups of these drugs: the sulfonylureas, which include acetohexamide, chlorpropamide, tolazamide, and tolbutamide; and the biguanide phenformin.

### SULFONYLUREAS

These drugs, it is thought, lower blood sugar levels by causing the pancreas to secrete more insulin. They may also potentiate the action of insulin throughout the body. They are effective only in the presence of some pancreatic function, and they do not affect the take-up and release of glucose by muscles. Their rate of breakdown in the body varies, and this affects their duration of action. Any of them may produce hypoglycemia, particularly in the elderly and those with impaired kidney or liver function. They should be used with caution, if at all, in these patients and also in patients with serious thyroid disorders, because they may affect thyroid function.

### BIGUANIDES

These drugs increase glucose uptake by muscles in the presence of insulin and inhibit the release of glucose by the liver. They may reduce absorption of carbohydrates from the gut, and therefore their effects may modify insulin requirements in diabetics. They also produce a loss of weight in overweight diabetics. They may have a role in preventing the onset of diabetes in certain individuals who show high blood sugar levels after meals.

Deaths have been reported due to alterations in the acidity of the blood in patients taking the biguanide phenformin, but no actual causative relationship has been proved. Phenformin should not be given to patients with congestive heart failure or to those with impaired kidney or liver function. It should not be used in pregnancy. Alcohol should be used with caution by patients taking this drug.

**The Use of Oral Antidiabetic Drugs**

A large long-term study in this country and additional studies elsewhere have indicated that oral antidiabetic drugs are no more effective than diet alone in prolonging life in diabetic patients. Indeed, the studies suggest that there may be an increased incidence among users of such drugs of abnormalities in electrical activity of the heart, heart attacks, and death.

While these findings are not uniformly accepted by the medical community, they have led to more stringent guidelines for the use of oral antidiabetic drugs. They should be used only in patients with diabetes of the maturity-onset type who cannot be treated with diet alone or who are unwilling or unable to take insulin if weight reduction and dietary control fail.

The sometimes high incidence of "secondary failure" (whereby an initially successful oral antidiabetic agent subsequently fails to maintain a low blood sugar) often responds to the addition of a different chemical class of oral antidiabetic drug. However, in light of the toxicities mentioned above, this practice has become questionable. These drugs should not be used in pregnancy or in a diabetic emergency, such as before surgery.

# DRUGS USED TO TREAT THYROID DISORDERS

The thyroid gland lies in the neck, in front of and on both sides of the windpipe. It produces two hormones, thyroxine and triiodothyronine. These hormones are responsible for speeding up the rate of metabolism (use of energy) of the cells in the body. The thyroid gland is under control of the pituitary gland, which produces a thyroid-stimulating hormone. If there is a deficiency of thyroid hormones in the blood, the pituitary increases its stimulation of the thyroid gland. The reverse happens if there is an excess of thyroid hormones in the blood.

Thyroid hormones are available in drug form either as extracts of thyroid glands obtained from slaughtered animals or as synthetic preparations of thyroxine or triiodothyronine. Because of their unpredictable strengths and the problems of standardization, the use of thyroid extracts has now largely given way to synthetic preparations. These are highly purified and standardized.

There are several disorders of the thyroid gland for which drug treatments are used: goiter, underworking of the gland (hypothyroidism, myxedema), overworking of the gland (hyperthyroidism, thyrotoxicosis), and other rare disorders such as thyroiditis.

## Goiter

Goiter is a simple enlargement of the thyroid gland. This enlargement may occur when the body lacks a supply of the chemical iodine. What happens is this: the pituitary gland, sensing a thyroid hormone shortage, produces an increased amount of thyroid-stimulating hormone. But because iodine is necessary for the production of thyroid hormones, the thyroid gland is frustrated in its efforts to comply. The gland keeps trying, with the result that it grows larger, forming a goiter. Goiter may occur in certain areas well away from the sea, where water supplies lack iodine and seafoods rich in iodine are scarce. Excessive calcium in hard water may interfere with the absorption of iodine from the gut. Rarely, there are genetic factors which interfere with the thyroid gland's manufacture of hormones. Thyroid enlargement may occur, though rarely, because certain foods contain substances which block thyroid hormone production. These substances, called goitrogens, are present in cabbage, Brussels sprouts, and turnips. Some drugs may also interfere with thyroid hormone production—for example, para-amino salicylic acid and sulfonamides. Iodine mixtures taken for coughs may produce thyroid enlargement, and the gland may enlarge during certain periods of increased demand—as in puberty, pregnancy, or breast feeding. Whatever the cause of simple goiter, the deficiency of thyroid hormone leads to an increase in size of the gland.

The drug treatment of goiter is to give a thyroid hormone. This reduces the amount of thyroid-stimulating hormone being produced by the pituitary and therefore reduces the size of the gland.

## Underworking of the Thyroid Gland

Underworking of the thyroid gland, or hypothyroidism, may be congenital. When a baby is born with some defect of the thyroid gland, the lack of thyroid hormones can retard mental and physical development, resulting in a group of characteristics called cretinism. In rare cases, underworking of the thyroid gland may occur during childhood. More frequently it occurs in adult life. Hypothyroidism results in a slowing down of all metabolic processes in the body. It may be associated with a thick, pale swelling of the skin called myxedema.

Thus, disorders of the thyroid gland associated with underproduction of thyroid hormones include cretinism, juvenile myxedema, adult hypothyroidism, and adult myxedema. The treatment of these disorders is administration of thyroid hormones, replacing the hormones which the gland is incapable of producing.

THYROID (thyroid extract, desiccated thyroid). Despite its variable composition, clinical results with thyroid are remarkably uniform and it is still widely used. It is the least expensive of the different thyroid preparations. It contains variable amounts of thyroxine and triiodothyronine. The extract is somewhat unstable and loses potency upon prolonged exposure to air.

THYROXINE (thyroxine sodium, levothyroxine). The sodium salt of thyroxine is soluble and may be given by mouth. It is considered by many to be the drug of choice in most thyroid deficiency disorders. Because of its delayed effects, the starting dose must be small and then slowly increased at two-week intervals until the required response is obtained. At the start of treatment thyroxine may produce rapid beating of the heart, anginal pain, and muscle cramps. Too large a dose may cause restlessness, excitement, irregular heart rhythm, headache, flushing, sweating, excessive loss of weight, and muscle weakness. It may also affect the heart. These effects are all usually temporary and related to dosage. Large doses may cause death in patients with myxedema and heart disease. Thyroxine should, therefore, be used with caution in patients with heart disease. It may increase the effects of anticoagulants and upset the stability of patients receiving antidiabetic drugs. Phenytoin and possibly aspirin may increase the effects of thyroxine.

TRIIODOTHYRONINE (liothyronine sodium) produces adverse effects similar to those of thyroxine. These disappear when the dose is reduced or the drug is stopped. The drug is used when a rapid effect is required. It should not be given to patients with angina or heart disorders. Because of its short duration of action, it is impractical for long-term use.

THYROGLOBULIN (thyroglobulin extract) is partly purified thyroid extract standardized to contain thyroxine and triiodothyronine in a ratio of 2.5 to 1. It is relatively expensive and offers no significant advantages.

## Overworking of the Thyroid Gland (Hyperthyroidism, Thyrotoxicosis)

Hyperthyroidism occurs more frequently in women than in men and usually in early adult life. But it is not uncommon in later life, when its features differ from those seen in the younger person. It is also known as toxic goiter, exophthalmic goiter (because the eyes appear prominent), Graves' disease, Parry's disease, and Basedow's disease. The cause of hyperthyroidism is unknown. It produces many symptoms, including nervousness, tiredness, sweating, trembling, breathlessness, enlargement of the thyroid gland in some patients but not in others, prominence of the eyes, heart disorders, increase of appetite and yet loss of weight.

The treatment of hyperthyroidism is to give antithyroid drugs, or to remove part of the gland by surgery, or to suppress its activity by using radioactive iodine. None of these treatments has any effect upon the underlying cause of the disorder, but they do effectively prevent the consequences of overstimulation of the gland, and therefore the body, until a natural remission occurs.

Drugs are of particular use in children, young adults, pregnant women, and patients with mild hyperthyroidism. Treatment should continue for up to two years.

Antithyroid drugs interfere with the production of thyroid hormones by the thyroid gland, and control may be achieved by observing changes in the patient's symptoms and by measuring the pulse rate and body weight. It is customary to start with high doses and then slowly reduce the daily dose to a satisfactory maintenance level. Three groups of drugs are used to suppress thyroid function: thioamides, including the thiouracils (methylthiouracil, propylthiouracil); the imidazoles (carbimazole, methimazole), which act by chemically blocking thyroid hormone synthesis; and iodine and iodides, which increase the storage and diminish the release of thyroid hormones.

Basically, there are four antithyroid drugs in common use: methylthiouracil and propylthiouracil; and carbimazole and methimazole. There is little to choose among these four drugs, and in equally effective dosage they vary little in adverse effects. Iodine and iodides cause shrinking of overworking goiters (toxic goiters), but this effect is transient and so these substances are used only before surgery and in emergencies. Except in its radioactive form, iodine is of no use in the *treatment* of hyperthyroidism.

Carbimazole produces adverse effects more frequently in the first two months of treatment. It should be given with utmost caution to patients in whom the thyroid enlargement is pressing on the windpipe (initially it may *increase* the enlargement, producing further pressure). Infants should not be breast-fed by mothers taking carbimazole. It should be used in the smallest doses possible during pregnancy and stopped about one month before the baby is due. Methimazole, methylthiouracil, and propylthiouracil produce adverse effects similar to those of carbimazole. A rare complication in the use of propylthiouracil is a tendency to bleed. All these drugs may produce blood disorders, and you should stop taking them immediately if you develop skin rashes, fever, and swollen glands. Blood disorders usually clear when the drug is stopped, but very occasionally deaths do occur. Adverse effects usually occur within the first month of treatment.

Carbimazole, methimazole, methylthiouracil, and propylthiouracil are absorbed and excreted quickly. Generally, they should be given three times daily and continued for at least one to two years. It takes up to two months before you feel the benefits of treatment. In too large a dose they can produce hypothyroidism, which may cause enlargement of the gland. They also increase the blood supply to the gland, which may produce problems if the gland is to be surgically removed.

# LOCAL ANESTHETICS

Local anesthetics are drugs which block the transmission of sensory impulses in nerve tissues when applied locally in appropriate concentrations. Their effects are reversible, and they are used to produce loss of pain without loss of nervous control. They could be called local pain relievers. However, they *can* produce loss of nervous control (paralysis) if injected directly into a nerve fiber. Those local anesthetics in common use have been selected because they do not irritate the tissues to which they are applied, nor do they cause permanent nerve damage. They are soluble in water and can be sterilized. Their choice depends upon the speed with which they work, their duration of action, and their potential adverse effects when absorbed into the bloodstream. The latter is important, since they can affect all nervous tissues, including the brain.

The effects of local anesthetics wear off quickly when removed from their site of action. For this reason, it is customary to mix a local anesthetic with a drug which closes off the blood supply (a vasoconstrictor). In this way, the local anesthetic is not "washed away" so rapidly into the bloodstream. The drugs used for this purpose are epinephrine and norepinephrine. Their use is not without danger. For example, if the mixtures are used to block pain in a finger, the constriction of blood vessels may so affect the circulation as to cause gangrene. Therefore, anesthetic/vasoconstrictor mixtures should not be used near terminal arteries—in the fingers, toes, ears, nose, and penis.

Local anesthetics may be absorbed into the bloodstream and produce stimulation and then depression of the brain. This can cause anxiety, restlessness, yawning, nausea, vomiting, twitching, convulsions, coma, and death. Pallor, sweating, a fall in blood pressure, irregular heart rhythm, heart failure, and respiratory failure may also occur, producing sudden collapse and death. Repeated local use may produce allergic reactions—skin rashes, asthma, anaphylactic shock. They should, therefore, be given with utmost caution to patients with impaired heart, kidney, or liver function. Such adverse effects are reduced by adding the vasoconstrictor drugs. Their repeated use in the eye may damage the cornea, and a protection should always be worn for half a day over an eye that has had anesthetic drops applied.

There are two chemical types of local anesthetics. The older compounds include tetracaine, benzocaine, cocaine, and procaine. The newer ones include bupivacaine, lidocaine, mepivacaine, and prilocaine. They may be administered in several different ways according to the drug being used. *Surface* or *topical anesthesia* (as a solution, jelly, or lozenge), because it blocks pain nerve endings in the skin or mucous membranes, must have good powers of penetration. Such anesthetics include tetracaine, benzocaine, cocaine, lidocaine, and prilocaine. Tetracaine and cocaine are used on the eye. *Local* or *infiltration anesthesia* is produced by *injection* into the area. To be effective the drug must not be absorbed into the bloodstream so quickly that its effects wear off. The local anesthetics used for this purpose include lidocaine, procaine, mepivacaine, and prilocaine. The latter two do not require the addition of a vasoconstrictor.

Injections of local anesthetics are also used to produce *regional nerve block* to cut off pain sensation in an area, for example by dentists. *Epidural anesthesia* is a nerve block produced by injecting the anesthetic into the space between the lining membranes of the spinal cord in order to produce anesthesia of a large area of the body—the legs, for example. *Caudal anesthesia* is an injection into the space between the lining membranes at the lower end of the spinal cord where the main nerves from the spinal cord run together before leaving the spine to supply the pelvis and legs. It may be used, for example, in childbirth. The drugs used for these purposes include bupivacaine, lidocaine, mepivacaine, prilocaine, and procaine.

*Spinal anesthesia* is produced by injecting the local anesthetic inside the covering membrane of the spinal cord, thereby causing temporary paralysis of the nerves with which it comes into contact. The area affected—which may range from the arms to the legs—is determined by the specific gravity of the drug (i.e., the rate at which it descends through fluid inside the spinal cord) and by the position of the patient, who may be tilted up or down according to the area meant to be anesthetized. Tetracaine and bupivacaine are used for this purpose. Lidocaine may be injected into a vein to produce a general anesthesia.

The choice of local anesthetic depends upon many factors but in particular upon the risk of absorption and the production of dangerous adverse effects. The concentrations used are absolutely critical, yet unfortunately their names often sound alike, which can lead to problems unless the label is read carefully.

# DRUGS USED
# TO TREAT SKIN DISORDERS

We know surprisingly little about the causes of many common skin disorders—eczema, psoriasis, acne, warts, and dandruff, for example. Against such a background of ignorance it is no wonder that there are many myths about treatment. As noted previously, when there are many claimed treatments for a particular disorder there often is no specific treatment—otherwise we would all know about it and use it. This applies particularly to skin disorders.

Thanks to the pharmaceutical industry we have seen great advances in the specific and effective cure of many infective skin disorders (see antibiotic and antifungal drugs, pp. 199 and 200). We have also seen the introduction of the corticosteroids, which have revolutionized the relief of many skin disorders. Such old-fashioned treatments as tar, sulfur, and resorcinol continue, and others, such as the antihistamines, have not produced the results that we hoped for, except in their specific and effective use by mouth in allergic rashes, particularly rashes due to drugs. Most skin treatments remain nonspecific. At the very least they should not make the disorder worse, yet the widespread uses of antihistamines, local anesthetics, antibiotics, and antiseptics in skin applications have led to the production of allergic rashes, and the generous use of corticosteroids (p. 197) has led to other problems.

In the treatment of skin disorders, the danger is that skin preparations containing too many potent drugs may be applied in too large a quantity to too large an area too often and over too long a period of time; even base creams may produce allergies. You should be as sensible about applying drugs to the skin as you are about taking drugs by mouth. Know what you are treating, know what you are applying, and know the benefits and risks. With longstanding skin disorders you can try different recommended preparations, but do not be conned into paying huge sums of money to private hair and skin clinics.

Numerous skin applications are available—creams, ointments, lotions, dusting powders, sprays, pastes. They are used for treating skin disorders in different stages of severity and in different areas of the body. For example, lotions are used in acute skin conditions and where the skin is unbroken. Watery lotions act by evaporation and cool the skin. When used, they should be applied frequently. The addition of alcohol to a skin lotion increases its cooling and drying effect. Where the skin is broken, an astringent (p. 205) may be included, as it helps to seal the weeping surface of the skin. Lotions are used for scabbed and dried skin disorders. They cool by evaporation and deposit a powder on the surface. Dusting powders (e.g., talc) are useful for treating skin disorders which affect skin folds—under the arms, in the groin, under the breasts. Creams and ointments are used on various skin disorders, and pastes are useful for dry scaly patches.

The choice of the base for creams and ointments and other skin applications is often of equal importance to the choice of active drug in the preparations. This is because the effectiveness of the active drug can be altered by the type of base used.

In this section are discussed the various groups of drugs most frequently included in skin applications.

## Soothing Skin Applications

### DEMULCENTS

These are usually gums from stems, roots, and branches of various plants, for example acacia (gum arabic), tragacanth (gum tragacanth), glycyrrhiza (licorice root), agar and sodium alginate (from algae). Synthetic drugs like methylcellulose are also used. Glycerin is a common constituent of skin applications, and mixed with starch it forms a jelly base called starch glycerite. Glycerin should be used only in small concentration because it can be irritant. Propylene glycol is related to glycerin and is used in lotions and ointments because it mixes with water and also dissolves in oils. Many other glycols are used to make water-soluble bases for ointments.

Demulcents are soothing because they coat the surface of the skin or mucous membranes (mouth, gums, and throat) and protect the underlying area from the air and other irritating agents.

### EMOLLIENTS

Emollients are fats and oils which are soothing when applied to the skin. They soften the skin and are chiefly used as a base to which other active drugs (e.g., antibiotics) are added. They soften the skin by forming an oily film over the surface of the skin, thus preventing water from evaporating from the surface cells and so keeping them moist.

Emollient skin applications contain vegetable oils, animal fats, paraffin and related chemicals, and waxes.

The vegetable oils are usually cottonseed oil, corn oil, peanut oil, almond oil, and cocoa-bean oil. Animal fats, from the wool of sheep, are of two types: wool fat (anhydrous lanolin) and hydrous wool fat (known simply as lanolin), which is wool fat mixed with 20 to 30 percent water. Wool fat can produce skin allergies. It is not used as often as it used to be.

Paraffin-related preparations include mineral oil, white petroleum, and yellow petroleum (e.g., Vaseline is a brand preparation of white and yellow petroleum jellies). Waxes are principally obtained from beeswax (yellow wax). White wax is bleached beeswax. Spermaceti is a waxy substance from the head of the sperm whale. It is used to raise the melting point of ointments, such as cold cream, so that they don't melt too easily when applied to warm skin, particularly in hot climates. Spermaceti is present in rose-water ointment along with white wax, almond oil, rose water, and rose oil. This mixture forms the basis of most commonly used cold creams.

## Protective Skin Applications

Protectives are used to cover the skin and mucous membranes in order to keep them from contact with an irritating agent. They are by definition insoluble and inactive and cover the skin physically rather than by means of any chemical effect. They include dusting powders used to protect the skin in certain areas (e.g., skin folds), and on the surfaces of ulcers and wounds. They are smooth and prevent friction; some absorb moisture from the surface of the area to which they are applied, and thus help to decrease friction and prevent infection (for example, protectives containing zinc oxide or starch). On open wounds they make a crust. Those containing starch must contain an antiseptic such as boric acid or salicylic acid to prevent the starch from fermenting. Dusting powders often contain talc (which is mainly magnesium silicate), and of course talc is widely available as talcum powders.

Mechanical protectives such as collodion were formerly used to close off small wounds, but it is now considered better to let the air get to a wound. Petroleum gauze and gauzes impregnated with antibiotics are useful as protective dressings to wounds, although the tendency now is to use dry nonadherent dressings. Barrier creams, ointments, and sprays, used to protect the skin against water-soluble irritants, usually contain dimethicone (silicone) or a related silicone oil. They adhere to the skin, have water-repellent properties, and provide protection against the irritating effects of soap, water, skin cleansing agents, and breakdown products from urine. They may be useful in preventing bedsores and diaper rash. They should not be used on inflamed or damaged skin or near the eyes because they may produce irritation. Numerous preparations containing silicone are available, and it is worth trying one of these preparations for prevention of bedsores or diaper rash. They are less effective in preventing industrial dermatitis. They may produce allergic skin reactions.

## Suntan and Sunburn Applications

Sunburn and suntan are caused by ultraviolet light in the sun's rays. The shorter ultraviolet light waves cause the burning, and the longer waves cause the tanning. Tanning results from migration of the brown pigment melanin from the base layer of the skin up into the surface cells. This provides some protection against sunburn, but the main protection comes from a thickening of the surface layer of cells. The effectiveness of suntan applications is therefore related to their ability to cut out the burning effects of the sun's rays while allowing the tanning rays to get through. Drugs which have this effect include para-aminobenzoic acid or its esters, and titanium dioxide. These preparations are the most effective sunscreens against the middle-wavelength ultraviolet light involved in sunburn. They include Pabanol and Pre-Sun (5 percent para-aminobenzoic acid in 50 to 70 percent ethyl alcohol); Block-Out, Pabafilm, and Spectraban (2.5 percent iso-amyl—p-N,N-dimethylaminobenzoate—PABA ester). Many other, often less effective preparations are available. Claims for vitamin A must be regarded with caution. General-purpose skin creams and oils often help to prevent the skin from getting burned but do not prevent its getting red.

There are many treatments for sunburn. Among the most common are calamine lotion and zinc lotion. Applications containing a corticosteroid (see p. 197) can be very effective. Most experts advise against using applications containing an antihistamine because they may produce sensitivity, and usually in sunburn there is a fairly large area of skin to be treated. Many preparations contain a local anesthetic such as lidocaine or benzocaine which can also irritate the skin.

A person with photosensitivity is excessively sensitive to sunlight; his skin gets red and burns very easily. The condition is usually caused by the use of a drug. For example, certain tetracycline antibiotics (p. 217), griseofulvin (an antifungal drug, pp. 200, 213), phenothiazine major tranquilizers (p. 53), oral antidiabetic drugs (p. 186), minor tranquilizers, thiazide diuretics (p. 104), oral contraceptive drugs (p. 173), gold (used to treat rheumatoid arthritis, p. 122), diphenhydramine (an antihistamine, p. 204), and, rarely, even saccharin and cyclamates, can all cause photosensitivity.

Drugs applied to the skin—for example, tar (the basis of tar and ultraviolet ray treatment of psoriasis) and hexachlorophene, an antiseptic present in numerous skin applications and toiletries (p. 202)—may also sensitize it to sunlight. Various deodorants (p. 206) may also sensitize the skin, and so too may suntan applications (e.g., para-aminobenzoic acid).

The important thing to remember, if you find yourself burning more quickly than usual, is that the reason might be a drug you are taking or a skin application you are using. Stop using it immediately to see whether it is what is causing your increased sensitivity.

Some people are actually allergic to sunlight and can develop severe dermatitis on exposed parts of their skin. They may get protection from taking an antimalarial drug such as chloroquine (Part III) by mouth and applying creams containing a drug such as sulisobenzone. Certain disorders may produce sunlight allergy—for example porphyria (a disorder of metabolism). If you develop a rash on the exposed parts of your skin always consult your doctor.

## Corticosteroid Skin Applications

Corticosteroids (see p. 159) reduce inflammatory and allergic reactions and are therefore widely used to treat many skin disorders, in order to reduce redness, soreness, swelling, pain, and irritation. Corticosteroids are present alone or in combination with other drugs in numerous skin, eye, and ear applications prescribed by doctors. They are very effective, particularly when an allergic factor is present. However, they do not cure but only suppress the symptoms, so that if the underlying skin disorder is not self-limiting, or if the causative agent is not removed (for example, contact dermatitis caused by an article worn on the body), it will flare up again when the corticosteroid preparation is stopped.

Corticosteroids available for use on the skin include hydrocortisone (in numerous preparations), triamcinolone, fluocinolone, betamethasone, fluocinonide, flumethasone, fluoromethalone, and flurandrenolide. These vary in potency, and so concentrations included in skin preparations vary from 0.025 percent for triamcinolone up to 2.5 percent for hydrocortisone. The popularity of any particular preparation may reflect the results of vigorous sales promotion more than any clear differences in effectiveness.

In using corticosteroid skin preparations it must be remembered that when inflammation is reduced, the resistance to infection is lowered and secondary infection may occur. This is particularly likely to happen when corticosteroids are used under airtight dressings (for instance plastic), causing boils, thrush, and other infections to develop. Allergy to corticosteroid applications may also occur, and this should always be considered if there is a poor response to treatment.

Long continued use of corticosteroids, particularly under plastic dressings, may cause a local wasting of the deep layers of the skin, producing a flattened, depressed, stripy-looking area that may not go away for years. Some corticosteroids applied to the skin may enter the blood circulation and have an effect on the pituitary gland (p. 162). This is particularly likely to happen to children (who may also lick the ointment off the skin) and in adults using very large amounts. Very rarely, hair may grow at the site of repeated applications of corticosteroids.

Some skin disorders can get infected (e.g., infected eczema) and become soggy with pus. In these infected skin disorders the use of an application containing a corticosteroid and an anti-infective drug (e.g., an antibiotic; see facing page) may be very effective. Such a combination is also useful on skin rashes in areas where infection is likely to occur, for example, in the groin or around the anus. But do not forget that there is a slight risk that an anti-infective drug may produce an allergic reaction which the corticosteroid will mask. Remember this if a skin rash seems to be getting worse despite the fact that initially it improved on such a preparation.

The wrong use of such combinations in primary infective skin disorders may produce very severe effects. For example, if they are used to treat impetigo, a small localized patch may be turned into a serious widespread skin infection; a simple fungus infection (e.g., athlete's foot) may spread over a large area; and herpes simplex (cold sores) may produce nasty ulcers.

Do not forget also that corticosteroids can delay the healing of ulcers (particularly leg ulcers). Finally, it is important that you should not borrow skin ointments containing a corticosteroid or anti-infective drug from a neighbor or friend—different disorders and different people respond differently.

Hydrocortisone is the drug of first choice among corticosteroid skin applications, particularly if given in appropriate strength—from 0.25 to 1 percent. Fluorinated corticosteroids (so called because they contain a fluorine side chain), which include fluocinolone and betamethasone, are effective, but if they are used excessively over prolonged periods they may produce wasting of the deep layer of the skin, particularly when used on the face, flexures (knees and elbows), and moist areas. They may also produce soreness and irritation at the site of application. Some experts say they should not be used in patients with acne rosacea of the face or in patients (usually children) with eczema of the flexures. They may be useful in skin disorders that do not respond well to hydrocortisone, e.g., psoriasis (see p. 209).

Corticosteroids mixed with an antibiotic (see facing page), antifungal drug (p. 200), or antiseptic (p. 201) may be used where the primary skin condition would be expected to respond to corticosteroids but where there is an added infection (e.g., infected eczema). To repeat my warning, such combinations should not be used where the skin disorder is primarily infective. The choice of preparation is not critical. Such simple principles as not too much for too long should apply, and if the disorder gets worse stop the treatment and see your doctor.

### Antibiotic Skin Applications

When a skin infection is superficial (for instance, impetigo), an antibiotic skin application can be dramatically effective. If the infection is deep under the skin surface (as an abscess), local applications of an antibiotic are useless and an antibiotic by mouth or injection is necessary.

When the sulfonamides and penicillin were introduced, doctors used them liberally in skin applications, and many patients had allergic reactions, inconvenient for some patients, but positively dangerous for others. The drugs sensitized the patient, with the consequent risk of a severe allergic reaction if that patient had to be given a sulfonamide or a penicillin for some more serious infection.

Because of these risks, do not use a skin application containing an antibiotic which is known to produce allergic reactions and which is also used to treat other infections by mouth or by injection. There is a useful range of antibiotic drugs available which rarely cause allergic reactions and are used only on the skin. They include neomycin, bacitracin, gentamicin, and polymyxin B. However, because of their widespread use, singly or in combination with other drugs, we are increasingly seeing allergic reactions to neomycin and bacitracin. Chlortetracycline is taken by mouth and seldom produces allergic skin reactions; it is useful for certain infections of the skin, but not the commonly occurring ones such as impetigo and infected wounds, which are caused by a group of bacteria resistant to chlortetracycline. Penicillin and sulfonamides should be completely avoided on the skin, and so too should chloramphenicol and streptomycin because of the risk of allergy. An exception is in the antibacterial therapy of severe burns, where special sulfonamides may be used as topical antibacterial drugs. In addition, the use of chloramphenicol and sulfacetamide applications in eye and ear infections is still recommended by some specialists.

Antibiotic skin applications should be used for as short a time as possible, and if the disorder gets worse they should be stopped immediately. For most commonly occurring infections of the skin and wounds, bacitracin and bacitracin plus neomycin or gentamicin are useful. For infections of the eyes and ears, chlortetracycline, sulfacetamide, and chloramphenicol may be added to the list.

### Antifungal Skin Applications

Before reading this section it may be useful to read the section on antifungal antibiotics (p. 212), which discusses the antifungal drugs used locally and by mouth. Some of these have revolutionized the treatment of fungus and yeast infections.

These include such drugs as: griseofulvin, used by mouth to treat fungus infections of the hair, skin, and nails (e.g., favus, ringworm, athlete's foot); amphotericin, given by mouth to treat severe fungus infections affecting internal organs but which may also be applied to the skin to treat fungus infections of the groin and nail beds; candicidin, clotrimazole, and miconazole, used to treat thrush infections of the skin and vagina in local applications; and chlordantoin, used to treat thrush infections of the vagina.

Nystatin is used to treat thrush and is available in powders, drops, ointments, vaginal suppositories, and tablets. Propionic acid (which is also used as a food preservative) and sodium propionate are weakly fungistatic and are included in some antifungal ointments. Tolnaftate is available in cream, solution, and powder to treat fungal skin infections. Undecylenic acid and calcium or zinc undecylenate are similarly available in creams and powders.

Nystatin is the drug most commonly used in treating thrush infections. Griseofulvin represents a big advance in the treatment of long-standing ringworm and other fungus infections of the hair, skin, and nails. It is taken by mouth and enters the infected tissues, but it has to be taken for a prolonged period of time—for up to one year, for example, in the treatment of fungus infections of the nails (see griseofulvin, p. 213). Amphotericin B, clotrimazole, miconazole, and tolnaftate are effective and can be applied locally. The selection of drug is not critical (e.g., for athlete's foot), provided treatment is carried out as directed by the doctor or pharmacist, and provided treatment is continued for a sufficient length of time.

### Antiparasitic Skin Applications

Benzyl benzoate and gamma benzene hexachloride are useful for treating scabies and lice. The applications for scabies should be used all over the body below the head after a bath; everyone in the family should be treated and all exposed clothes and bedding should be washed. Three successive treatments at about twelve-hour intervals should be applied. A single application is usually sufficient for lice. Crotamiton is also effective against scabies and lice. Chlorophenothane (DDT) is useful for treating head lice, but it does not destroy the fertile eggs. Chlorophenothane is not effective against scabies. Gamma benzene hexachloride head lotion is also available for treating head lice. For treating body lice, a cream or powder may be used. Chlorophenothane dusting powder may also be used for body lice. Everyone in the household must be treated, and all clothes and bedclothes must be washed.

## Antiseptics and Disinfectants

There is great confusion over the use of the terms "antiseptic" and "disinfectant." In general "antiseptic" usually refers to those drugs applied to the skin or other parts of the body in an attempt to prevent infection. We use the term "disinfectant" to describe a chemical applied to objects in order to destroy germs. Antiseptic preparations applied to the skin are sometimes called germicides. Antiseptics may kill or prevent the growth of bacteria, fungi, and viruses. Some disinfectants are used as antiseptics in reduced strengths, but some disinfectants are too irritant to use as antiseptics and some antiseptics are not strong enough to use as disinfectants.

Antiseptics and disinfectants belong to various chemical groups which can make the choice look very complex and confusing. In fact most doctors learn to use one or two preparations (often by their brand name), and I think this is the best advice I can give you. The choice is not critical, and the need to use such preparations is greatly overemphasized in the advertising media.

Some main chemical groups to which antiseptics and disinfectants belong are the following:

CHLORINE AND CHLORINE-RELEASING SUBSTANCES. Chlorine kills germs, and the most commonly used chlorine-releasing chemical is sodium hypochlorite. This is present in many commonly used preparations. Others include chlorinated lime solution (Dakin's solution) and chlorinated lime (often mixed with boric acid solution, as in eusol).

DETERGENTS. These include complex ammonia compounds such as benzalkonium, benzethonium, cetylpyridinium, and domiphen. These last two are used as antiseptics in throat lozenges. An important point to remember about these preparations is that soap can reduce their activity. They are also prescribed by doctors as shampoos for the treatment of dandruff.

PHENOL AND RELATED DRUGS. These lose their effects fairly quickly when diluted. They include phenol, cresol, and thymol. Solutions of these should not be applied to large wounds, since they can be absorbed into the bloodstream and can be very toxic. Most phenol skin preparations contain a wax or petrolatum base which prevents the antiseptic from reaching the bacteria. Other preparations have too low a concentration of phenol.

CHLORINATED PHENOLS. The most widely used of these have included a mixture of chlorinated phenols, and hexachlorophene. Hexachlorophene was widely used in the sixties in numerous skin applications and toilet preparations, even in toothpaste. A preparation probably includes an antiseptic if it is termed "medicated." Most of this "medication" was and is totally unnecessary. Following reports that hexachlorophene produced brain damage when applied extensively to the skin of premature babies, its use became restricted and its concentration in skin preparations was reduced. Hexachlorophene is effective only when allowed to accumulate on skin over several days with repeated applications. It may produce skin sensitivity and also make the skin sensitive to sunlight. Chlorocresol and chloroxylenol are other examples of chlorinated phenols.

DYES. Two types of dyes are used as antiseptics. Acridines, which include acriflavine, aminacrine, proflavine, and ethacridine, are slow-acting but work in the presence of pus and damaged tissues, which inhibit the effects of some antiseptics. In high concentration they may delay wound healing and produce skin sensitivity. Dyes such as brilliant green, crystal violet, and malachite green are derivatives of triphenylmethane and were widely used before the introduction of antibiotics and antifungal drugs.

FORMALDEHYDE. Formaldehyde and related drugs may be used as disinfectants, but not as antiseptics because they irritate the skin. Glutaraldehyde is superior to formaldehyde as a sterilizing agent. It lacks formaldehyde's disagreeable odor.

OTHER CHEMICAL GROUPS include alcohol, oxidizing compounds such as hydrogen peroxide, iodine and iodophors (complexes of iodine), and salts of heavy metals such as mercury and silver. Merbromin (Mercurochrome), an organic mercurial salt which is of little use, is present in many first-aid kits.

Chlorine-releasing substances such as sodium hypochlorite or chlorinated phenols are perfectly suitable as disinfectants, but do not forget that chlorine acts as a bleach. For cleaning the skin povidone-iodine is useful, and so are chlorinated phenols such as chloroxylenol and hexachlorophene.

## Irritant Skin Applications

These are drugs which are applied to the skin to produce "inflammation." They cause dilation of the blood vessels in the skin, resulting in redness and warmth. This reaction is used to bring relief from a deep-seated pain by the process known as counterirritation: by producing increased circulation in a part of the skin, a similar effect may be produced in a deeper-lying tissue which shares the same nerve supply from the spinal cord as that area of skin. For example, applying a counterirritant to the abdominal wall may relieve underlying gut pain. This is the principle behind the old-fashioned treatment for pleurisy —a hot poultice.

A commonly used counterirritant is heat from a hot-water bottle, a heat lamp, or a diathermy machine. Many drugs are also used as counterirritants in rheumatic liniments, rubs, and other applications. They include methylsalicylate (related to aspirin), camphor oil, menthol, and methyl nicotinate. Rheumatic liniments also have various aromatic oils added to make their smell distinctive.

The choice of a rheumatic liniment is not critical; one may smell nicer than another. Rubbing and massaging is often more important.

## Anti-itching Skin Applications and Drugs

There are many causes of itching (called pruritus by doctors), including allergic skin rashes, eczema, nervous rashes, scabies, body lice, and insect bites. In these disorders scratching may give relief, but it often leads to skin damage and further itching. In elderly patients the skin itself may degenerate to produce itching. Some drugs—aspirin, carbromal, and morphinelike drugs, for example may produce itching. Kidney disorders, liver and gall bladder disorders, and diabetes may also be responsible. It is therefore important for you to be examined properly by your doctor if you have an itching disorder, because it is better to treat the cause than to treat the itch. There are two main approaches to the drug treatment of itching: skin applications and oral drugs.

Skin applications to treat itching may contain such antiseptics as phenol, benzyl alcohol, balsam of Peru, and chlorbutol in small concentrations. These can, however, irritate the skin and produce allergic rashes. Local anesthetics (p. 204) are often used in small concentrations in skin applications, but again these may irritate the skin and produce skin allergies. Antihistamine creams (p. 204) are useful for small areas (e.g., insect bites) but are not recommended for large areas—they too may produce allergic skin rashes. Other drugs such as menthol and camphor are also used.

A useful drug to kill scabies, crotamiton, should be applied with caution to inflamed skin because it may make the inflammation worse. Corticosteroid skin applications (p. 197) are now probably the most widely used and most effective, particularly in treating itching and inflamed skin disorders. The fluorinated corticosteroids are the most effective for relieving itching (see p. 198). Other drugs used to treat itching include titanium dioxide (which is also used as a suntan application, p. 196). It is present in some face powders and cosmetics.

Two main groups of drugs are taken by mouth to relieve itching: antihistamines (pp. 130–1) and major tranquilizers (p. 53). One commonly used drug from the antihistamine group is chlorpheniramine.

The severe itching which accompanies obstructed gall bladder disease may be relieved by such male sex hormones as testosterone (Part III), which may also be helpful in senile pruritus and obstructive jaundice. Cholestyramine (p. 99) may help in liver and gall bladder disease because it reduces the blood level of bile salts, which is high in these disorders; it is thought that they are the cause of the itching.

Sedatives (p. 45) and minor tranquilizers (p. 51) are also used, but these must be given with caution to the elderly. The same caution should apply to the use of antihistamines and major tranquilizers in the elderly, who can quickly become confused under an apparently "normal" dose of any of these drugs. Simple skin applications should be tried first, such as a small volume of liquefied phenol added to calamine lotion or some other mixture. Discuss this with your doctor or pharmacist.

Irritation of the anus and vaginal area is not uncommon and may be caused by diabetes, threadworms, vaginal discharge, athlete's foot fungus, and thrush (particularly after a course of antibiotics by mouth). Vaginal deodorant sprays and wipes may also produce vaginal irritation. As with general itching, it is important to attempt to diagnose the cause and treat it. Sometimes this is difficult because of complex social, psychological, and sexual factors. The most effective applications to use in the treatment of pruritus ani and/or vulvae are those which contain a corticosteroid (p. 197) combined with an antifungal drug (p. 200) and an antiseptic (p. 201).

Estrogen creams may help the elderly patient with pruritus vulvae.

### Antihistamine Skin Applications

Numerous available skin applications contain antihistamines. These are sometimes of use in treating small, acutely irritating, and painful skin lesions such as an insect bite, nettle rash, or poison ivy. Their regular use and their use on large areas should be avoided because they can produce allergic skin rashes. Antihistamine skin applications available include pyrilamine, diphenhydramine, tripelennamine, and chlorpheniramine.

The choice of antihistamine preparation is not critical, but their use is very limited; always read the instructions on the package.

### Local Anesthetic Skin Applications

Numerous skin applications contain a local anesthetic. Their widespread or regular use is not recommended because of the risk of producing irritation of the skin and allergic rashes.

Preparations available include benzocaine, dibucaine, lidocaine, cyclomethycaine, promoxine, and tetracaine.

Choice of preparation is not critical, but it is very important always to read the instructions on the package.

## Caustic and Keratolytic Skin Applications

Caustics are drugs used to destroy tissue at the site of application. If the drug causes a scab by precipitating protein from the damaged cells, it is also called a cauterizant or an escharotic. Surgeons use electric needles to burn (or cauterize) the ends of small bleeding blood vessels.

Some commonly used caustics are acetic acid, phenol, podophyllum, trichloracetic acid, and silver nitrate. They are used to treat warts and corns.

Keratolytics are included in some skin applications because they loosen the surface cells of the skin and cause them to swell and soften so that they can be cut off easily. They are used to treat warts, corns, and acne and include benzoic acid, salicylic acid, and resorcinol.

## Astringent Skin Applications

Astringents are drugs which act on the surface of cells to precipitate protein. They do not enter the cell and therefore do not kill the cell, but they make its surface less permeable to water and other liquids, causing it to dry up and shrink. They are included in skin applications and have the effect of hardening the skin, drying up soggy areas of damaged skin, and reducing minor bleeding from skin abrasions. Astringents in various dilutions may be used in throat lozenges, mouth washes, eye drops, ear drops, treatment for hemorrhoids, and as caustics (for burning off dead tissue, etc.). In the past they have been used to treat diarrhea and other disorders of the gut. They are now widely used in antiperspirant sprays and applications (p. 206). The main ones used are salts of zinc and aluminum.

Aluminum sulfate, aluminum hydroxychloride, aluminum chloride, and aluminum chlorhydroxide are strong astringents and may be used as mild caustics. Bismuth subgallate and bismuth subcarbonate are used as astringents to shrink hemorrhoids. Hamamelis is another astringent used to shrink hemorrhoids, and hamamelis water (witch hazel) is used as a cooling application for sprains and bruises. Zinc chloride is used as a caustic, astringent, and deodorant. Zinc sulfate is used as an astringent, particularly in eye drops.

Aluminum acetate and zinc acetate are mild astringents of choice, but it really depends on what is being treated—sweating feet or a small abrasion, hemorrhoids or a leg ulcer. Aluminum chlorhydroxide is the most common astringent in antiperspirant preparations. If in doubt always consult your doctor or pharmacist.

### Antiperspirant Skin Applications

These are available in every size, shape, and color of container, as pads, sprays, roll-ons, and creams, and with numerous fragrances, to be applied to an ever-increasing number of parts of the body.

The drugs most commonly used as antiperspirants include salts of aluminum and zinc. Some may stain fabric, some are acidic and irritate the skin, and some are soluble in alcohol and may be used in sprays and aerosols. Antiperspirants which contain an aluminum salt may produce an allergic skin rash on sensitive skins. The mechanism of action of antiperspirants is unknown, but some experts consider them to be astringents (see p. 205).

### Deodorant Skin Applications

Like antiperspirants, the market is flooded with deodorant preparations. They reduce the number of bacteria that live on the skin. Since these bacteria break down sweat, their reduction produces a reduction in body odor. Antiseptics such as hexachlorophene (p. 202 and Part III) and benzalkonium (p. 201 and Part III) are frequently used in deodorant preparations. Hexachlorophene may produce allergic skin rashes on sensitive skins, and benzalkonium and related complex ammonia compounds are inactivated by soap and can irritate the skin in concentrations above 1 percent. Some deodorants contain antibiotics which can also cause allergic reactions and sensitize the individual to their future use. In addition, people may become allergic to the perfume used in these preparations.

If you develop a rash in the areas where you apply a deodorant or antiperspirant, consider that it may be an allergic reaction and stop using it immediately.

It is a sad consequence of contemporary marketing that women (particularly young women) are persuaded to feel unclean if they do not use vaginal deodorants (feminine sprays and wipes). Such deodorants may mask uncleanliness and are potentially harmful. There is gathering evidence that pregnant women may run a risk from such applications. Drugs enter the bloodstream more easily from mucous surfaces such as the mouth, rectum, and vagina than they do from the skin. In pregnant women these drugs can enter the developing baby, and experiments have shown that hexachlorophene applied to rats' vaginas can damage unborn rats. Vaginal deodorants, particularly sprays, are best avoided because they may in addition cause irritation and bladder trouble (urethritis and cystitis). Stick to soap and water. Furthermore, we do not know enough about the long-term effects of the propellants used in such sprays.

## Other Drugs Used in Skin Applications

ALLANTOIN is used in preparations to treat psoriasis (Alphosyl lotion contains allantoin and coal tar extract in a nongreasy base). It is also used in Masse cream to treat diaper rash and cracked nipples.

CALAMINE is used as a mild astringent in creams, lotions, and dusting powder.

ANTHRALIN (dithranol) kills parasites and is used in small concentrations in ointments and pastes to treat psoriasis and other longstanding skin disorders. It can burn and stain the skin brown and cause allergic rashes in sensitized patients.

ICHTHAMMOL is slightly antibacterial and it irritates the skin. It has been used in skin applications to treat chronic skin disorders (e.g., eczema). Mixed with glycerin it was formerly in fashion as an application on superficial thrombophlebitis, and before antibiotics as a topical dressing on abscesses, and in infections of the ears.

IODOCHLORHYDROXYQUIN is used to treat bacterial and fungal infections of the skin. It has been used as a deodorant and for treating acne.

SALICYLIC ACID is used to treat hardened skin and corns.

SELENIUM SULFIDE is used to treat dandruff and other scalp disorders.

STARCH is used in dusting powders.

SULFUR is a mild antiseptic and has been used to treat acne and other disorders.

TALC is used as a dusting powder.

TAR is used to treat eczema and psoriasis.

ZINC OXIDE is used as a mild astringent (p. 205) and as a soothing agent and protective (pp. 194, 195).

These drugs appear in numerous proprietary preparations for the treatment of many skin disorders.

## Drugs Used to Treat Some Common Skin Disorders

If you have read this section very carefully you should be in a position to understand the treatment of most common skin disorders. However, I will give you a list of some commonly self-treated skin disorders and mention some (not all) of the various drugs which doctors use, bearing in mind that this book is about drugs and not specifically a book about treatments, although of course in many cases the drugs mentioned are the specific treatment.

ACNE (acne vulgaris). There is no specific treatment for acne, and it is best to use what suits you or to keep trying different preparations at intervals. Doctors often prescribe acne treatments which contain keratolytics (p. 205) to peel off the skin—sulfur, resorcinol, salicylic acid. Ultraviolet light may be used for this purpose, and some applications contain an abrasive. Many acne applications contain detergent antiseptics such as benzalkonium (see p. 201). These have been recommended for cleaning the face at night, as has hexachlorophene (p. 202). Antibiotics (e.g., erythromycin and neomycin) are also used (p. 199), and corticosteroids (p. 197) are often tried, especially mixed with an antibiotic (p. 198). A daily dose of a tetracycline antibiotic (p. 217) by mouth for several weeks is said to help, and trimethoprim-sulfamethoxazole and clindamycin have also been tried in a similar way.

ALLERGIC DRUG RASHES. Antihistamines by mouth (pp. 130–1) are effective with eruptions of the nettle-rash (urticaria) type. If the rash is severe, corticosteroids by mouth (p. 197) are indicated. Local soothing applications (p. 194) and cooling lotions are all that should be applied to the skin. Of course any drug should be stopped immediately if a skin rash develops.

ATHLETE'S FOOT *(Tinea pedis).* Read section on antifungal skin applications (p. 200) and, depending on how severe the case is, discuss treatment with your doctor. Athlete's foot can sometimes develop like an infected eczema (pp. 198, 209).

CHILBLAINS. Drugs used to increase the circulation (p. 94) are often not effective and not indicated. Local ointments containing irritants (p. 202) are of doubtful value; so too are vitamins, high doses of calcium, and high doses of calciferol (vitamin $D_2$) (Part III). Warm clothing is important. The best treatment has been preventative—central heating.

COLD SORES (herpes simplex). Treatment is usually disappointing. Local anesthetics (p. 204) and astringents (p. 205) have been tried. Antibiotics are of little effect. Claims have been made for idoxuridine (Part III), an antivirus drug used to treat eye ulcers. See warning about using corticosteroid applications (p. 197). A combination of a topical red dye and irradiation has been successful in some cases, but in animal tests the combination has resulted in the occurrence of precancerous cells, limiting its use.

CORNS. Applications used to treat corns usually contain a caustic or keratolytic (p. 205) such as salicylic acid, alum, acetic acid. Lead plaster mass is sometimes used as a protective.

CUTS AND ABRASIONS. Ordinary soap and water are satisfactory, but if you wish you may use an antiseptic cleaning preparation (p. 201).

DANDRUFF. Any detergent shampoo is of use, and there is no evidence that "medication" (p. 202) is of value. Doctors try keratolytics (p. 205) such as coal tar, sulfur, salicylic acid, and selenium sulfide. Detergent antiseptics such as benzalkonium are also used.

DIAPER RASH. Prevention is better than cure. Wash and rinse diapers well and periodically expose the baby's bottom to the fresh air for an hour or so. Any protective (p. 195) or soothing application (p. 194) may help prevent the rash—zinc cream and castor oil, or a barrier cream containing a silicone (p. 195). Detergent antiseptics such as benzalkonium (p. 201) may help if a rash has developed. For severe cases a preparation containing a corticosteroid and an anti-infective drug is useful (p. 198).

ECZEMA. Depending upon the acuteness, doctors use lotions, ointments, creams, or pastes. Soothing applications (p. 194), mild astringents (p. 205), mild keratolytics (p. 205), corticosteroids (p. 197), antibiotics (p. 199), and antifungal drugs (p. 200) may be used.

HAIR LOSS *(alopecia)*. There is no specific treatment. The vast majority of patients get better regardless of treatment.

HEMORRHOIDS. Preparations usually contain a mixture of an astringent (p. 205), a soothing application (p. 194), a local anesthetic (p. 204), and a local antiseptic (p. 201). Some contain a corticosteroid (p. 197). The choice is not critical. Sprays should be avoided. Read warning about using over-the-counter preparations (p. 38) before a definite diagnosis has been made by your doctor.

IMPETIGO. Treatment is specific. See p. 199.

INSECT BITES AND STINGS. Usually all that is needed is a cooling or soothing application (p. 194). An antihistamine cream (p. 204) may help, and a corticosteroid application (p. 197) is very effective. An antibiotic needs to be given by mouth if infection develops. If you are allergic to insect bites try an insect repellent containing diethyltoluamide alone or in combination with ethohexadiol, dimethylcarbate, butopyronoxyl, or dimethylphthalate, and carry antihistamine tablets (p. 131) with you.

MOUTH ULCERS. There are numerous nonspecific, ineffective treatments available. Doctors use applications containing a corticosteroid (p. 197) such as hydrocortisone, local anesthetic applications (p. 204), and local antiseptic applications (p. 201). Soothing applications (p. 194), astringents (p. 205), protectives (p. 195), antibiotics (p. 199), and antifungal applications (p. 200) have been tried. For thrush, nystatin is effective, and so is amphotericin. For a severe ulcerative condition of the mouth called herpes stomatitis (Vincent's disease), metronidazole (see Part III) is effective in tablet form.

PLANTAR WARTS. These are warts on the soles of the feet, and caustics (p. 205) are usually used to treat them. Three percent formalin solution foot soaks may be useful. Sometimes plantar warts must be removed surgically.

PSORIASIS. Depending upon the severity, acuteness, and extent of the rash, doctors use lotions, ointments, creams, and pastes. These may be soothing applications (p. 194), astringents (p. 205), keratolytics (p. 205), and corticosteroids (of the fluorinated type, p. 198). After the corticosteroids, tar (p. 207) and anthralin (p. 207) are the most commonly used drugs. Coal tar, which sensitizes the skin to ultraviolet light, is the basis of tar baths and sun-ray treatment in psoriasis. Airtight plastic dressings over corticosteroid creams have produced damage to the skin and other complications (p. 197).

SCABIES. See antiparasitic drug preparations (p. 200).

SUNBURN. See p. 196. These usually consist of cooling and/or soothing lotions (p. 194) such as calamine lotion and zinc lotion. Corticosteroid creams are effective (p. 197).

WARTS. If you believe a treatment will make a wart disappear, it may well do so. Most applications contain caustics or keratolytics (p. 205), e.g., acetic acid, salicylic acid, nitric acid, formaldehyde, and podophyllum. Skin specialists freeze warts off with liquid nitrogen or solid carbon dioxide, and some are removed surgically.

# ANTIBIOTICS

The term "anti-infective therapy" is used to describe drug treatment of infections by microorganisms (bacteria, viruses, and fungi), protozoa, and worms. Drugs from *all* sources (including synthetic) used to treat microorganic infection may be called antimicrobial drugs. Antibiotics are included in this group. Technically speaking, the term "antibiotic" (literally "a life-destroying substance") refers to drugs *obtained* from microorganisms, but in common use it is synonymous with antimicrobial, and will be so used here.

Antibiotics may be antibacterial and/or antifungal. They are chemicals which stop the growth of microorganisms (bacteriostatic) and/or eventually kill them (bactericidal). The numerous available antibiotics vary in structure, actions, effects, and the type of bacteria which are sensitive to them. They are produced by various microorganisms such as fungi and bacteria and have been obtained from molds, soil, and other sources. The chemical structure of some of them is known, and a few have been synthesized. Those produced from molds may be called biosynthetic, and those whose structure is modified by the addition of other chemicals to the growing medium are called semisynthetic.

An antibiotic may be tested by placing microorganisms in a liquid culture medium containing varying dilutions of the drug. Antibiotics are not effective against all microorganisms; some are effective against bacteria, others against fungi, some against many bacteria, some against only a few. The number of types of bacteria (or fungi) against which a particular antibiotic is effective is called its antibacterial (or antifungal) spectrum. If it is active against many types of bacteria, it is called a broad-spectrum antibiotic.

Bacteria may become resistant to an antibiotic even when it is used correctly. Generally, if resistance to one antibiotic from a group of antibiotics develops, there is a cross-resistance to other antibiotics in that group. The use of two or more antibiotics together may help to prevent the development of resistance. This is a technique frequently used in the treatment of tuberculosis, but not normally recommended in treating other disorders except where the two drugs act synergistically. Fixed-dose combination preparations are not recommended and can give a false sense of security when the dose of the effective drug is not sufficient.

Drug resistance may also be developed by microorganisms because of improper treatment. This may be the result of inappropriate doses and/or inappropriate intervals between doses, of failing to continue treatment long enough, and of inappropriate antibiotic combinations. Delay in starting antibiotics may affect response, and so will the response of the body to the infecting microorganism and to the drug. For example, pus cells destroy the antibiotic effects of sulfonamides, the acidity of the urine may change the effectiveness of certain antibiotics given to treat urinary infections, an abscess with tough walls will prevent antibiotics from getting into the abscess, and antibiotics may not be able to pass certain tissue barriers (for example, into the brain and eye). The drugs may also fail to be absorbed from the gut.

The "condition" of the patient will affect the choice of drug, as will the risk of allergic reactions in certain individuals. Factors such as age, genetic characteristics, general physical conditions (e.g., liver and kidney function), pregnancy, and other concurrent infections present may also affect the choice of an antibiotic drug. Furthermore, the patient's response to treatment and in particular his "defense mechanisms" against infections are very important; even when the antibiotics work, the body must eliminate the microorganisms.

Antibiotics may be used effectively to prevent the development of an infection if given just after exposure (e.g., high doses of penicillin after running the risk of getting gonorrhea) or if given to prevent recurrence of infection with a particular organism (e.g., to prevent certain types of tonsillitis). However, they have often been used for wrong reasons, causing many complications, as in their use to sterilize the gut before abdominal surgery, their use in premature babies, and their use to "prevent" bacterial infections in patients with virus infections.

Adverse effects produced by antibiotics are on the increase. This may be related to the increasing number of preparations available, and the increasing number of patients being treated. Antibiotics may produce specific adverse effects (for example, chloramphenicol may damage the bone marrow, neomycin may damage the kidneys), but in addition all antibiotics share two additional major adverse effects: the risk of allergic reactions and the risk of superinfections with other microorganisms.

Allergic reactions include anaphylactic shock, skin rashes, swollen face, fever and painful joints, bone marrow damage, and jaundice. Superinfections occur because many microorganisms live together in a balanced community in many parts of our bodies (nose, mouth, gut, skin, lungs, bladder, vagina). Any disturbance in this balance (as when an antibiotic knocks out a group of organisms) may lead to an overgrowth (superinfection) of other microorganisms—yeasts, fungi, bacteria, viruses. These are usually minor but may occasionally be very serious and on rare occasions fatal. They are difficult to treat and are more likely to occur with broad-spectrum antibiotics, in children under three years old, the elderly and/or debilitated, and patients with disorders such as diabetes and pulmonary infections.

Remember: Antibiotics are valuable drugs if used appropriately. Their effectiveness in treating some infections, however, does not mean that they should be used to treat all infections. They should not be used for minor self-limiting infections; they should be used in appropriate doses at appropriate intervals and for an appropriate length of time. They should not be used simply because they are new, particularly when safe, effective established alternatives are available. Finally, they should never be taken without medical advice. Never take antibiotics because "there were a few left in the house," or "because they did my neighbor good." Unless you and your doctor have decided that self-treatment with an antibiotic is appropriate for you, do not take them without advice and do not always expect them from your doctor.

## Antifungal Antibiotics

Most fungi in and on the body are harmless, but sometimes they may increase and spread to cause infections. For example, *Candida albicans* (which causes thrush in the mouth) lives "normally" on the skin, in the mouth, and in the gut alongside bacteria without causing any trouble—unless the bacteria happen to be killed off by antibiotics. Under these circumstances the fungus multiplies and the patient may develop thrush of the mouth, gut, anus, and vagina. Occasionally, in severely ill patients, this can spread to the lungs. Other factors may help to trigger fungal infections: diabetes, alcoholism, the use of steroids, and X-ray treatment.

Airborne spores (e.g., aspergillosis) may infect the lungs, and very rarely fungi may affect other organs. More commonly they may infect the scalp (scalp ringworm), groin *(Tinea cruris)*, feet (athlete's foot: *Finea pedis*), nails, and skin (ringworm: *Tinea circinata*).

A few antibiotics have antifungal effects. The three in common use are nystatin, griseofulvin, and amphotericin.

NYSTATIN stops the growth of fungi and is particularly effective against *Candida albicans*, but it has no effect on bacteria. Absorption from the gut is negligible, and it has few adverse effects.

GRISEOFULVIN stops the growth of most fungi. It is given by mouth, in a fine powdered form (in tablets), and it is fairly well absorbed from the gut. After absorption it is deposited in skin, hair, and nails and is effective in treating fungal infections of these tissues, particularly ringworm. Since it does not kill but simply stops growth, it has to be given for prolonged periods (up to one year in some cases) to treat infections of hair and nails. Its use should therefore be appropriate; it should not be used to treat minor infections. It should not be taken by patients with latent porphyria, and it is important to remember that it may increase the effects of alcohol.

AMPHOTERICIN is active against a range of fungi similar to that of nystatin, but it is more active against yeastlike fungi. It is poorly absorbed from the gut. Its use is reserved for severe fungal infections, when it is given by slow intravenous infusion. The injection site should be changed frequently, and tests of kidney function should be carried out at frequent intervals. It may be used in ointments, which occasionally cause irritation, itching, and skin rash. It is also available as lozenges for fungal mouth and throat infections.

Other antifungal drugs include candicidin, chlordantoin, chlorphenesin, miconazole, benzoic acid, flucytosine, glyceryl triacetate, acrisorcin, diiodochlorhydroxyquin, nitrofurazone, gentian violet, propionic acid (used in foods as a preservative), sodium propionate, tolnaftate, and undecylenic acid and clotrimazole. These are all mainly used for local applications as powders, sprays, creams, drops, and vaginal suppositories.

## Penicillins

Penicillin was the first antibiotic to be produced, by growing *Penicillium* mold on broth. It became available for use in 1941. The original crude extracts of the fermentation of the mold contained several penicillins. By adding various chemicals to the fermentation, several naturally produced penicillins have been developed. These include benzathine penicillin G, penicillin G (benzylpenicillin), and procaine penicillin G. In addition the chemical structure of the penicillin may be altered to produce what are called *semisynthetic* penicillins. They are not wholly synthetic; the basic penicillin structure is still obtained from molds by fermentation. These include amoxicillin, ampicillin, carbenicillin, cloxacillin, dicloxacillin, methicillin, nafcillin, oxacillin, penicillin V (phenoxymethylpenicillin), phenethicillin, and several others.

These products are all known as penicillins, and benzylpenicillin is often taken as the main example of the group. The semisynthetic penicillins have an advantage over penicillin G because most of them are more resistant to the acid in the stomach and are more effective by mouth; some of them are active against many more types of bacteria (broad-spectrum), and some are effective against bacteria which have developed a resistance to benzylpenicillin. However, it is important to remember that when bacteria *are* sensitive to penicillin G or penicillin V, the other semisynthetic penicillins are *not* as effective. Furthermore, they are usually more expensive—an important point to remember when treating tonsillitis.

Penicillins damage the developing cell walls of multiplying bacteria, making them burst. They therefore kill bacteria (they are *bactericidal*), but only when the bacteria are multiplying. Other antibiotics (for example, tetracyclines) interfere with bacterial growth and are called *bacteriostatic*. It follows that if a tetracycline and a penicillin are given together they will *antagonize* each other, theoretically making each other less effective. However, depending on its concentration, any penicillin or other antibiotic may be both bacteriostatic and bactericidal.

Bacteria may become resistant to the effects of penicillin in two ways. They may produce enzymes which inactivate the penicillin—the best known of these is called *penicillinase*. In addition, some bacteria develop a tolerance to penicillin (resistance) and just go on multiplying in the presence of doses which would previously have killed them. Development of resistance has often been related to the indiscriminate use of penicillins, and it is a serious risk, particularly in surgical wards of hospitals. Fortunately, some of the semisynthetic penicillins— methicillin, cloxacillin, and dicloxacillin, for instance—are resistant to penicillinase.

Allergic reactions to penicillin are not uncommon. When penicillin is given to a patient who has become hypersensitive, an allergic reaction may occur—skin rashes, swelling of the face and throat, fever, and swollen joints. Anaphylactic shock (see p. 128), which is very rare, may be followed by death. It is more common after injections and in patients who have previously had an allergic reaction to oral or parenteral

penicillin. Penicillin sensitivity may also be produced by skin ointments, ear drops, eye drops, and throat lozenges, although most of
these preparations are no longer available. It may follow the handling
of penicillin, breathing it, and drinking milk from cows treated with
penicillin for mastitis. For these reasons, penicillin should not be used
in topical applications or throat lozenges. The latter may also produce
a sore tongue, mouth, and lips and also a black furry coating on the
tongue. Ampicillin produces a skin rash in patients suffering from
glandular fever or chronic lymphatic leukemia. All penicillins may
cause diarrhea, nausea, heartburn, or pruritus ani.

Penicillins are incredibly safe drugs. Adverse effects are more likely
to occur because of errors in prescribing than from any other cause.
Remember that cross-allergy to penicillin occurs, and if you are allergic
to one (say, penicillin V) you may be allergic to another (e.g., ampicillin). Skin testing for allergy is not always useful because the allergy
is thought (at least in some cases) to be due to the breakdown products
of penicillin in the body rather than to the penicillin drug. Also some
people consider the substances produced during manufacturing (and
included in the preparation) to be a cause of allergy to a penicillin
preparation. The proper combination of skin tests is probably useful
in detecting those patients who are likely to have a life-threatening
anaphylactic reaction. Manufacturing-process contaminants may also
have accounted for other symptoms such as diarrhea.

Penicillins should not be taken for trivial infections or by patients
who have had a previous allergic reaction. They should be taken with
caution by patients who have had an allergic reaction to any other
drug. They provide us with a range of very valuable antibiotics which
if used appropriately are very effective.

The dosage varies according to the penicillin used, the route of
administration, the disorder being treated, and the patient. Penicillin
G is best given by injection, procaine penicillin G (which is longer-
acting) is given by intramuscular injection, penicillin V by mouth.
Methicillin, cloxacillin, and dicloxacillin are active against penicillinase-producing resistant bacteria; they may be given by injection
(cloxacillin and dicloxacillin may be given by mouth) but should be
strictly reserved for treating such resistant infections. Ampicillin is
usually taken by mouth except in serious infections when it is given
intravenously. It has become widely prescribed for upper and lower
respiratory infections, urinary infections such as cystitis, and other
infections.

## Cephalosporins

The cephalosporins are produced from a basic penicillinlike nucleus. Several of them are in use—cephaloridine, cephapirin, cephradine, cephalothin, cefazolin, cephaloglycin, and cephalexin. They act on the same groups of bacteria as do the natural penicillins, but so far they are relatively resistant to penicillinase. They also act on a broad spectrum of bacteria in the same way as does ampicillin, and are effective against some bacteria which are resistant to ampicillin. They may produce allergic reactions, and in some patients cross-allergy may occur between cephalosporins and some penicillins. Cross-resistance may be shown to cephalosporins by bacteria resistant to methicillin and cloxacillin.

Cephalexin and cephradine may be given by mouth. Their absorption from the stomach and gut may be delayed by food. Cephaloglycin is taken by mouth and has been used principally to treat urinary infections. This preparation is no longer recommended. Cephaloridine, cephalothin, cefazolin, and cephapirin are given by injection. They all may produce blood disorders; cephaloridine may cause kidney damage and is seldom used.

Some cephalosporins are being extensively promoted. Their use should, nevertheless, be restricted to selected cases in which sensitivity tests have been carried out on the infecting organisms.

## Macrolide Antibiotics and the Lincomycin Series

These include erythromycin, oleandomycin, lincomycin, and clindamycin. The first two are known as macrolide antibiotics. They are active against roughly the same narrow group of bacteria sensitive to the natural penicillins. They are bacteriostatic. They may be of use in treating tissue infections caused by bacteria resistant to the natural penicillins, or in cases in which the patient is allergic to penicillins. Erythromycin has been the most widely used of the group, but bacteria quickly became resistant to it, especially if it is given for more than one week. Its use has been replaced by other antibiotics in many cases.

The macrolide and lincomycin series of antibiotics may cause diarrhea (particularly lincomycin and clindamycin), liver damage, blood disorders, and allergy (fever and skin rashes). Erythromycin estolate may cause liver damage with jaundice and fever if it is given for more than two weeks, particularly with a second course of treatment. This adverse effect is thought to be allergic, and clears up when the drug is stopped. Bacteria may develop some cross-resistance to these drugs. The macrolide antibiotics are inactivated by the acid in the stomach and have to be given in acid-resistant capsules, as specially covered (enteric-coated) tablets, as their esters (e.g., erythromycin estolate), or as their stearate. Oleandomycin is more toxic and seldom used. Lincomycin and clindamycin may cause a potentially life-threatening inflammation of the bowel. While this occurs with other antibiotics as well, the incidence appears to be higher with these two, and their use should be restricted to the limited number of infections for which they are clearly the drugs of choice. Taken orally, lincomycin is poorly absorbed, while clindamycin is almost completely absorbed.

## Tetracyclines

The first tetracycline to be discovered was aureomycin, in 1948. It was grown from molds. Another one, called terramycin, was discovered in 1950. Two years later their chemical structure was determined and it was found to consist of a basic structure of four rings (tetracyclic). They were therefore called tetracyclines, and the generic name chlortetracycline was given to aureomycin, and oxytetracycline to terramycin. Aureomycin and Terramycin remained as brand names. Oxytetracycline is also available under numerous other brand names. Since the fifties numerous tetracyclines have been produced and tested, but only a few have proved to be of value. These include demeclocycline (demethylchlortetracycline), tetracycline, doxycycline, methacycline, and minocycline.

The tetracyclines have the broadest spectrum of activity against bacteria of any antibiotics, but some bacteria are now resistant to them. One of the problems with the tetracyclines is that they are only partially absorbed from the gut and enough goes on to reach the lower bowel and affect the normal organisms which live there. This may alter the balance between bacteria and fungi and lead to a superinfection with thrush which can affect the mouth, bowel, anus, and vulva, producing soreness and irritation. A more serious risk in hospitals is the development of tetracycline-resistant bacteria, which may cause severe enteritis and, in rare cases, death. This complication is more likely to follow the use of tetracycline during abdominal operations. These superinfections may also affect the lungs.

Absorption of tetracyclines from the gut may be decreased by interaction with calcium, iron, and magnesium salts when these are taken at the same time. Milk, alkalis, and aluminum hydroxide (as found in many antacid preparations) have the same effect—none should be taken at the same time as tetracycline, or its absorption will be decreased and the desired therapeutic effects will not be achieved. Absorption is similarly reduced by food, with the exceptions of doxycycline and minocycline. *Every container of tetracyclines should carry a date beyond which the capsules should not be used,* due to the toxicity of tetracycline breakdown products. Demeclocycline (demethylchlortetracycline), doxycycline, and minocycline are better absorbed than the other tetracyclines. Tetracyclines are excreted in the urine and in the bile. Doxycycline is excreted primarily via the bile and hence is the safest tetracycline to use in case of renal failure. Since its excretory products are largely inactive, it has less effect on the natural bowel bacteria than other tetracyclines, and accordingly a lesser incidence of superinfection.

Very rarely, tetracyclines given by injection may produce severe liver damage (sometimes fatal), particularly when given to pregnant women with infections of their kidneys. Tetracyclines are deposited in growing teeth, producing discoloration and staining in young children. Not only the first set of teeth is affected; the adult teeth may also be stained for life, and there is an added risk of tooth decay. They are also deposited in bone, and bone growth stops during tetracycline treatment. These effects on teeth and bone may occur before the baby is born (if the mother is given tetracyclines) and right on into childhood. Therefore they should be avoided in pregnancy and preferably not given to children under seven or eight years of age. They may discolor nails at any age if taken over a prolonged period. Allergic reactions, including blood disorders, to tetracycline drugs are rare. Sensitivity of the skin to sunlight may occur in patients receiving demeclocycline; this is less likely with the others. A delay in blood coagulation has been noted in some patients.

Tetracyclines may affect protein production in the body, and also kidney function. These are indicated by a rise in the blood levels of breakdown products of proteins (e.g., as estimated by blood urea levels). Urea and other waste products are excreted by the kidneys, and this may have no consequence if the kidneys are healthy. However, if their function is impaired, these waste products may accumulate in the blood, producing loss of appetite, vomiting, and weakness. This is called kidney failure, and it may occur unexpectedly in elderly patients who are given tetracycline, usually for a chest infection. Doxycycline, which needs to be given only once a day, is said to affect impaired kidneys less than other tetracyclines.

## Streptomycin and Other Aminoglycosides

Streptomycin was discovered in soil in 1944. Other, less toxic, chemically related antibiotics have since been discovered. They include gentamicin, neomycin, tobramycin, kanamycin, and paromomycin. They are bactericidal against a wide spectrum of bacteria responsible for serious infections. Bacteria quickly develop resistance to streptomycin and less quickly to its relatives. Those bacteria resistant to neomycin and kanamycin are also resistant to streptomycin, but the reverse is not necessarily true.

These antibiotics are poorly absorbed from the gut and have to be given by intramuscular or intravenous injection. They are quickly excreted by the kidneys, and impaired kidney function may lead to dangerously high blood levels. They are painful when given by injection, and their principal adverse effects include deafness (which may be permanent) and disorders of the organ of balance due to damage to the main nerve which supplies the ear and organ of balance. They may also damage the kidneys and affect nerve muscle junctions, producing muscle weakness and depression of respiration.

These adverse effects are more likely to occur with high doses, prolonged courses of treatment, in patients over middle age, and in patients with impaired kidney function. Allergic reactions may occur, particularly with streptomycin, which may also cause severe allergic skin reactions in those handling the drug (for example, nurses). Anyone handling the drug should be very cautious and wear gloves.

Streptomycin is used to treat tuberculosis in combination with other drugs such as ethambutol and/or isoniazid. It is also used to treat plague. Kanamycin has been used to treat tuberculosis but is now generally reserved for other serious infections. Neomycin, streptomycin, and kanamycin, because they are not significantly absorbed from the gut, are also used orally to treat gastroenteritis. However, their use should be restricted to specific infections, and their widespread use in antidiarrheal mixtures is not recommended (see "Anti-infective Drugs," p. 81, under Drugs Used to Treat Diarrhea). Neomycin is present in numerous eye, ear, and skin applications, and as such is frequently a cause of allergic reactions, primarily skin rashes.

Gentamicin may be related to neomycin. It is active against a wide spectrum of bacteria, has to be given by intramuscular injection, and may damage the kidneys and the main nerves to the ear, causing disorders of balance. It is also used in local applications. Tobramycin is a new antibiotic similar to gentamicin. It is primarily reserved for infections resistant to gentamicin.

## Polypeptide Antibiotics

POLYMYXINS are a group of antibiotics including polymyxin A, B, C, D, and E (colistin). Two are in use, polymyxin B and colistin (polymyxin E). They are not yet available in a pure state, and therefore the dose is measured in units of activity per milligram of weight. They are used to treat certain infections and in skin applications. Polymyxins are poorly absorbed from the gut, and even with injections it is difficult to get a high blood level. Therefore, large doses must be used. They may produce kidney damage and affect nerve muscle junctions, producing muscle weakness and depression of respiration. After injection, polymyxin B may produce mild adverse effects on the nervous system —dizziness and sensory disturbances over the face, hands, and feet.

BACITRACIN is chemically related to the polymyxins. It is mainly used in eye, ear, and skin applications. It may be used to prepare the gut for surgical operations. Bacitracin is usually combined with other antibiotics (see under Drugs Used to Treat Skin Disorders, p. 199). It is not absorbed from the gut, and like the polymyxins it may produce serious kidney damage if given by injection. Kidney damage has also occurred when bacitracin has been used locally in abdominal operations. Very rarely, it may produce allergic reactions after application to the skin.

## Other Antibiotics

RIFAMYCINS. Several have been produced, but only one, rifampin, is used. Rifampin is used primarily to treat tuberculosis. It has also (because it is excreted in the bile) been used to treat gall bladder infections. Adverse effects include nausea and occasionally jaundice, blood disorders, and allergic reactions. It should not be used during the first three months of pregnancy. Rifampin is taken orally, preferably on an empty stomach.

CHLORAMPHENICOL was the first broad-spectrum antibiotic to be discovered. It was introduced in 1947 and soon became widely promoted and prescribed. Its indiscriminate use for minor infections has led to unnecessary deaths from bone marrow damage. It is a valuable drug for treating typhoid fever and certain types of meningitis. Its potentially fatal toxicity precludes its use in all but serious infections resistant to other, less toxic antibiotics. It is also used in eye, ear, and skin applications.

VANCOMYCIN is too toxic to be used routinely and should be reserved for treating serious infections resistant to other antibiotics. It is not absorbed from the gut and has to be given by intravenous injections which may be painful and produce thrombophlebitis. Average doses may produce fever and skin rashes. Large doses or prolonged doses may produce irreversible deafness and kidney damage.

## Sulfonamides

Sulfonamides are synthetic antimicrobial drugs and by technical definition not antibiotics. However, they are usually discussed along with antibiotics.

In 1935 it was found that the dye prontosil red protected mice from streptococcal infections and that the active antibacterial agent in the body was a breakdown product of the red dye called sulfanilamide.

Following this discovery hundreds of similar drugs have been produced and tested for antibacterial activity. They belong to the sulfonamide group and they prevent bacteria from multiplying by competing with them for a vitamin called folic acid which is essential for their cell nutrition. The most frequently used are sulfadiazine, sulfisoxazole, sulfamethoxazole, sulfathiazole, and a combination of a sulfonamide (sulfamethoxazole) with trimethoprim.

The sulfa drugs, as they are colloquially called, do not differ very much from one another in their antibacterial effects upon particular bacteria. However, their effects in the body vary quite substantially according to how well they are absorbed from the gut, their distribution throughout the body, and the rate at which they are excreted in the urine. They reach a high concentration in the urine, and some are very useful for treating urinary infections, particularly since they may be given in a smaller dosage than that required for other infections.

They have a wide range of antibacterial activity, but sulfonamide-resistant strains of bacteria are frequent, particularly in hospitals. They are made ineffective by pus and dead tissue. Except for succinylsulfathiazole and phthalylsulfathiazole, they are well absorbed from the gut. Their rates of excretion in the urine determine the intervals of time between doses. According to their degree of absorption from the gut and the rate of excretion in the urine, they may be divided into several groups.

Those that are poorly absorbed from the gut and are used to treat infections of the gut include phthalylsulfathiazole and succinylsulfathiazole. Development of bacterial-resistant strains, systemic side effects, and interference with the synthesis of clotting factors limits their usefulness.

Long-acting types which may be given just once a day are sulfadimethoxine, sulfamethoxydiazine, and sulfamethoxypyridazine.

Those which are well absorbed and need to be given every 8 to 12 hours are sulfamethoxazole and sulfaphenazole.

Those which are well absorbed and rapidly excreted in the urine and need to be given every 6 to 8 hours include sulfadiazine, sulfamethazine, sulfisoxazole, sulfamethiazole, and sulfathiazole.

Adverse effects from sulfonamides are common and vary according to the particular drug used. They are more related to duration of treatment than to the dosage used. They include loss of appetite, nausea, vomiting, fever, drowsiness, and a decline in mental alertness. Alteration of the respiratory pigment in red blood cells may occur, producing blueness (cyanosis) and headache, mental depression, and diarrhea. Some older sulfonamides may form crystals in the urine (crystalluria) and produce kidney damage. Initially, this may cause pain in the kidneys, pain on passing urine, and blood in the urine. In some cases it may completely knock out the production of urine by the kidneys. This is a rare complication with the newer, more soluble sulfonamides. Allergic reactions are common and include skin rashes, fever, and aching joints. Sulfonamides should not be applied to the skin, because they easily produce sensitization. Allergic reactions are more likely to occur late in treatment or when starting a repeat course of a sulfonamide. You should be cautious about taking another sulfonamide if you have had a previous reaction, even though cross-sensitization between the various sulfonamides does not always occur. Continued treatment in someone who is allergic may produce serious artery damage (polyarteritis nodosa). Sulfonamides may also produce sensitivity of the skin to sunshine, which may cause a severe dermatitis. Sulfonamides (particularly long-acting ones) in rare cases produce a serious disorder, with skin rashes and ulcers of the mouth (Stevens-Johnson syndrome), which may be fatal. In view of this toxicity, the long-acting sulfonamides should be used with caution. Rarely, liver damage may occur and prove fatal. With courses of treatment extending for more than seven to ten days blood disorders due to bone marrow damage may occur. Therefore, it is advisable to have frequent blood tests when on prolonged treatment with sulfonamides.

Because of the risk of kidney damage from crystalluria, it is necessary to drink plenty of fluids when on sulfonamides. This is particularly true if you are in the tropics where you lose a lot of fluid through sweating. It also helps if the urine is kept alkaline by taking sodium citrate or sodium bicarbonate solution. There is less risk of crystalluria with the slowly excreted sulfonamides. Sulfonamides should not be used in patients with impaired kidney function. Their use should be avoided in premature babies and in babies during their first few weeks of life because they displace bile pigments from the blood proteins to produce jaundice. They should also be avoided when childbirth is a few days off.

With the newer sulfonamides, adverse reactions are fewer, but kidney damage, allergic reactions, and blood disorders may be produced by any of them.

### Combinations of Sulfamethoxazole with Trimethoprim

Trimethoprim is a wide-spectrum antibacterial drug which interferes with the metabolism of bacterial cells at a stage just after the one which sulfonamides block. The use of trimethoprim and a sulfonamide (sulfamethoxazole) together, therefore, successfully blocks two vital processes in the cellular development of bacteria. This is an example of one drug potentiating the action of another by acting synergistically.

While sulfonamides alone are bacteriostatic, this combination is bactericidal. It is well absorbed when taken by mouth. Sulfamethoxazole is absorbed and excreted at a rate similar to that of trimethoprim, so that after a few days the ratio of the two drugs in the bloodstream and urine is kept relatively constant. The combination reaches satisfactory blood levels about one hour after absorption, reaching a peak in two to four hours, which lasts for up to seven or eight hours and then tapers off by the time about 24 hours has elapsed. One important point about this combination is that the tissue levels in target organs such as the kidneys or lungs are higher than the blood levels. It is of particular use in treating urinary infections, and it may be used in typhoid fever. Trimethoprim-sulfamethoxazole contains two drugs, so bacterial sensitivity to *each* drug should be tested. It should be used only if the bacteria are sensitive to *both* drugs.

# DRUGS USED
# TO TREAT INFECTIONS
# OF THE URINARY SYSTEM

A wide range of bacteria may infect the urinary tract to produce infection of the kidneys (pyelonephritis), the bladder (cystitis), and the outlet from the bladder (urethritis). Equally, there is a wide range of effective drugs available to treat these infections—sulfonamides, trimethoprim-sulfamethoxazole, cephalosporins, tetracyclines, and semisynthetic penicillins such as ampicillin. For infections resistant to these there are the other reserve antibiotics discussed earlier. The dose will depend on many factors: the severity of the infection, the type of infecting bacteria, the condition of the patient, and particularly the state of the patient's kidney function. Doses of antibiotics needed to treat lower urinary tract infections (urethritis and cystitis) will be smaller than those needed for general infections, because the drugs selected are those that concentrate in the urine. Doses to treat infection in the kidneys need to be the same as those used in treating general infections.

With urinary tract infections it helps to drink plenty of fluids (two quarts a day) and urinate often. Also, the acidity of the urine may affect the effectiveness of an antibiotic. It is worth making the urine acid if you are taking tetracyclines, nitrofurantoin, or semisynthetic penicillins. Urine should preferably be made alkaline if you are taking (for example) streptomycin, erythromycin, lincomycin, or gentamicin. The decision to make your urine acid or alkaline (by taking certain acid or alkaline salts) depends upon how well your kidneys are functioning. This is a decision for your doctor.

Much trouble is caused through inadequate treatment of urinary infections. With first attacks a full course of appropriate antibiotic should be taken for ten days, after the urine has been examined. With the second and all subsequent attacks, the urine should be reexamined to determine the infecting organism and the appropriate antibiotic should be selected and taken for at least two to three weeks. With recurrent attacks (chronic cystitis) full investigations are necessary, as well as obvious precautions such as not using such potential irritants as vaginal deodorants, particularly sprays. In chronic cystitis, treatment after relief of acute symptoms should continue for up to three months or more, usually at a reduced maintenance dose of the antibiotic used to treat the acute attack or in selected cases by using a urinary antiseptic such as nitrofurantoin, methenamine, or one of its salts. (See individual drugs in Part III.) These urinary antiseptics are generally active only in acidic urine.

# DRUGS USED
# TO TREAT TUBERCULOSIS

The drug treatment of tuberculosis has taught doctors a lot about how to use antibiotics and other anti-infective drugs, especially in terms of effectiveness tests and an understanding of the dangers involved in long-term drug use. In particular, through the efforts of tuberculosis specialists—and their mistakes—we have learned much about how infecting organisms can develop resistance to drugs and how individuals and groups of people can vary in their response to drug treatment.

The bacteria which cause tuberculosis can easily develop resistance to antituberculosis drugs, so treatment is now considered in two separate categories—*before* the development of bacterial resistance, and *after*.

The drugs used in initial treatment are often referred to as primary antituberculosis drugs. Because resistance develops to all antituberculosis drugs if they are given singly, initial treatment in severe infections always involves the use of three drugs in combination followed by two drugs in combination for continuing long-term treatment. Two-drug combination treatment begins after tests show which two drugs are most effective against the organisms. But these sensitivity tests may take up to three months. For safety during this period, three drugs in combination are nearly always used as an interim treatment. For mild infections, two drugs in combination are often considered adequate.

The primary drugs used to treat tuberculosis are ethambutol, isoniazid (INH, isonicotinic acid hydrazide) and rifampin.

If there is evidence that the infecting bacteria are developing resistance to the primary drugs, secondary (reserve) drug treatment becomes necessary. Since secondary drugs usually produce more adverse effects than the primary ones, the decision on which ones to use requires great knowledge about the patient, the stage of his illness, and the drugs to be used. Secondary antituberculosis drugs include streptomycin (see p. 218), capreomycin, cycloserine, aminosalicylic acid (para-aminosalicylic acid, PAS; or its calcium or sodium salts), ethionamide, kanamycin, pyrazinamide, and viomycin. Isoniazid may also be used in conjunction with secondary drugs.

A common regimen in tuberculosis of the lung starts with an INH ethambutol or INH rifampin combination, although some doctors prefer to reserve rifampin for resistant cases. Streptomycin is usually added as a third drug in more serious infections until the infection is under control. In some cases, INH alone may be the initial treatment.

Modifications of such regimens are necessary according to the resistance patterns, type of tuberculosis bacterium, and condition of the patient.

# DRUGS USED
# TO TREAT CANCER

Cancer is a disorder of cell growth which may affect any tissue or organ. Treatment of cancer is aimed at reducing or stopping this disordered growth. Drugs are becoming increasingly useful for this purpose because not only is it possible to prolong the life of many patients suffering from various types of cancer but drugs can also make life much more comfortable. There are many different types and stages of cancer, so it is difficult to generalize about treatment. Furthermore, the drugs are very complex and their use is always changing as new advances are made. Drug treatment of cancer should always be in the hands of experts who understand the disorder being treated and the effects of the drugs being used.

Anticancer drug treatment (often called chemotherapy) does not attack cancer cells selectively and may damage noncancer cells. Therefore, in no drug treatment is it more important to balance the expected benefits with the predictable risks. Naturally, all the basic principles of drug use apply to the treatment of cancer—the results of treatment will depend upon the physical and psychological state of the patient and upon the functioning of such vital organs as the kidneys and liver. In addition, many anticancer drugs damage the bone marrow, thus affecting red and white blood cell production. The condition of the blood and bone marrow must be watched carefully while the patient is being treated with such drugs, and special facilities for extra support may be needed—for example, blood transfusions in case of anemia and special precautions against infection if the drugs damage the production of white blood cells. These contingencies indicate even more strongly the need for highly specialized care.

There are several groups of anticancer drugs which interfere with cell division. One commonly used group called alkylating agents produces a chemical effect inside cells, interfering with cell division and thus causing serious damage to actively dividing noncancer cells, particularly in the bone marrow, skin, the cells lining the stomach and gut, and in the unborn baby. Many of them (e.g., cyclophosphamide) reduce the body's resistance to infection, and so special precautions against infection are necessary. Different alkylating agents act differently on different cells, thus producing a great deal of variation in susceptibility to them.

Alkylating anticancer drugs include busulfan, carmustine (BCNU), chlorambucil, dacarbazine, melphalan, streptozotocin, thiotepa, and uracil mustard.

Another group of anticancer drugs are called antimetabolites because they interfere with the normal chemical processes inside cells by combining with enzymes. Enzymes are substances produced by living cells which promote chemical changes, and by combining with them the drugs thus block cell functions—including cell division. Drugs are available which block the effect of any one of three enzymes which use either folic acid, purine, or pyrimidine as building blocks. They are therefore known as folic acid antagonists, purine antagonists, and pyrimidine antagonists. They are used to treat leukemias and have produced dramatic and long-lasting cures in the treatment of choriocarcinoma (a cancer which develops from the tissues of an unborn baby). They may damage actively dividing noncancer cells, producing damage to bone marrow, to the gut lining, and to the unborn baby. Pyrimidine antagonists may also damage the lining of the mouth, damage the nails, and produce loss of hair. Folic acid antagonists may interfere with the body's immune response to infection and to the introduction of foreign tissue. Because of the latter characteristic they are used to help prevent rejection of organ transplants.

Antimetabolites include folic acid antagonists (methotrexate); purine antagonists (mercaptopurine, azathioprine, and thioguanine); and pyrimidine antagonists (fluorouracil, floxuridine, and cytarabine).

Other anticancer drugs are natural products. Extracts from the periwinkle plant yield two of them—vinblastine and vincristine. Their action is probably connected with their tendency to bind with a key protein, interfering with cell division and thus reducing the growth of certain cancers. They can damage bone marrow and cause loss of hair, and both may damage nerve tissue. Vincristine is less toxic than vinblastine. Another naturally occurring product is called l-asparaginase. It is found in guinea pig serum and is also produced by bacteria called *E. coli*. It may cause fever, allergic reactions, liver damage, blood clotting disorders, and nerve damage. It is used to treat leukemia. Some antibiotics have a controlling effect on certain cancers; these drugs include dactinomycin (actinomycin D), daunorubicin (daunomycin), doxorubicin, mithramycin, and bleomycin.

Various other anticancer agents include hydroxyurea, mitotane, and procarbazine. In addition, corticosteroids (p. 159) and sex hormones (pp. 163, 166) are used for certain cancers; so also are radioactive isotopes such as that of iodine.

Certain anticancer drugs, including azathioprine, cyclophosphamide, dactinomycin, mercaptopurine, and thioguanine, are also (or even mainly) immunosuppressants and are used to suppress rejection after organ transplants and in the treatment of other disorders.

# DRUGS USED
# TO TREAT MALARIA

Malaria is caused by four species of *Plasmodium* protozoa: *P. vivax, P. falciparum, P. malariae,* and *P. ovale.* These parasites are spread by certain female mosquitoes that feed on human blood. The mosquito picks up the infection by drinking blood from an infected person in whom both female and male parasite sporelike bodies are present. These become fertilized in the stomach of the mosquito and then find their way to its salivary gland. When a mosquito with developing "spores" in its salivary glands bites a human, that person is in turn infected with malaria.

The parasites enter the human bloodstream, quickly settling in the liver, where they multiply and grow. After a period of five and a half to sixteen days hundreds of new baby parasites are released into the bloodstream. They enter the red blood cells, and here they continue to divide. Finally the infected red cells burst, releasing hundreds more baby parasites which again enter further red cells and the cycle continues. Some of these parasites develop into sexual forms, both female and male, and then circulate in the bloodstream. When a mosquito bites that person, the blood containing female and male "spores" enters its stomach and the cycle begins again.

After infection from a mosquito "bite" the individual feels no symptoms while the parasites are dividing and growing in the liver. As they are released into the bloodstream (the so-called "blood stage"), the patient develops shivering, fever, and headaches. In *vivax* infections these fevers occur every 48 hours (benign tertian malaria), in *falciparum* the fever is usually continuous, and in *malariae* malaria it recurs every 72 hours (quartan malaria). Between the fevers the patient often feels well, except for weakness.

CAUSAL PROPHYLAXIS. The aim is to try to kill the parasites as soon after infection as possible and before they enter the liver. This means that drugs have to be taken continuously whenever an individual is in an infected area. However, there are no drugs safe enough to do this. The drugs used, chloroguanide and pyrimethamine, are markedly effective against *falciparum* parasites, but only partially effective against *vivax*.

SUPPRESSIVE TREATMENT. The aim of suppressive drug treatment is to try to stop the "blood stage" development of the parasites, thus keeping the individual free from chills and fevers. Suppressive treatment does not stop infection and drugs have to be taken during the period of exposure to infection and for several weeks afterward. *Falciparum* infections usually respond well to suppressive drugs, whereas *vivax* may relapse when the drugs are stopped. The drugs most commonly used for suppression of symptoms are chloroquine, chloroguanide, and pyrimethamine. Quinine is also effective in relieving symptoms.

CLINICAL CURE. The two drugs most commonly used in treating symptoms are chloroquine and amodiaquine. These are very effective against *vivax* and *falciparum*.

RADICAL CURE. A combination of chloroquine and primaquine is used to get a radical cure from *vivax* malaria, but only when the individual has left the infected area and is free from the risk of reinfection. To produce a radical cure of *falciparum* malaria, suppressive drugs (e.g., chloroquine, chloroguanide, or pyrimethamine) should be continued for at least one week after exposure to malaria. The use of pyrimethamine for ten weeks after exposure can cure *vivax* malaria.

# DRUGS USED TO TREAT WORM INFECTIONS

Some worm infections (such as pinworm infections) may be harmless and produce nothing more than an itchy anus, while others may be very serious and produce convulsions by invading the brain (as in the case of tapeworm). Parasitic worms (or helminths) may infect the gut and many tissues throughout the body. Thus, while pinworm infection is easy to diagnose and treat, some infections are very difficult to diagnose. For this reason people with the more serious forms of worm infection should always be in the hands of experts experienced in diagnosis and treatment. Furthermore, some of the drugs used to treat worm infections can produce serious adverse effects.

Drugs used to treat patients suffering from worm infections are usually referred to as antihelmintics. Other anti-infective drugs may also be used in treatment.

There have been many advances in drug treatment of worm and fluke infections in recent years, and the drugs commonly used include bephenium, dichlorophen, diethylcarbamazine, bycanthone, levamisole, mebendazole, niclosamide, niridazole, piperazine, pyrantel, pyrvinium, tetrachloroethylene, thiabendazole, and antimony compounds.

In the event of less serious infections, piperazine or pyrantel is used to treat roundworm; mebendazole or thiabendazole to treat whipworm; bephenium, pyrantel, or thiabendazole to treat hookworm; thiabendazole or pyrvinium to treat threadworm; and pyrantel, piperazine, or pyrvinium to treat pinworm.

# DRUGS USED
# TO TREAT AMEBIASIS

Amebiasis is caused by infection with organisms called *Entamoeba histolytica*. These organisms secrete a substance which forms a protective envelope (cyst) around themselves. Inside these cysts the cells divide usually into four cells. When the cysts are swallowed they burst, releasing their cells, which continue to live and divide inside the large bowel, where they form further cysts. It is estimated that about one in every ten people throughout the world has amoebic cysts in his gut. Infection is associated with poverty and poor sanitation. The cysts, which may survive for months in water, are passed on from human to human. Food is the most common vehicle of infection, and only the cystic stage is infective. It is spread principally by human feces, but waterborne infections do occur.

Infections may cause dysentery, ulcers of the bowel, and peritonitis, and the infection may invade the liver to produce hepatitis and liver abscesses. Patients who are pregnant are very susceptible to invasion of the tissues by amoebic organisms, and so also are patients on anticancer drugs and corticosteroids.

Drugs used to treat amebiasis include emetine, dehydroemetine, and metronidazole (which has revolutionized treatment). Other drugs used are antibiotics, chloroquine, organic arsenics, diiodohydroxyquin, and iodochlorhydroxyquin.

Cure of amebiasis means not only relief from symptoms but also the total absence of cysts from the feces for a period of at least six weeks with weekly tests, then six months with monthly tests, then two years with six-month tests.

Other drugs used to treat parasitic infections include suramin, pentamidine, melarsoprol, and melarsonyl.

# PART III

# PHARMACOPEIA

In this section, drugs are listed in alphabetical order by their brand names and by their generic or chemical names. The list includes both the most frequently prescribed drugs and the most common nonprescription drugs. Brand-named drugs are listed in small capitals; generics appear in normal text type. All the drugs mentioned in Parts I and II of this book will be found here.

Drug preparations available only on a doctor's prescription are marked with an asterisk. Some of these may be available over the counter in certain reduced strengths (for example, antihistamines), and some may be available in different forms (for example, as nose drops but not as eye drops). Therefore, if in doubt always check with your pharmacist.

To look up a description of effects, adverse effects, precautions, and dosage for a given drug, find it in the list. If it is a brand-named drug, you will be referred to its generic name. Following the generic name, before the description, the most commonly used brand-named equivalents, and the full chemical name for the generic, are given in parentheses. You should understand that the brand-named drugs listed after a generic name will not necessarily have effects—desired or undesired —identical to those of the generic. The brand-named drugs may vary in their rate and extent of absorption, and in other ways. This can affect their availability to the body—and hence their ultimate effectiveness. You should also keep in mind that it is not possible in a book of this size to list every brand name of each generic; therefore, only a few of the more common brand names are given as examples. The important idea here is always to make a point of looking up the generic name of the brand-named preparation you will know about.

The most detailed descriptions of effects, adverse effects, precautions, and dosage will be found under the entry for that drug which is the principal member of a given group of drugs. Cross-referencing makes it easy to locate these key entries. When a brand-named drug contains more than one active drug agent, you are given the name of each. Some of these constituent drugs are seldom used alone, so their descriptions are very brief.

The dosages listed here are intended only as a general guide. Always check the dose of any drug preparation with your doctor or pharmacist, or against information supplied with the package. Dosages of nonprescription drugs are not provided here; refer to instructions on the package. Dosages for children are also deliberately omitted here, because they vary, depending on the child's age, weight, and other factors. Dosage indications are given in two different ways: Sometimes the entry will state that a certain dose is to be taken a certain number of times a day (e.g., 100 mg. two to three times daily). Sometimes it will state that a total amount is to be taken over the course of the day in divided doses according to the instructions of a physician or pharmacist (e.g., 1200 mg. in divided doses).

Note that a comprehensive danger list of drugs to be avoided during pregnancy has *not* been included, although in many cases such precautions are noted for individual drugs. This is because such a list will always be growing as researchers keep adding more drugs to it, and there is a tendency to assume, quite wrongly, that a drug must be safe if it isn't on the list. If you are pregnant, ask your doctor or pharmacist for advice about drug use.

The general term "blood disorder" mentioned frequently among possible adverse effects refers to disorders of the red or white blood cells caused by drugs acting upon the blood-forming tissues in bone marrow, or upon the blood cells themselves.

Certain drugs enhance the effects of alcohol. This enhancement may be pharmacologically complex, but for simplicity's sake only the term "increase" is used here.

Information about adverse effects of specific drugs, treated only in general in Part II, is given here in detail. However, if every reported adverse effect of each drug were to be listed, this book would run to several volumes; therefore, only the more commonly recognized or particularly harmful of such effects are given. A description usually starts with mild adverse effects (such as nausea and dizziness), which are often related to amount and frequency of dosage and can be reduced or stopped by reducing the dose or stopping the drug. Next come moderate to severe adverse effects, including allergic effects. Finally, some serious reported adverse effects are noted.

Adverse effects may start with mild symptoms, so be on your guard with certain drugs, particularly those that are known to cause serious blood disorders. The warning signal may be a sore throat and fever. Also, severe allergic reactions may occur in someone who has previously experienced a mild reaction to a different drug.

The purpose of listing adverse effects is not to alarm you but to alert you to the possibility that the development of any new symptom may be due to the drug you are taking. Also, it will help you to weigh the benefits and risks of a particular drug. Do not make up your mind against a prescribed drug just because its list of adverse effects is longer than that of another drug. The important point is its benefit/risk ratio for *you*. This must be discussed with your doctor. Remember, considering the quantity of drugs swallowed every day, the majority of them are incredibly safe.

*AARANE   See cromolyn sodium.

acacia (gum arabic)   A gummy exudate from species of African *Acacia*. It is used in the preparation of emulsions and lozenges.

*acenocoumarol (SINTROM)   An anticoagulant drug. Read Drugs Used to Prevent Blood from Clotting, p. 90. It has effects and uses similar to those described under phenindione. *Adverse effects* May cause nausea, loss of appetite, and dizziness. *Dose* By mouth, 8 to 16 mg. initially; maintenance: 4 to 12 mg. daily according to blood tests.

acetaminophen (TYLENOL)   A mild pain reliever. It also reduces fever. Unlike aspirin, it has no anti-inflammatory properties. It is a suitable non-inflammatory pain reliever for patients sensitive to aspirin. Read Aspirin, Nonnarcotic Pain Relievers, and Drugs Used to Treat Rheumatism and Arthritis, p. 118. *Adverse effects* Skin rashes and blood disorders have been reported. Overdose may cause liver damage, and therefore acetaminophen is more dangerous, weight for weight, when taken in overdose than is aspirin. Prolonged use of large doses may cause kidney damage. *Precautions* Acetaminophen should be taken with caution by patients with impaired kidney or liver function. *Dose* By mouth, 500 to 1000 mg. Maximum in 24 hours is 2600 mg.

*acetanilid   A more toxic form of phenacetin. Read Aspirin, Nonnarcotic Pain Relievers, and Drugs Used to Treat Rheumatism and Arthritis, p. 118.

*acetazolamide (DIAMOX)   A diuretic. Used to reduce the pressure inside the eye in the treatment of glaucoma. Read Diuretics, p. 103. It is occasionally used to treat epilepsy. Read Drugs Used to Treat Epilepsy, p. 142. *Adverse effects* These are frequent but mild, and may be reversed by stopping or reducing the dose. They include drowsiness, and numbness and tingling of the face, hands, and feet. Fatigue, excitement, and thirst may occur and—rarely—skin rashes. Liver, kidney, and blood disorders have been reported, and on rare occasions have caused death. The water-salt balance of the body may be disturbed. If given with potassium bicarbonate, it may cause kidney stones. *Precautions* Should not be given to patients who have a low blood potassium level (e.g., patients with Addison's disease). *Dose* By mouth, for glaucoma, 500 mg. initially, then 250 mg. every six hours.

**acetic acid** Used in some cough medicines. it is also used as a skin irritant in rheumatic liniments (see p. 202), and in antiseptic skin applications (p. 201).

*****acetohexamide (DYMELOR)** An oral antidiabetic drug. Read Drugs Used to Treat Diabetes, p. 182, and see chlorpropamide. *Adverse effects* May produce headaches, stomach upsets, vertigo, and nervousness; occasionally it disturbs liver function tests. *Dose* By mouth, 500 to 1500 mg. daily in divided doses.

**acetone** Used as a solvent for fats, resins, and other chemicals.

**acetophenetidin** See phenacetin.

**acetylcholine** A parasympathomimetic drug. Read Drugs Which Act on the Autonomic Nervous System, p. 145.

*****acetylcysteine (MUCOMYST)** Used to dissolve sputum. Read Drugs Used to Treat Coughs, p. 135. It may produce bronchospasm, nausea, vomiting, sore lips, runny nose, and fever. It should be used with caution in elderly and/or debilitated patients who have difficulty in breathing and coughing. *Dose* By inhalation, a nebulized solution, 3 to 5 ml. of a 20% solution or 6 to 10 ml. of a 10% solution, three to four times daily. By direct instillation, 1 or 2 ml. of a 10 or 20% solution every one to four hours.

**acetylsalicylic acid** See aspirin.

*****ACHROMYCIN** See tetracycline.

*****ACHROMYCIN V** See tetracycline.

**acriflavine** Used in antiseptic skin applications (see p. 201). It may produce sensitivity of the skin to sunlight.

*****acrisorcin** See aminacrine hexylresorcinate.

*****ACTH and ACTH gel** See corticotropin.

*****ACTHAR and ACTHAR gel** See corticotropin.

*****ACTIDIL** See triprolidine.

*****ACTIFED** Contains triprolidine hydrochloride 2.5 mg. and pseudo-ephedrine hydrochloride 60 mg. in each tablet; 1.25 mg. and 30 mg. respectively in each 5 ml. of syrup. See triprolidine and pseudoephedrine. Read Drugs Used to Treat Common Colds, p. 132, Drugs Used to Treat Coughs, p. 135, and Antihistamine Drugs, p. 127. *Dose* By mouth, 1 tablet or 2 teaspoonfuls (10 ml.) three times daily.

*****ACTIFED C** An expectorant. Contains codeine phosphate 10 mg., triprolidine hydrochloride 2 mg., pseudoephedrine hydrochloride 30 mg., and glyceryl guaiacolate 100 mg. See codeine, triprolidine, and pseudoephedrine. Read Drugs Used to Treat Coughs, p. 135. *Dose* By mouth, 2 teaspoonfuls (10 ml.) four times daily.

*****ACTINOMYCIN D** See dactinomycin.

**activated attapulgite**  A highly absorbent mineral. Read Drugs Used to Treat Diarrhea, p. 80.

**activated charcoal**  Read Drugs Used to Treat Diarrhea, p. 80.

*****adiphenine (TRASENTINE)**  Used alone or in combination with phenobarbital to relieve spasm in the stomach or gut and also renal (kidney) colic. It has effects, uses, and adverse effects similar to those described under atropine. Read Drugs Which Act on the Autonomic Nervous System, p. 145, and Drugs Used to Treat Indigestion and Peptic Ulcers, p. 74.

**adrenaline**  See epinephrine.

**adrenocorticotropic hormone (ACTH)**  See corticotropin.

**adrenocorticotropin**  See corticotropin.

*****ADRIAMYCIN**  See doxorubicin.

*****ADROCAINE**  See procaine.

*****ADROYD**  See oxymetholone.

*****AEROSPORIN**  See polymyxin B.

*****AFRIN**  A nasal decongestant spray containing oxymetazoline, benzalkonium, sorbitol, glycine, and phenylmercuric acetate. Look up constituent drugs, and read Drugs Used to Treat Common Colds, p. 132. *Dose* Spray twice daily, in the morning and at bedtime.

**agar**  Obtained from algae and other sources. It is soluble in boiling water and swells to form a solid jellylike mass on cooling. As it is not absorbed from the gut and takes up water when it swells, it is therefore sometimes used in mixtures to treat constipation. Agar is also used as a thickener in various manufactured foods. Read Drugs Used to Treat Constipation, p. 82.

**AGAROL emulsion**  Contains mineral oil and agar. Read Drugs Used to Treat Constipation, p. 82. *Dose* By mouth, ½ to 1 tablespoonful (7.5 to 15 ml.).

**AGAROL with phenolphthalein**  See agar and phenolphthalein. Read Drugs Used to Treat Constipation, p. 82. *Dose* By mouth, ½ to 1 tablespoonful (7.5 to 15 ml.).

*****AKINETON**  See biperiden.

*****ALBAMYCIN**  See novobiocin.

**alcohol (ethyl alcohol)**  Used as a solvent and preservative in drug preparations. It has been used to treat circulatory disorders.

*****ALCOPARA**  See bephenium.

*****ALDACTAZIDE**  Each tablet contains 25 mg. hydrochlorothiazide and 25 mg. spironolactone. See constituent drugs. Read Diuretics, p. 103. *Dose* By mouth, 1 to 4 tablets daily.

*****ALDACTONE**  See spironolactone.

*****ALDOMET**  See methyldopa.

*****ALDORIL-15**  Contains methyldopa 250 mg. and hydrochlorothiazide

15 mg. in each tablet. See methyldopa, and read Drugs Used to Treat Raised Blood Pressure, p. 108. See hydrochlorothiazide and read Diuretics, p. 103. *Dose* By mouth, dependent on the individual's response. Maximum recommended daily dose, 12 tablets.

\*ALDORIL-25   See Aldoril-15. This preparation contains 25 mg. of the diuretic hydrochlorothiazide.

**alginic acid**   A substance obtained from algae. It is included in tablets to make them break up and disperse readily when they enter the stomach. Sodium alginate is one of its salts.

ALKA SELTZER   Each tablet contains aspirin 324 mg. with monocalcium phosphate 200 mg., citric acid 1.055 G., and sodium bicarbonate 1.904 G. See aspirin and sodium bicarbonate.

\*ALKERAN   See melphalan.

**allantoin**   A substance that occurs naturally in comfrey root but is also manufactured. It has been used to encourage wound-healing and in preparations used to treat psoriasis and other skin disorders.

ALLEREST TABLETS   Each adult tablet contains phenylpropanolamine hydrochloride 25 mg., chlorpheniramine maleate 1 mg., and methapyrilene fumarate 5 mg. See phenylpropanolamine, chlorpheniramine, and methapyrilene. Read Drugs Used to Treat Common Colds, p. 132, and Antihistamine Drugs, p. 127.

ALLEREST TIME-RELEASE CAPSULES   Each capsule contains phenylpropanolamine hydrochloride 50 mg., pyrilamine maleate 15 mg., methapyrilene fumarate 10 mg. See phenylpropanolamine, pyrilamine, and methapyrilene, and read Drugs Used to Treat Common Colds, p. 132, and Antihistamine Drugs, p. 127.

\*allopurinol (ZYLOPRIM)   Reduces the formation of uric acid and is used in the treatment of gout. In the early stages of treatment acute attacks of gout may occur, but after several weeks of continuous treatment these become less frequent and stop. Deposits of urate crystals in the skin (tophi) diminish in size. Allopurinol reduces the risk that patients with gout will develop kidney stones, and it may prevent kidney damage. Unlike other drugs used to treat gout, it may be used in the presence of kidney damage and it may also be used to prevent a rise in plasma uric acid which can occur in some patients treated with certain diuretics. It may therefore be used along with a diuretic in patients suffering from gout and congestive heart failure. Read Drugs Used to Treat Gout, p. 124. *Adverse effects* Include nausea, vomiting, diarrhea, headaches, fever, abdominal pains, and skin rashes. Nerve damage (peripheral neuritis) and enlargement of the liver have occasionally been reported. *Dose* By mouth, a starting dose of 100 mg. once a day, increasing slowly to a maintenance dose of between 300 and 600 mg.

**almond oil** Obtained from the bitter or sweet almond. Used in skin applications.

**aloe** Obtained from cut leaves of various species of aloe. It is an irritant laxative. Large doses may damage the kidney.

*ALPEN See ampicillin.

*ALPHADROL See fluprednisolone.

*alphaprodine (NISENTIL; alphaprodine hydrochloride) An analgesic with actions and effects similar to those described for meperidine. *Dose* By subcutaneous injection, 20 to 60 mg. By intravenous injection, 20 to 30 mg.

*ALPHOSYL lotion Used to treat psoriasis. It contains allantoin 2% and refined coal tar extract 5% in a nongreasy base. See allantoin and coal tar.

ALUDROX (aluminum hydroxide with magnesium hydroxide) Available as gel and as tablets. Read Drugs Used to Treat Indigestion and Peptic Ulcers, p. 74.

**aluminum acetate** In solution (Burow's solution), used as an antiseptic and as an astringent (see pp. 201, 205). Domeboro tablets, dissolved in water, have the same effect.

**aluminum chlorhydroxide** An astringent and antiperspirant (see p. 205).

**aluminum chloride** An astringent and antiperspirant (see p. 205).

**aluminum glycinate** Used as an antacid. Read Drugs Used to Treat Indigestion and Peptic Ulcers, p. 74.

**aluminum hydroxide (AMPHOJEL)** A useful slow-acting antacid. *Adverse effects* May cause constipation and may interfere with the absorption of digoxin and phosphates and vitamins. Aluminum hydroxide decreases the absorption of digoxin and tetracycline antibiotics from the gut and therefore reduces their effectiveness. These drugs should not be given together. Read Drugs Used to Treat Indigestion and Peptic Ulcers, p. 74. *Dose* By mouth, aluminum hydroxide gel, 7.5 to 15 ml. as needed. Dried aluminum hydroxide gel, 0.3 to 1.2 G. as needed.

**aluminum hydroxychloride** An astringent and antiperspirant (see p. 205).

**aluminum magnesium silicate** Used as a thickening agent, as a binder, and as a disintegrating agent in various drug preparations.

**aluminum oxide particles** Used as a cleansing base in Epi-Clear Scrub Cleanser.

**aluminum phosphate gel (PHOSPHALJEL)** An alternative to aluminum hydroxide, since it does not interfere with the absorption of phosphates. *Dose* By mouth, 5 to 15 ml. as needed. Another alternative is dried aluminum phosphate gel. *Dose* By mouth, 400 to 800 mg. as needed.

**aluminum sulfate solution** An astringent.

**aluminum silicate** Used as an inert filler in making drug preparations.

\*ALUPENT See metaproterenol.

\*amantadine (SYMMETREL; amantadine hydrochloride) An antiviral drug used to prevent influenza A infections. It is also used to treat Parkinsonism. Read Drugs Used to Treat Parkinsonism, p. 149. *Adverse effects* May cause indigestion, dizziness, slurred speech, insomnia, and lethargy. Occasionally it may cause nausea, anorexia, vomiting, and skin rash. These effects are dose-related. Very high doses may cause convulsions. *Precautions* Should not be given to patients with epilepsy, and should be given with caution to the elderly and patients receiving stimulants. It may increase the effects of trihexyphenidyl, benztropine, and orphenadrine, drugs also used to treat Parkinsonism. Dosage of these drugs should be reduced if amantadine is also given. *Dose* By mouth, 200 mg. daily for 10 days following exposure to influenza. For Parkinsonism, 100 mg. daily for one week followed by 100 mg. twice daily.

\*AMBENYL Expectorant containing bromodiphenhydramine hydrochloride 3.75 mg.; diphenhydramine hydrochloride 8.75 mg.; codeine sulfate 10 mg.; ammonium chloride 80 mg.; potassium guaiacolsulfonate 80 mg.; menthol 0.5 mg.; and alcohol 5 percent per 5 ml. See constituent drugs and read Antihistamine Drugs, p. 127, and Drugs Used to Treat Coughs, p. 135. *Dose* By mouth, 1 or 2 teaspoonfuls (5 to 10 ml.) four times daily.

\*AMBODRYL See bromodiphenhydramine.

\*AMCILL See ampicillin.

\*AMESEC Each tablet contains aminophylline 130 mg., ephedrine hydrochloride 25 mg., and amobarbital 25 mg. See aminophylline and ephedrine. Read Drugs Used to Treat Bronchial Asthma, p. 138. See amobarbital sodium and read Sleeping Drugs and Sedatives, p. 43. *Dose* By mouth, 1 to 5 capsules or 1 to 3 tablets every 24 hours.

\*amethocaine See tetracaine.

\*aminacrine (aminacrine hydrochloride; aminoacridine hydrochloride) Used as a skin antiseptic. It is related to proflavine but is less likely to stain the skin.

\*aminacrine hexylresorcinate (acrisorcin) An antiseptic used in skin applications.

**aminoacetic acid (glycine, glycocoll)** Sometimes included in indigestion mixtures and combined with aspirin in order to reduce chances of gastric irritation.

\*aminoacridine See aminacrine.

*aminophylline (theophylline and ethylenediamine) Relaxes involuntary muscles and is used to relieve spasm of the bronchi as in asthma or bronchitis. Read Drugs Used to Treat Bronchial Asthma, p. 138. It also works as a diuretic, increases the heart rate, and stimulates respiration. *Adverse effects* Causes nausea and vomiting. It may be given by injection or by rectum in suppositories. Rapid injection of aminophylline may cause nausea, vomiting, restlessness, dizziness, rapid heart rate, and fall in blood pressure. Similar effects occasionally occur with the suppositories, which may also irritate the rectum. Intramuscular injections are painful. *Precautions* Injections should be given slowly. In children, the dose must be adjusted according to age, weight, and disease severity. *Dose* By mouth, 100 to 300 mg. in one dose. Intravenously, 250 to 500 mg. in one dose. By rectum, 360 mg. once or twice a day.

aminopyrine Formerly used as a pain reliever. Because it may produce severe blood disorders, it should *not* be used.

*aminosalicylic acid (para-aminosalicylic acid; PAS) Used to treat tuberculosis. See sodium aminosalicylate.

*amitriptyline (ELAVIL; amitriptyline hydrochloride) A tricyclic antidepressant drug. Read Antidepressants, p. 56. *Adverse effects* Similar to those described under imipramine. In the first few weeks of treatment adverse effects—including dryness of the mouth, blurred vision, drowsiness, and constipation—may dominate desired effects. Trembling, rapid beating of the heart, and a fall in blood pressure may also occur. *Precautions* Should not be given to patients with glaucoma or patients likely to develop urinary retention. It should be given with caution to patients who have received monoamine oxidase inhibitors in the previous ten days or who are presently taking them. It should preferably be avoided in patients with heart disease, particularly those with disorders of heart rhythm. It antagonizes the action of several antihypertensive drugs, including guanethedine and bethanidine. *Dose* By mouth, initial dose, 30 to 50 mg. daily (at night or in divided doses). Maintenance dose, 20 to 100 mg. daily (at night or in divided doses).

ammonium alum Used as an astringent.

ammonium chloride Used to make the urine acid. It is also present in many cough medicines, in which it is irritant and of doubtful value. Read Drugs Used to Treat Coughs, p. 135.

amobarbital (AMYTAL) An intermediate-acting barbiturate used as a sedative and hypnotic. Read Sleeping Drugs and Sedatives, p. 43. *Adverse effects, precautions, and drug dependence* See Phenobarbital. *Dose* By mouth, sleeping dose, 100 to 200 mg. at night. Sedative dose, 20 to 30 mg.

amobarbital sodium (AMYTAL sodium) An intermediate-acting barbiturate used as a sedative and hypnotic. Read Sleeping Drugs and Sedatives, p. 43. *Adverse effects, precautions, and drug dependence* See phenobarbital. *Dose* By mouth, sleeping dose, 100 to 200 mg. at night. Sedative dose, 20 to 30 mg. three times a day.

*amodiaquine (CAMOQUIN)  An antimalarial drug with effects and uses similar to those described under chloroquine. Read Drugs Used to Treat Malaria, p. 227. *Adverse effects* Long-continued use may cause blue-gray deposits in the cornea of the eyes, fingernails, and hard palate. *Dose* By mouth for suppression of malaria, 200 to 400 mg. once weekly. To control an attack, a single dose of 600 mg. or 400 to 600 mg. daily for three days.

*amorphous IZS  An insulin preparation. Read Drugs Used to Treat Diabetes, p. 182.

*amoxicillin (LAROCIN)  Very similar in its actions to ampicillin, except that it is more rapidly and completely absorbed. See ampicillin. *Dose* By mouth, 250 to 500 mg. three times daily.

*amphetamine sulfate (dextroamphetamine sulfate)  A stimulant which produces increased activity and mental alertness. Read Stimulants: Amphetamines, p. 64. It lifts mood, diminishes the sense of fatigue, and produces wakefulness. Some people develop headaches, restlessness, and insomnia. Large doses produce a lift in mood followed by a fall, at which time the patient may feel exhausted and depressed. It was previously widely prescribed for the treatment of depression and obesity. However, because of its abuse potential and risk of dependence the prescribing of amphetamine for these problems is no longer recommended. It is still used for such rare disorders as hyperkinetic syndrome in children and narcolepsy. *Adverse effects* Dry mouth, nausea, difficulty in urinating, agitation, restlessness, trembling, loss of appetite, and constipation. Rapid beating of the heart with disordered rhythm may also occur. Prolonged use in children depresses growth. Larger doses produce fatigue, depression, fever, hallucinations, convulsions, and coma. *Drug dependence* Amphetamine is a drug of dependence and produces characteristic symptoms. Read Dependence on Drugs, p. 23. *Dose* By mouth: for narcolepsy, 30 to 50 mg. two to three times daily; for hyperkinesis, 5 to 10 mg. three times daily.

*AMPHICOL  See chloramphenicol.

AMPHOJEL  See aluminum hydroxide.

*amphotericin B (FUNGIZONE)  An antibiotic related to nystatin. It has an antifungal action against a wide range of yeasts and fungi (e.g., thrush). Read about antifungal antibiotics in Antibiotics, p. 210. *Adverse effects* Unpleasant and potentially dangerous adverse effects are common because high doses have to be used. These include headache, loss of appetite, and fever which passes after the first few days. Debility, muscle and joint pains, sweating, flushing, loss of appetite, and diarrhea may occur. Low blood pressure, blurred vision, and convulsions have been reported. Application to the skin may produce local irritation, itchiness, and skin rash. The most serious adverse effects are on the kidneys. *Precautions* Should be injected slowly into a vein. Tests of kidney function should be frequently carried out and the drug stopped at the first sign of kidney damage. *Dose* Initially up to 250 mcg. per kg. of body weight daily, increased to 1 mg. per kg. on alternate days by slow intravenous injection.

*ampicillin (AMCILL; ALPEN; PRINCIPEN; TOTACILLIN; OMNIPEN; PENBRITIN; POLYCILLIN; anhydrous ampicillin; ampicillin trihydrate; ampicillin sodium [for injections])** A semisynthetic penicillin. It is widely prescribed. Read about penicillins in Antibiotics, p. 210. *Adverse effects* May cause diarrhea, nausea, and vomiting. Allergic reactions such as itching skin, fever, and swelling of the throat may occur. Ampicillin can cause two types of skin rash. The first is a nettle rash (urticaria); this is a sign of penicillin allergy and indicates the drug should be stopped immediately. The other is a red rash that looks a bit like measles, and occurs particularly in patients suffering from infective mononucleosis. This rash can develop 10 to 20 days after starting the drug (even if the course of treatment has finished) but will eventually go away after the drug is stopped, and a subsequent course will not necessarily cause it to recur. The measlelike rash is therefore not thought to be a true penicillin allergy. *Precautions* Patients allergic to penicillin must be assumed to be allergic to ampicillin. *Dose* By mouth, 1 to 6 G. daily in divided doses every six hours. By intramuscular injection, 1 G. twice daily. By intravenous injection, solution of 250 to 500 mg. of ampicillin in 20 to 40 ml.

*amyl nitrite (isoamyl nitrite)** Relaxes involuntary muscles, particularly those in blood vessels. It is used to relieve angina and may also be used to relieve kidney pain (renal colic) and gall-bladder colic. Read Drugs Used to Treat Angina, p. 100. *Adverse effects* Flushing of the face, throbbing headache, and faintness are the commonest adverse effects. Restlessness, vomiting, and a blue skin coloration may occur with high doses. *Precautions* Should not be used in patients who have had a coronary thrombosis. It should be used with caution in patients with glaucoma, head injury, brain hemorrhage, or marked anemia. *Dose* By inhalation, 0.12 to 0.3 ml.

*AMYTAL** See amobarbital.

*AMYTAL SODIUM** See amobarbital sodium.

*ANABOL** See methandriol.

ANACIN** Each tablet contains aspirin 400 mg. and caffeine 32.5 mg. See aspirin and caffeine.

*ANADROL  See oxymetholone.

ANAHIST  An over-the-counter cough remedy. Each 10 ml. contains dextromethorphan hydrobromide 10 mg., thonzylamine hydrochloride 12.5 mg., ammonium chloride 100 mg., sodium citrate 270 mg., and alcohol 0.5%. See each constituent drug, and read Drugs Used to Treat Coughs, p. 135.

*ANAVAR  See oxandrolone.

*ANCEF  See cefazolin.

*ANCOBON  See flucytosine.

*ANDROID  See methyltestosterone.

*anhydrohydroxyprogesterone  See ethisterone.

*anileridine (LERITINE; anileridine hydrochloride)  A narcotic pain reliever with uses and effects similar to those of morphine. Read Morphine and Narcotic Pain Relievers, p. 115. It may be given by mouth or injection. It produces less constipation, sedation, nausea, and vomiting than morphine. *Dose* By mouth, anileridine hydrochloride, 25 to 50 mg. repeated every six hours if necessary. Anileridine, by subcutaneous or intramuscular injection, 25 to 75 mg. repeated every six hours if necessary.

*anisindione (MIRADON)  An orally administered anticoagulant drug with actions and effects similar to those described under phenindione. Read Drugs Used to Prevent Blood from Clotting, p. 90. It may color the urine red. *Dose* By mouth, 25 to 250 mg. daily.

*ANSOLYSEN  See pentolinium.

*ANSPOR  See cephradine.

*ANTABUSE  See disulfiram.

antazoline (ARITHMIN; antazoline hydrochloride; in NASOCON NASAL SPRAY; antazoline phosphate; antazoline mesylate)  A weak and short-acting antihistamine. It may cause nausea and vomiting. *Adverse effects, precautions* Read Antihistamine Drugs, p. 127. *Dose* By mouth, antazoline hydrochloride, 100 to 300 mg. daily in divided doses. Antazoline mesylate, by intramuscular injection, 500 to 1000 mg.

*ANTEPAR  See piperazine.

anthralin  See dithranol.

*ANTIBASON  See methylthiouracil.

antipyrine  Effects, uses, and adverse effects similar to those described under phenacetin. It may cause skin rashes. Large doses may cause nausea, drowsiness, coma, and convulsions. Prolonged use may cause blood disorders.

*ANTIVERT  Each tablet contains meclizine 12.5 mg. (or 25 mg.) and nicotinic acid 50 mg. See meclizine and read Drugs Used to Treat Nausea, Vomiting, and Motion Sickness, p. 71. *Dose* By mouth, 25 to 50 mg. one hour before traveling; may be repeated once every 24 hours for the duration of the journey. Up to 100 mg. daily may be taken for vertigo.

*ANTURANE See sulfinpyrazone.

ANUSOL Suppositories and ointment for treating hemorrhoids. Contains bismuth subgallate 2.25%, bismuth rescorcin compound 1.75%, zinc oxide 11%, boric acid 5%, benzyl benzoate 1.2%, balsam of Peru 1.8%, cocoa butter, and vegetable oil base. See constituent drugs, and read about treatment of hemorrhoids in section on Drugs Used to Treat Skin Disorders, p. 193.

*apomorphine (apomorphine hydrochloride) Causes vomiting by stimulating the vomiting center in the brain. Used to treat noncorrosive poisonings by mouth. Read Morphine and Narcotic Pain Relievers, p. 115. *Adverse effects* Persistent vomiting and drowsiness, weakness, and dizziness. Apomorphine may increase the rate of breathing, increase heart rate, and reduce blood pressure. *Precautions* Should be used with caution in children, the elderly, the debilitated, and those with heart disorders. It should not be used in patients who are unconscious or in cases of poisoning by corrosive substances. *Dose* By injection, under skin or into muscle, 2 to 8 mg.

*APRESOLINE See hydralazine.

AQUA-BAN Tablets contain ammonium chloride, which acts as a short-term diuretic. Read Diuretics, p. 103. It is claimed to be of use in treating premenstrual tension thought to be caused by excess fluid retention.

*AQUEX See clopamide.

*ARALEN See chloroquine.

*ARAMINE See metaraminol.

*ARFONAD See trimethaphan.

*ARISTOCORT See triamcinolone.

*ARISTOSPAN See triamcinolone.

*ARITHMIN See antazoline.

*ARLIDIN See nylidrin.

*ARTANE See trihexyphenidyl.

ARTHRITIS PAIN FORMULA Tablets contain aspirin with antacids— dried aluminum hydroxide gel and magnesium hydroxide. See aspirin, aluminum hydroxide, and magnesium hydroxide.

ARTHRITIS STRENGTH BUFFERIN Each tablet contains aspirin 486 mg. with antacids—aluminum glycinate 73.5 mg. and magnesium carbonate 140.5 mg. See aspirin, aluminum glycinate, and magnesium carbonate.

A.S.A. ENSEALS Enteric-coated aspirin tablets containing 325 mg. or 650 mg. of aspirin. See aspirin.

ascorbic acid (vitamin C) Read Vitamins, p. 155.

**ASCRIPTIN** Each tablet contains aspirin 300 mg. with added antacids —magnesium hydroxide and aluminum hydroxide. See aspirin, magnesium hydroxide, and aluminum hydroxide.

**ASPERGUM** Chewing gum contains 228 mg. aspirin in each piece. See aspirin.

**aspirin (acetylsalicylic acid)** Discussed at length in the section Aspirin, Nonnarcotic Pain Relievers, and Drugs Used to Treat Rheumatism and Arthritis, p. 118. Aspirin is an effective mild pain reliever and reduces fever and inflammation. *Adverse effects* May produce irritation of the lining of the stomach and may cause nausea, vomiting, pain, and bleeding from the stomach. Bleeding may occur despite changes in formulation and may be unaccompanied by symptoms of indigestion. Some people are allergic to aspirin and develop skin rashes and symptoms like those seen in hay fever or asthma. Aspirin increases blood clotting time, and it may produce swelling of the throat (angioneurotic edema), nettle rash (urticaria), and inflammation of the heart muscle (myocarditis). High doses produce dizziness, noises in the ear (tinnitus), sweating, nausea, vomiting, mental confusion, and overbreathing. *Precautions* Should not be taken by anyone with a stomach upset or a disorder such as peptic ulcer. It should never be taken on an empty stomach or with alcohol. Always take aspirin with a long drink of fluid. Never give aspirin to a child who is feverish and vomiting. It should only be given to feverish children along with plenty of fluids. Aspirin should be given with utmost caution to children under one year of age. It should not be given to people who suffer from hemophilia or are on anticoagulant drugs. Aspirin may increase the effects of drugs used to treat diabetes. It increases the toxicity of sulfonamides and decreases the effects of some drugs used to treat gout. It should be given with caution to the elderly and debilitated who may be anemic and to people who are anemic or suffer from impaired kidney function. Combination with other pain relievers may produce kidney damage if such a mixture is taken regularly for many years. Never take aspirin or any other pain reliever daily without medical advice. Aspirin is a drug, and the consequences of overdose are serious, but it is a most valuable drug if used sensibly. *Dose* By mouth, for pain, 300 to 900 mg. in one dose, up to 3.6 G. daily in divided doses. Higher doses are used in acute rheumatic disorders.

*ATABRINE See quinacrine.

*ATARAX See hydroxyzine.

*ATROMID-S See clofibrate.

*atropine Acts on the brain and nerves, initially stimulating the brain, producing excitement and restlessness. In large doses it causes depression, drowsiness, delirium, and coma. It reduces the muscular rigidity and salivation of Parkinsonism. It diminishes the production of saliva by the salivary glands and sweat by the sweat glands. It also reduces secretions produced by the bronchial tubes, stomach, and gut. It relaxes involuntary muscles when they are in spasm and increases the heart rate and dilates small blood vessels. Atropine has three effects on the eyes: it dilates the pupils, paralyzes the muscles that make the eye focus, and increases the pressure of the fluid inside the eye. Atropine is used to dry up secretion in the lungs before a general anesthetic, to treat renal colic or colic from the gall bladder, and to treat asthma. It is included in mixtures used to treat peptic ulcers and Parkinsonism. Atropine should not be used to dilate the pupils because of its prolonged action, which may trigger an attack of glaucoma. Read Drugs Used to Treat Indigestion and Peptic Ulcers, p. 74, and Drugs Used to Treat Parkinsonism, p. 149. *Adverse effects* Dryness of the mouth, thirst, dilation of the pupils, dry skin, rapid beating of the heart, flushing, difficulty in urinating, and constipation. Dizziness, vomiting, and ataxia may occasionally occur. Toxic doses cause rapid heartbeat, increased breathing, high temperature, rash, hallucinations, and delirium. Allergy to atropine is common—it causes skin rashes and red eyes (conjunctivitis). *Precautions* Should not be given to patients with glaucoma (closed angle or narrow angle). It should be given with caution to patients with enlarged prostate glands (it can cause retention of urine) or heart disorders. Its effects may be increased by other drugs, e.g., major tranquilizers, antidepressants, and antihistamines. It should not be given to patients who have received in the previous ten days, or who are currently receiving, a monoamine oxidase inhibitor antidepressant drug. *Dose* Atropine methylnitrate is used mainly to treat congenital pyloric stenosis (narrowing of the outlet of the stomach). By mouth, 200 to 600 mcg. half an hour before meals. Atropine sulfate by mouth, 0.25 to 2 mg. daily in single or divided doses. By injection (subcutaneous, intramuscular, or intravenous), 0.25 to 2 mg.

*AUREOMYCIN See chlortetracycline.

*AVENTYL See nortriptyline.

AYDS Contains corn syrup, vegetable oils, sweetened condensed whole milk, and vitamins. It is used as a dieting aid (25 calories per candy cube). Read Reducing Drugs, p. 68.

*azathioprine (IMURAN) Principally used as an immunosuppressant, but also belongs to a group of drugs used to treat cancer (see p. 227). *Adverse effects* May damage the bone marrow, producing blood disorders, and cause muscle wasting and skin rashes. For other adverse effects, see mercaptopurine. *Precautions* Should not be used in patients with impaired liver function and probably not in pregnancy. *Dose* By mouth or injection, 2 to 5 mg. per kg. of body weight daily according to needs.

*AZO GANTRISIN Each tablet contains sulfisoxazole 500 mg. and phenazopyridine hydrochloride 50 mg. See sulfisoxazole and phenazopyridine and read Drugs Used to Treat Infections of the Urinary System, p. 223. *Dose* By mouth, 4 to 6 tablets initially, followed by 2 tablets four times daily.

*AZOLID See phenylbutazone.

*AZULFIDINE See sulfasalazine.

*bacitracin An antibiotic used mainly for application to the skin. Read Antibiotics, p. 210, and Drugs Used to Treat Skin Disorders, p. 193.

BACTOCILL See oxacillin.

*BACTRIM Tablets contain sulfamethoxazole 400 mg. and trimethoprim 80 mg. See each drug and read Sulfonamides, p. 220.

balsam of Peru Used in skin applications as a mild antiseptic. Continued use may cause allergic skin rashes.

*BANTHINE See methantheline.

*barbital A long-acting barbiturate. It was formerly used as a sedative and hypnotic. Read Sleeping Drugs and Sedatives, p. 43.

*barbital sodium A long-acting barbiturate. It was formerly used as a sedative and hypnotic. Read Sleeping Drugs and Sedatives, p. 43.

basic fuchsin See carbol-fuchsin.

BAYER ASPIRIN Each tablet contains 325 mg. aspirin. See aspirin.

BAYER CHILDREN'S ASPIRIN Each tablet contains 75 mg. aspirin in an orange-flavored base. See aspirin.

BAYER TIMED-RELEASE ASPIRIN Each tablet contains 650 mg. aspirin. See aspirin.

*beclamethasone (beclamethasone dipropionate; Vanceril) A steroid used to treat bronchial asthma, in the form of a new inhalation preparation which avoids the substantial side effects of oral steroids. It represents an important advance in asthma therapy. Read Drugs Used to Treat Bronchial Asthma, p. 138. *Adverse effects* Minor. Primarily fungal infections of the throat and bronchial irritation. Toxicity from long-term use has not been established. *Precautions* During stress or an asthma attack, patients who have changed over from oral steroids will require oral steroids in large doses in addition to the beclamethasone inhalations. This transitional requirement may continue for from several months to a year. Such conditions can be life-threatening, and patients should carry a warning card to indicate this requirement. *Dose* Two inhalations (100 mcg. total) three to four times daily in adults. Maximum daily dose for adults is 20 inhalations (1000 mcg., or 1 mg.), and for children aged 6–12, 10 inhalations (0.5 mg.). Data for children under age 6 is insufficient.

**beeswax** Used in skin applications. Yellow beeswax may produce allergic reactions. So-called white beeswax has been bleached.

**belladonna alkaloids and extracts** See atropine, and read Drugs Which Act on the Autonomic Nervous System, p. 145.

\*BELLAFOLINE See belladonna alkaloids.

\*BELLERGAL SPACETABS Each tablet contains 0.2 mg. belladonna alkaloids, 0.6 mg. ergotamine tartrate, and 40 mg. phenobarbital. See belladonna and ergotamine, and read Drugs Used to Treat Migraine, p. 125. See phenobarbital, and read Sleeping Drugs and Sedatives, p. 43. *Dose* By mouth, 1 tablet in the morning and 1 tablet in the evening.

BENADRYL See diphenhydramine.

BENADRYL COUGH PREP See Benylin Syrup.

BENDECTIN Each capsule contains Bentyl hydrochloride 10 mg., Decapryn succinate 10 mg., and pyridoxine hydrochloride 10 mg. For Bentyl see dicyclomine; for Decapryn see doxylamine. Read Drugs Used to Treat Nausea, Vomiting and Motion Sickness, p. 71. For pyridoxine see Vitamins, p. 155. *Dose* By mouth, 2 tablets at bedtime. In severe cases of daytime nausea 1 tablet may also be taken in the morning and afternoon.

\*BENDOPA See levodopa.

\*bendroflumethiazide (NATURETIN) A diuretic; see p. 103. It has effects, uses, and adverse effects similar to those described under chlorothiazide. It is long-acting (about 18 hours). *Dose* By mouth, 5 to 20 mg. once a day, reducing to a maintenance dose of 2.5 to 10 mg. daily or on alternate days.

\*BENEMID See probenecid.

BEN GAY A pain-relieving application containing methylsalicylate and menthol. See methylsalicylate and menthol, and read Irritant Skin Applications, p. 202.

**bentonite** A soapy clay used to make suspensions semi-solid.

\*BENTYL See dicyclomine.

\*BENTYL **with phenobarbital** Syrup, tablets, and capsules contain various strengths of dicyclomine and phenobarbital. See dicyclomine, and read Antihistamine Drugs, p. 127. See phenobarbital, and read Sleeping Drugs and Sedatives, p. 43. *Dose* By mouth, 1 to 2 tablets or teaspoonfuls (5 ml.) three to four times daily.

BENYLIN SYRUP Each 5 ml. contains diphenhydramine hydrochloride 12.5 mg., ammonium chloride 125 mg., sodium citrate 50 mg., chloroform 20 mg., menthol 1 mg., and alcohol 5%. See diphenhydramine, and read Antihistamine Drugs, p. 127, and Drugs Used to Treat Coughs, p. 135. *Dose* By mouth, 1 or 2 teaspoonfuls (5 ml.) four times daily.

**benzalkonium (ZEPHIRAN)** Used as an antiseptic (see p. 201).

\*benzathine penicillin G (BICILLIN, PERMAPEN) A long-acting penicillin given by intramuscular injection. Read Penicillins, p. 213.

BENZEDREX See propylhexedrine.

**benzene hexachloride** See gamma benzene hexachloride.

\*benzestrol (CHEMESTROGEN) A synthetic estrogen. Read Female Sex Hormones, p. 166. *Dose* By mouth, 2 to 3 mg. daily or 2 to 5 mg. by intramuscular injection.

\*benzethonium (benzethonium hydrochloride) A detergent disinfectant with effects and uses similar to those of cetrimide. Read Drugs Used to Treat Skin Disorders, p. 193.

**benzocaine (ethyl aminobenzoate)** A local anesthetic much less toxic than cocaine. It is available in lozenges to relieve pain in the mouth and throat and also in an ointment for local application. Read Local Anesthetics, p. 191.

**benzoic acid** Used as an antiseptic, antifungal agent, and preservative. Read Drugs Used to Treat Skin Disorders, p. 193. Benzoic acid compound mixture contains benzoic acid and salicylic acid. Whitfield's ointment contains benzoic acid, salicylic acid, and emulsifying agent.

**benzoin** A balsamic resin used in inhalations.

\*benzphetamine (DIDREX) An amphetaminelike drug used for dieting. Read Reducing Drugs, p. 68.

\*benzquinamide (EMETE-CON; QUANTRIL) An anti-anxiety drug. Read Minor Tranquilizers, p. 51. It is also used to treat nausea and vomiting. Read Drugs Used to Treat Nausea, Vomiting, and Motion Sickness, p. 71.

\*benzthiazide A diuretic drug. See chlorothiazide, and read Diuretics, p. 103. *Dose* By mouth, 50 to 150 mg. daily in divided doses.

\*benztropine (COGENTIN; benztropine mesylate) Produces effects similar to those described under atropine. It also has some antihistamine properties (see p. 129) and ganglion-blocking properties. Read Drugs Which Act on the Autonomic Nervous System, p. 145. *Dose* By mouth, 0.5 mg. at bedtime, initially. Increase to 1 to 2 mg. in two divided doses.

**benzyl alcohol** Used as an antiseptic and as a weak local anesthetic in various skin applications.

**benzyl benzoate** Used to treat scabies, p. 200.

\*benzyl penicillin See penicillin G.

\*bephenium (ALCOPARA; bephenium hydroxynaphthoate) Used to treat worm infections (see p. 229). It is effective against hookworms and roundworms. *Adverse effects* It may cause nausea, dizziness, vomiting, headaches, and diarrhea. *Dose* By mouth, 5 G. as a single dose.

**berberine sulfate** Taken by mouth as a bitter tonic.

*BEROCCA Contains vitamin $B_1$ 15 mg., vitamin $B_2$ 15 mg., vitamin $B_6$ 5 mg., niacinamide 100 mg., calcium pantothenate 20 mg., vitamin $B_{12}$ 5 mcg., and folic acid 0.5 mg. Read Vitamins, p. 155.

*BETA-CHLOR See chloral betaine.

BETADINE Aerosol sprays, vaginal douches, shampoos, skin cleansers. See povidone iodine.

*betamethasone (CELESTONE; VALISONE) A corticosteroid (see p. 160). It has effects and uses similar to those of prednisolone.

*betamethasone valerate (VALISONE) Available in creams and ointments. It is used as an anti-inflammatory and anti-allergic agent. It has effects and uses similar to prednisolone. See Corticosteroids, p. 160, and read Drugs Used to Treat Skin Disorders, p. 193.

*bethanechol (URECHOLINE; bethanechol chloride) A parasympathomimetic drug. Read Drugs Which Act on the Autonomic Nervous System, p. 145. *Dose* By mouth, 5 to 30 mg. three to four times daily. By subcutaneous injection, 2.5 to 10 mg. three to four times daily.

*BICILLIN See benzathine penicillin G.

*BICILLIN CR Contains benzathine penicillin G 150,000 units and procaine penicillin G 150,000 units per ml. See benzathine penicillin G and procaine penicillin G. Read Penicillins, p. 213.

*biperiden (AKINETON) Produces atropinelike effects and is used to treat Parkinsonism. See atropine, and read Drugs Used to Treat Parkinsonism, p. 149. *Dose* By mouth, 2 mg. three or four times daily.

*biphasic insulin An insulin preparation. Read Drugs Used to Treat Diabetes, p. 182.

bisacodyl (DULCOLAX) A laxative. Read Drugs Used to Treat Constipation, p. 82. It may cause abdominal cramps, and suppositories may produce local rectal irritation. *Dose* By mouth, 5 to 10 mg. daily; tablets must be swallowed (without chewing or crushing) with a full glass of water. By rectum, 5 to 10 mg. daily.

*bishydroxycoumarin See dicoumarol.

bismuth carbonate Used as an antacid. Read Drugs Used to Treat Indigestion and Peptic Ulcers, p. 74.

bismuth resorcin compound Used in anti-itching skin applications and as a keratolytic. Read Drugs Used to Treat Skin Disorders, p. 193.

bismuth salts Once widely used to treat syphilis. They are used in some antacid mixtures (see p. 76), as antidiarrheals (see p. 80), and as protectives (see p. 195) in some skin powders, pastes, and suppositories.

bismuth subcarbonate A very weak antacid. There is little justification for its use. Read Drugs Used to Treat Indigestion and Peptic Ulcers, p. 74.

**bismuth subgallate** Used as a mild astringent in skin applications. Read Drugs Used to Treat Skin Disorders, p. 193.

BISODOL An antacid powder containing magnesium carbonate, sodium bicarbonate, and bismuth carbonate with a peppermint flavor. See Antacids, p. 76.

*BLENOXANE See bleomycin.

*bleomycin (BLENOXANE) A mixture of anti-cancer antibiotics obtained from the growth of *Streptomyces verticullus.* Read Drugs Used to Treat Cancer, p. 225. *Adverse effects* Nausea, vomiting, skin rashes, high temperatures and sores in the mouth. *Dose* 10 to 20 mg. per square meter of body surface daily by intravenous or intramuscular injection, or by regional intra-arterial perfusion.

BLOCK-OUT See Suntan and Sunburn Applications, p. 196.

BONINE See meclizine.

**boracic acid** See borax.

**borax (sodium borate; sodium tetraborate; boric acid; boracic acid)** Has feeble antibacterial and antifungal properties. It is used in solutions, dusting powders, mouthwashes, and lotions. *Adverse effects* Repeated use of boric acid (in any way) may lead to accumulation of the drug in the body. Poisoning can result in skin rashes, vomiting, diarrhea, coma, and death. Convulsions, kidney failure, and alterations in body temperature may occur. Deaths of children have occurred after application of boric acid solution or powder to damaged skin surfaces. Deaths have also followed the washing out of internal organs (such as the bladder) with boric acid solution. Boric acid has been excluded from most reputable baby dusting powders for many years. Never use preparations which contain borax or boric acid (boracic acid).

**boric acid** See borax.

BRASIVOL A skin-cleansing application containing aluminum oxide and a neutral soap base. It is presented in fine, medium, and rough forms for the treatment of acne (see p. 207).

*BRETHINE See terbutaline.

*bretylium (bretylium tosylate) Effects and uses similar to those described under guanethidine. Read Drugs Used to Treat Raised Blood Pressure, p. 108. *Dose* By mouth, 100 to 400 mg. daily in divided doses.

*BRICANYL See terbutaline.

**brilliant green** Used as an antiseptic. It may produce sensitivity of the skin.

*BRISTAMYCIN See erythromycin.

**bromide** See potassium bromide.

**bromodiphenhydramine (AMBODRYL)** An antihistamine drug. Read Antihistamine Drugs, p. 127.

**BROMO-SELTZER** Granules contain phenacetin 130 mg., potassium bromide 162.5 mg., caffeine 32.5 mg., and acetaminophen 195 mg. in each cupful along with sodium bicarbonate and citric acid. See phenacetin, potassium bromide, acetaminophen, and sodium bicarbonate.

**brompheniramine (DIMETANE)** An antihistamine drug. Read Antihistamine Drugs, p. 127.

**BRONKAID** Each tablet contains ephedrine sulfate 24 mg., guaiaphenesin 100 mg.,and theophylline 100 mg. See ephedrine, guaiaphenesin, and theophylline. Read Drugs Used to Treat Bronchial Asthma, p. 138, and Drugs Used to Treat Coughs, p. 135.

**BUFFERIN** Each tablet contains 324 mg. aspirin with added antacids —aluminum glycinate 49 mg. and magnesium carbonate 97 mg. See aspirin, aluminum glycinate, and magnesium carbonate.

**\*bupivacaine (MARCAINE; bupivacaine hydrochloride)** A local anesthetic (see p. 191) with effects and uses similar to lidocaine, but it works for a longer duration. Overdose may cause a fall in blood pressure, muscle twitching, depression of respiration, and convulsions. Its use in childbirth may cause the baby's heart to slow down.

**Burow's solution** See aluminum acetate.

**\*busulfan (MYLERAN)** An anticancer drug (see p. 226). *Adverse effects* May cause blood disorders, producing hemorrhages and bone marrow damage (this may be irreversible and begin several months after treatment is stopped). Loss of menstrual periods (amenorrhea) may occur as long as six months after the drug is stopped. It may also produce an "Addison's-like" disease of underworking of the adrenal glands (see p. 163). *Precautions* It should not be used in pregnancy, by breast-feeding mothers, or where there is a risk that bone marrow function has been weakened by radiotherapy. Concurrent administration of allopurinol to prevent formation of too much uric acid in the body is recommended. *Dose* By mouth, 2 to 12 mg. daily initially, reducing to a maintenance of 0.5 to 3 mg.

**\*butabarbital (BUTISOL)** An intermediate-acting barbiturate. It is used as a hypnotic. Read Sleeping Drugs and Sedatives, p. 43. *Dose* By mouth, 100 to 200 mg. at night.

**\*butabarbital sodium (BUTISOL sodium)** An intermediate-acting barbiturate. It is used as a hypnotic. Read Sleeping Drugs and Sedatives, p. 43. *Dose* By mouth, 100 to 200 mg. at night.

**\*butalbital (LOTUSATE)** A barbiturate. Read Sleeping Drugs and Sedatives, p. 43.

\*BUTAZOLIDIN  See phenylbutazone.

\*BUTAZOLIDIN ALKA  Butazolidin with added antacids—aluminum hydroxide gel 100 mg. and magnesium trisilicate 150 mg.

\*BUTISOL  See butabarbital.

butopyronoxyl  Used as an insect repellent.

CAFERGOT  Each tablet contains ergotamine tartrate 1 mg. and caffeine 100 mg. Suppositories contain ergotamine tartrate 2 mg. and caffeine 100 mg. See ergotamine and caffeine, and read Drugs Used to Treat Migraine, p. 125. Dose By mouth, 2 tablets at onset of migraine symptoms; 1 additional tablet every ½ hour if needed (maximum 6 tablets per attack, 10 tablets per week). Suppositories: 1 suppository at start of attack; 1 additional suppository one hour later if needed (maximum 2 suppositories per attack, 5 suppositories per week).

caffeine  Has a stimulating effect on the central nervous system and a weak diuretic effect. It is present in many over-the-counter pain relievers, tonics, and pick-me-ups. Read Stimulants: Caffeine, p. 63. Caffeine is found in tea, coffee, cocoa, and cola.

calamine  A zinc salt (zinc carbonate) mixed with an iron salt (ferric oxide). It is a mild astringent and is used in various skin applications. Read Drugs Used to Treat Skin Disorders, p. 193.

\*calciferol (ergocalciferol; vitamin D₂; DELTALIN; DRISDOL)  The same effects and uses as vitamin D. Deficiency in vitamin D causes rickets in children and osteomalacia (bone softening) in adults. Read Vitamins, p. 155. Adverse effects Excessive daily doses (150,000 units or more) may produce loss of appetite, nausea, vomiting, diarrhea, loss of weight, headache, dizziness, and thirst. The amount of calcium in the urine is raised, and kidney stones and calcification of arteries may develop. Dose By mouth, to treat rickets etc., up to 4000 units daily.

\*calcium aminosalicylate (PARASAL calcium)  Used to treat tuberculosis (see p. 224), it has effects and uses similar to those described under sodium aminosalicylate.

calcium carbonate (chalk)  An antacid present in many antacid mixtures. Read Drugs Used to Treat Indigestion and Peptic Ulcers, p. 74. Adverse effects May cause constipation. Its regular use may increase the blood calcium level and result in calcium being laid down in blood vessels and the kidneys. This is more likely to happen if it is taken with quantities of milk or cream, which leads to what is called the "milk-alkali syndrome." The symptoms produced include headache, weakness, loss of appetite, nausea, vomiting, abdominal pains, constipation, thirst, and frequent urination. These symptoms are associated with temporary or, rarely, permanent kidney damage. Calcium carbonate is one of the most effective and cheap antacids, but like any other drug it needs to be taken responsibly. *Dose* By mouth, 1 G. to 5 G. according to needs. Avoid prolonged or excessive dosage along with an increased intake of milk or cream.

**calcium hydroxide (slaked lime)** Used in solution as an antacid and as an astringent. In emulsion it is used in skin applications.

**calcium undecylenate** Used in antifungal skin preparations. Read Drugs Used to Treat Skin Disorders, p. 193.

*CAMOQUIN See amodiaquine.

**camphor** Used in cough medicines and to treat flatulence. It is also used in rheumatic liniments. See Drugs Used to Treat Skin Disorders, p. 193.

*CANDEPTIN See candicidin.

*candicidin (CANDEPTIN; VANOBID) An antifungal drug (see p. 212).

**cannabis sativa** See marijuana.

*CAPASTAT See capreomycin.

*capreomycin (CAPASTAT) An antibiotic used to treat tuberculosis (see p. 224). It is a reserve drug and should be used only along with other antituberculous drugs in order to reduce the development of resistant bacteria. It is not absorbed from the gut and has to be given by intramuscular injection. *Adverse effects* May produce vertigo and noises in the ears, and disturbances of salt and water balance in the body. The most serious adverse effects are irreversible deafness and progressive kidney damage. Allergic skin rashes, fever, and transient liver abnormalities have been reported. *Precautions* Should be given with caution to patients with impaired kidney function or a history of allergy and sensitivity reaction to drugs. *Dose* 1 G. daily by intramuscular injection.

*caramiphen (caramiphen hydrochloride) Has atropinelike effects and has been used to treat Parkinsonism. See atropine, and read Drugs Used to Treat Parkinsonism, p. 149. Caramiphen ethanedisulfonate is used in nasal decongestion preparations. Read Drugs Used to Treat Common Colds, p. 132.

*carbachol Shares some of the actions of acetycholine and is called a parasympathomimetic drug. It is used in eye drops to reduce the pressure inside the eye in patients with glaucoma. Read Drugs Which Act on the Autonomic Nervous System, p. 145. *Precautions* Should not be applied to the eyes of patients with corneal abrasions because it may be absorbed.

*carbamazepine (TEGRETOL) An anticonvulsant drug. Read Drugs Used to Treat Epilepsy, p. 142. It has been used to treat facial nerve pain (trigeminal neuralgia). *Adverse effects* Dryness of the mouth, nausea, diarrhea, dizziness, and double vision may occur. Skin rashes, blood disorders, and jaundice may rarely occur. *Precautions* It should not be given to patients who are taking monoamine oxidase inhibitor antidepressant drugs. It should preferably not be given during the first three months of pregnancy. *Dose* By mouth, 200 to 1200 mg. daily in divided doses.

\*carbenicillin (PYOPEN, GEOCILLIN, GEOPEN) Carbenicillin sodium is a semisynthetic penicillin. Read Penicillins, p. 213. To prevent the development of resistant bacteria its use is restricted to treating serious infections. *Adverse effects and precautions* Similar to those described under penicillin G. It should not be used in ointments and drops or for infections that would respond to other penicillins. *Dose* By mouth, 500 to 1000 mg. every six hours. By intravenous injection, 25 to 30 G. daily in divided doses, usually by injection into a saline infusion apparatus.

\*carbenoxolone sodium Used in Great Britain to treat benign gastric ulcers. Read Drugs Used to Treat Indigestion and Peptic Ulcers, p. 74. It seems to work better in patients who are up and about. Its value in the treatment of duodenal ulcer has not been proved. *Adverse effects* May cause salt and water retention in the body, leading to swelling (edema) and an increase in weight and blood pressure. This may trigger heart failure in patients with underlying heart disorders. It also reduces the blood potassium level, which may cause weakness and damage to muscles. It may affect enzyme actions in the liver. *Precautions* Should be used with caution in patients with heart disease or high blood pressure. Treatment should never be continued for more than four or six weeks. Potassium usually must be added to the diet. *Dose* By mouth, initially 50 mg. three times daily, increasing to 100 mg. three times daily for no more than six weeks.

\*carbidopa Blocks the breakdown of levodopa in the body. Read Drugs Used to Treat Parkinsonism, p. 149.

\*carbimazole (NEO-MERCAZOLE) An antithyroid drug. Read Drugs Used to Treat Thyroid Disorders, p. 187. It reduces the production of thyroid hormone and therefore reduces the rate at which the body burns up energy. *Adverse effects* Usually occurring in the first few months of treatment, these include nausea, headache, skin rashes, joint swelling and fever, blood disorders and hair loss. *Precautions* Infants should not be breast-fed by mothers taking carbimazole. Patients should report sore throats, skin rashes, or fever immediately, since these may be the first signs of a blood disorder. Caution is necessary when using this drug during pregnancy and in patients with any evidence that the thyroid gland is pressing on the windpipe. In high doses, the drug may produce enlargement of the thyroid gland. *Dose* By mouth, 10 to 60 mg. daily in divided doses, followed by a maintenance dose of 5 to 20 mg. daily for several months.

**carbinoxamine (CLISTIN-D; carbinoxamine maleate)** An antihistamine drug. Read Antihistamine Drugs, p. 127. *Dose* By mouth, 4 to 8 mg. three to four times daily.

*CARBOCAINE See mepivacaine.

**carbol-fuchsin solution (CASTELLANI'S PAINT)** Used as a skin antiseptic. It contains magenta 300 mg., phenol 4–5 G., resorcinol 10 G., acetone 5 ml., alcohol 10 ml., and water to 100 ml.

*carbon dioxide snow Used to destroy warts.

*CARBRITAL Each kapseal contains pentobarbital sodium 100 mg. and carbromal 250 mg. See pentobarbital and carbromal, and read Sleeping Drugs and Sedatives, p. 43.

*carbromal A hypnotic sedative. Read Sleeping Drugs and Sedatives, p. 43. *Adverse effects* Can release sufficient bromide to affect persons who are allergic to bromides. Chronic toxicity resembles bromide intoxication (bromism), with irritability, depression, and slurring of speech. Skin rashes (purpura) may develop, particularly on the lower legs and abdomen. High doses may produce acute toxic effects resembling those seen with chloral hydrate. *Drug dependence* May produce drug dependence of the barbiturate/alcohol type. Read Dependence on Drugs, p. 23. Carbromal (whether prescribed alone or in combination with a barbiturate) should be regarded as obsolete because of its toxicity.

*CARDILATE See erythritol.

*CARDOPHYLLIN See aminophylline.

*carisoprodol (RELA; SOMA) An anti-anxiety drug related to meprobamate. Read Minor Tranquilizers, p. 51.

CARTER'S LITTLE PILLS Contain aloe 16 mg. and podophyllum 4.5 G. See aloe and podophyllum, and read Drugs Used to Treat Constipation, p. 82.

CASAFRU LIQUID Contains 30% senna fruit extracts. See senna, and read Drugs Used to Treat Constipation, p. 82.

casanthranol (PERISTIM) A purified mixture obtained from cascara. Read Drugs Used to Treat Constipation, p. 82.

cascara sagrada Obtained from the dried bark of *Rhamnus purshiana*. Read Drugs Used to Treat Constipation, p. 82.

CASTELLANI'S PAINT See carbol-fuchsin.

castor oil Used as an irritant laxative. Large doses may produce nausea, vomiting, colic, and severe loss of fluid with purgation. Read Drugs Used to Treat Constipation, p. 82.

*CATAPRES See clonidine.

*CEDILANID See lanatoside C.

*CEFADYL See cephapirin.

*cefazolin (KEFZOL; ANCEF) See cephalosporin antibiotics. *Dose* By mouth, 250 to 1000 mg. every six to eight hours.

*CELBENIN See methicillin.

*CELESTONE See betamethasone.

*CELONTIN See methsuximide.

cephaeline See ipecac.

*cephalexin (KEFLEX) See cephalosporin antibiotics. *Dose* By mouth, 1 to 4 G. daily in divided doses.

*cephaloglycin (KAFOCIN) See cephalosporin antibiotics. This preparation is not recommended for use.

*cephaloridine (LORIDINE) See cephalosporin antibiotics. *Dose* By intramuscular injection, 0.5 to 1 G. every eight to twelve hours.

*cephalosporin antibiotics Read Antibiotics, p. 210. They are similar to penicillins, but they kill bacteria (bactericidal) and are active against more organisms. *Adverse effects* Nausea, vomiting, loss of appetite, and diarrhea have been reported. Skin rashes may occur, particularly in patients who are allergic to penicillin. High doses may produce kidney damage, convulsions, and a bleeding type of anemia. They may interfere with certain blood tests used to cross-match blood for patients requiring a blood transfusion. *Precautions* Should be used with caution in patients who are allergic to penicillin. Diuretics increase their toxicity. They should be given with caution to patients with impaired kidney function. These drugs are being intensively promoted to doctors.

*cephalothin (KEFLIN) See cephalosporin antibiotics. *Dose* By injection, 2 to 6 G. daily in divided doses.

*cephapirin (CEFADYL; cephapirin sodium) See cephalosporin antibiotics. *Dose* By intravenous or intramuscular injection, 500 mg. to 1 G. every four to six hours. Up to 12 G. daily may be given in very serious infections.

*cephradine (ANSPOR; VELOSEF) See cephalosporin antibiotics. *Dose* By mouth, 1 to 4 G. daily in divided doses.

*CERUBIDIN See daunorubicin.

cetrimide An antiseptic and detergent with emulsifying properties. Used as a skin-cleansing agent in numerous preparations and in shampoos. *Adverse effects* Some patients may develop sensitivity after repeated applications. It may cause the skin of the scalp to become very dry.

cetylpyridinium Used as a detergent antiseptic (see p. 201).

chalk See calcium carbonate.

*CHEMESTROGEN See benzestrol.

*chloral betaine (BETA-CHLOR) A nonbarbiturate sleeping drug with effects similar to those of chloral hydrate. See chloral hydrate and read Sleeping Drugs and Sedatives, p. 43.

*chloral hydrate (NOCTEC; SOMNOS)  A sleeping drug used mainly in children and the elderly. Read Sleeping Drugs and Sedatives, p. 43. *Adverse effects* It is a gastric irritant and must be taken well diluted. Chloral hydrate should not be used in patients with impaired liver, heart, or kidney function, or peptic ulcers. Some patients may develop drowsiness, disorientation, and paranoid ideas. If the patient takes chloral hydrate regularly, then has a drink of alcohol, he may experience flushing, rapid beating of the heart, and faintness due to a fall in blood pressure. *Drug dependence* Produces drug dependence of the barbiturate/alcohol type and increases the effects of alcohol. *Dose* By mouth, 300 to 2000 mg.

*chlorambucil (LEUKERAN)  An anticancer drug (see p. 225). *Adverse effects* Large doses can produce nausea and vomiting. Prolonged large doses can produce irreversible damage to the bone marrow, producing severe blood disorders. *Precautions* Should not be used in pregnancy and not when there is a risk that bone marrow function is weak (e.g., within four weeks of radiotherapy or treatment with another anticancer drug). *Dose* By mouth, 5 to 10 mg. daily initially, reducing to 2 to 4 mg. daily for maintenance.

*chloramphenicol (AMPHICOL; CHLOROMYCETIN; CHLOROPTIC; MYCHEL; OPHTHOCHLOR)  A valuable antibiotic with a wide range of activity against infecting organisms. Read Antibiotics, p. 210. It is a drug of choice in treating typhoid and paratyphoid fever, and meningitis due to *Hemophilus influenzae*. Chloramphenicol eye drops and ear drops are used for superficial infections. *Adverse effects* Serious effects include blood disorders which may be fatal, kidney damage, jaundice, inflammation of the main nerves of the eye (optic neuritis), and ulcers in the mouth with skin lesions (Stevens-Johnson syndrome). Ointments and drops may cause allergic skin rashes which may be serious in people sensitive to this drug. Dryness of the mouth, nausea, vomiting, diarrhea, and fungus infection (e.g., thrush—*Candida albicans*) of the gut may rarely occur; this causes a sore tongue and mouth, irritation and soreness in the anus and vagina, and, very rarely, pneumonia. Many of the serious adverse effects have been due to its careless use by doctors, e.g., high dosage, prolonged treatment, repeated use, and prescription for trivial disorders. Blood disorders may, however, occur with relatively small dosage and develop up to several months after treatment is stopped. *Precautions* Should not be used as a drug of first choice in bacterial infections, except in typhoid and paratyphoid fever, and in *Hemophilus influenzae* meningitis. *Dose* By mouth, 1.5 to 3 G. daily in divided doses. Chloramphenicol palmitate is used in mixtures, and chloramphenicol succinate for injections.

*chlorbutanol  See chlorbutol.

*chlorbutol (chlorbutanol)  A mild sedative with effects similar to chloral hydrate. It is also a local pain reliever, and has antibacterial and antifungal properties. It is used in nose sprays and ointments and also as a preservative in eye drops. It has been used to treat motion sickness but is less effective for this purpose than other preparations. *Dose* By mouth, 300 to 1200 mg. daily.

*chlorcyclizine (PERAZIL; chlorcyclizine hydrochloride)  An antihistimine. Read Antihistamine Drugs, p. 127. *Dose* By mouth, 50 mg. to 200 mg. daily in divided doses.

*chlordantoin (SPOROSTACIN)  An antifungal drug. It is used as a cream. Read Antifungal Drugs, p. 212.

*chlordiazepoxide (LIBRITABS; LIBRIUM; chlordiazepoxide hydrochloride)  A minor tranquilizer. Read Minor Tranquilizers, p. 51. *Adverse effects* May produce drowsiness, dizziness, fatigue, apathy, irritability, and unsteady walking (ataxia). It may also cause depression, indigestion, and changes in libido. Large doses may cause faintness. Rarely it may produce skin rashes, headache, nausea, constipation, frequent urination, and irregularities of menstruation. Blood and liver disorders have very occasionally been reported. Sometimes chlordiazepoxide may make patients very excited and restless instead of sedated (what is called a paradoxical reaction). *Precautions* Should be given with caution to patients with impaired kidney or liver function and to the elderly or debilitated, in whom "normal" doses may cause unsteadiness on the feet, drowsiness, and confusion. Its effects are increased by alcohol, barbiturates, narcotics, or any other drug that depresses brain function. Chlordiazepoxide may interfere with ability to drive motor vehicles or operate moving machinery. *Drug dependence* May rarely produce dependence of the barbiturate/alcohol type. Read Dependence on Drugs, p. 23. *Dose* By mouth, 30 to 100 mg. daily in divided doses.

chlorinated lime  A mixture of calcium chloride and calcium hypochlorite which releases chlorine. Used as a disinfectant (see p. 201).

chlorine  A germicide. It is used in the form of liquid chlorine for the chlorination of water and in the form of hypochlorates or other compounds as a disinfectant and antiseptic.

*chlormadinone (NORMENON, chlormadinone acetate)  A progestogen. Read Female Sex Hormones, p. 166, and Oral Contraceptive Drugs, p. 173.

*chlormethazanone  See chlormezanone.

*chlormezanone (TRANCOPAL; chlormethazanone)  Has effects and uses similar to meprobamate. Read Minor Tranquilizers, p. 51. *Adverse effects* May cause drowsiness, nausea, dizziness, skin rash, and dry mouth. Flushing of the skin and difficult urination may rarely occur, and very occasionally jaundice. *Precautions* May increase the effects of alcohol, and should not be given with other tranquilizers or monoamine oxidase inhibitor antidepressant drugs. It may interfere with the ability to operate moving machinery or drive motor vehicles. *Dose* By mouth, 300 to 800 mg. daily in divided doses.

**chlorocresol** An antiseptic, disinfectant, and preservative.

**chloroform** Used as an anesthetic. It has also been used as a flavoring agent and preservative (though these uses have now been banned because of its cancer-producing risks), and in rheumatic liniments. Regular daily doses of chloroform lead to drug dependence of the morphine type. Read Dependence on Drugs, p. 23.

*****chloroguanide (chloroguanide hydrochloride, proguanil hydrochloride)** An antimalarial drug. Read Drugs Used to Treat Malaria, p. 227. *Adverse effects* Large doses may cause vomiting and kidney discomfort. It should always be taken after meals. *Dose* By mouth, 100 to 200 mg. daily for 4 weeks after leaving an area where malaria is prevalent.

*****chloromycetin** See chloramphenicol.

**chlorophenothane (DDT; dicophane)** An insecticide. It is stored in the body fat and may cause chronic poisoning.

*****CHLOROPTIC** See chloramphenicol.

*****chloroquine (ARALEN; chloroquine phosphate)** Used to prevent and treat malaria (see p. 228) and amebiasis of the liver (see p. 230). It is also used to treat rheumatoid arthritis and similar disorders (see p. 122). *Adverse effects* Itching (pruritis), headache, and disturbances in vision may occur. Large doses over long periods may produce damage to the eyes (degeneration of the retina and opacities of the cornea). White patches on the skin due to loss of pigment may occur, and it may cause whitening of the hair. Rarely, wasting of muscles and mental breakdown may occur. These adverse effects are very rare with doses used to treat malaria. *Dose* By mouth, malaria prevention, 500 mg. weekly. Treatment, 1000 mg. daily, reducing to 500 mg. daily. Hepatic amebiasis, 0.5 to 1 G. daily. Rheumatoid arthritis, 120 to 900 mg. daily in divided doses. Can also be given by injection.

*****chlorothiazide (DIURIL)** A diuretic (see p. 103). Increases the water in urine by increasing the excretion of sodium, potassium, and chloride by the kidneys. These salts take water with them into the urine by a process of osmosis. Chlorothiazide works in about two hours and lasts from six to twelve hours. It does not lose its effect over time. It is used to treat an increase of body fluids (edema). It is also used to treat patients with raised blood pressure (see p. 112). *Adverse effects* Occasionally causes allergies, skin rashes, nausea, dizziness, pains in the stomach, sensitivity of the skin to sunlight, and weakness. It may rarely cause an acute disorder of the pancreas (acute pancreatitis) and blood disorders. Chlorothiazide and other thiazide diuretics may trigger an attack of gout or diabetes in some patients. Prolonged use results in a fall in blood potassium which can sensitize the heart to digitalis (see p. 86). *Precautions* Should be used with caution in patients with impaired kidney or liver function and in patients with diabetes. During prolonged treatment a high potassium diet or potassium supplements should be taken. *Dose* By mouth, 1 to 2 G. daily, reducing to a maintenance dose of 500 mg. to 1 G. two or three times weekly.

*chlorotrianisene (TACE)  A synthetic female sex hormone (estrogen) which is stored in the body fat, from which it is gradually released. It has the general effects of estrogens. Read Female Sex Hormones, p. 166. It is used to treat menopausal disturbances in a dosage of 12 to 24 mg. daily; to treat cancer of the prostate gland in a dosage of 24 mg. daily; to suppress milk production in a dosage of 48 mg. daily for seven days. Rarely, may produce nausea, vomiting, and withdrawal bleeding.

chloroxylenol  Used as an antiseptic and disinfectant. It is less toxic than phenol. Wet chloroxylenol dressings in contact with the skin may produce sensitivity reactions. Read Drugs Used to Treat Skin Disorders, p. 193.

chlorphenesin (MYCIL)  An antibacterial, antifungal drug used to treat fungus infections of the skin such as athlete's foot. Read Drugs Used to Treat Skin Disorders, p. 193.

chlorpheniramine (chlorprophenpyridamine maleate)  An antihistamine. Read Antihistamine Drugs, p. 127. *Dose* By mouth, 2 to 4 mg. three or four times daily. Also available as an elixir and injection.

*chlorphenoxamine (PHENOXENE; chlorphenoxamine hydrochloride)  Produces some atropinelike, antihistamine, and local anesthetic effects. See atropine and read Antihistamines, p. 129. It is used to treat Parkinsonism (see p. 149). *Dose* By mouth, 50 to 100 mg. three to four times daily.

*chlorphentermine (PRE-SATE; chlorphentermine hydrochloride)  Used as a reducing drug (see p. 70). It produces less stimulation than amphetamine. *Adverse effects* May cause dizziness, insomnia, and drowsiness; dryness of the mouth, nausea, constipation, diarrhea, difficult urination, delayed ejaculation, headache, sweating, skin rashes, and changes in mood. *Precautions* Should be used with caution by patients with heart disease, high blood pressure, glaucoma, overworking of the thyroid gland, or psychological disorders. It should not be taken by women who are breast-feeding, and it should not be given to patients who are being treated with monoamine oxidase inhibitor antidepressant drugs or within two weeks of stopping them. *Dose* By mouth, 65 mg. daily.

*chlorpromazine (LARGACTIL, THORAZINE; chlorpromazine hydrochloride) A phenothiazine major tranquilizer (neuroleptic). Read Major Tranquilizers, p. 53. It is also used to prevent nausea and vomiting. Read Drugs Used to Treat Nausea, Vomiting, and Motion Sickness, p. 71. *Adverse effects* May cause a fall in blood pressure, disorders of heart rate, drowsiness, depression, indifference, dry mouth, pallor, weakness, nightmares, and insomnia. Agitation may occur. Chlorpromazine may also cause disorders of the breasts in both men and women (enlargement and production of milk—gynecomastia and galactorrhea), absence of menstrual periods (amenorrhea), visional disturbances (opacities in the lens and cornea), and pigmentation of the skin and eyes. High doses may cause a fall in body temperature, or sometimes an increase. The drug may also cause jaundice that mimics blockage of the bile ducts in the liver (cholestatic jaundice), blood disorders, skin rashes, sensitivity of the skin to sunlight, and muscle tremblings (Parkinsonism and dystonias). *Precautions* May cause severe dermatitis in sensitized people. Chlorpromazine should never be given to unconscious patients and should be used with caution in the elderly and debilitated, in patients with impaired heart function, and in those with certain blood disorders. It should not be given to patients who have impaired liver function. It increases the effects of alcohol, barbiturates, narcotics, atropinelike drugs, and other drugs which depress brain function. It also increases the effects of drugs used to treat high blood pressure, and it should not be given along with drugs known to have a potential for producing blood disorders (e.g., phenylbutazone, thiouracil, amidopyrine). *Dose* By mouth or intramuscular injection, 25 to 50 mg. to prevent vomiting. By mouth, 75 to 300 mg. daily in divided doses in psychotic disorders.

*chlorpropamide (DIABINESE) Used to treat mild diabetes. Read Oral Antidiabetic Drugs, p. 186. It should not be used in obese people to replace diet control. *Adverse effects* Weakness, headache, skin rashes, blood disorders, and jaundice may occur. A person on chlorpropamide may get intolerance to alcohol and develop flushing of his face after a drink. *Precautions* Chlorpropamide should not be used by patients with impaired liver or kidney function or serious thyroid disorders. It should never be used during pregnancy. The blood sugar lowering effects may be increased by dicoumarol, monoamine oxidase inhibitor antidepressants, propranolol and other beta blockers, and aspirin. Its effects may be decreased by adrenaline, corticosteroids, oral contraceptives, and thiazide diuretics. *Dose* By mouth, 100 to 1000 mg. daily.

*chlorprophenpyridamine  See chlorpheniramine.

*chlorprothixene (TARACTAN)  A major tranquilizer (see p. 53). *Adverse effects* May cause dryness of the mouth, drowsiness, rapid heartbeat, fall in blood pressure, and vertigo. It may also cause skin rashes, fluid retention (edema), nasal congestion, constipation, convulsions, insomnia, and fainting. Large doses may cause Parkinsonism effects and fits. Blood disorders, nerve damage, and milk from the breasts have been reported as well as changes in liver function tests. *Precautions* Should not be given to patients with heart failure, coronary artery disease, or disorders of the blood vessels supplying the brain. It should be given with caution to patients with epilepsy or impaired liver or kidney function. It may increase the effects of alcohol, barbiturates, narcotics, and other depressant drugs and also drugs used to treat raised blood pressure. *Dose* By mouth, 30 to 600 mg. daily in divided doses.

*chlortetracycline (AUREOMYCIN)  See tetracycline.

*chlorthalidone (HYGROTON)  A thiazide diuretic. Read Diuretics, p. 103. It is effective for up to 48 hours. *Dose* By mouth, 100 to 400 mg. initially, then reduction to a maintenance dose of 100 to 200 mg. daily on alternate days.

CHLOR-TRIMETON  Nasal preparations, cough medicines, and oral antihistamine preparations contain chlorpheniramine. See chlorpheniramine and read Antihistamine Drugs, p. 127.

*chlorzoxazone (PARAFLEX)  A muscle relaxant. *Adverse effects* May produce nausea, vomiting, constipation, drowsiness, headache, and dizziness. It has been suspected of causing liver damage. It should not be used by patients with impaired liver function. *Dose* By mouth, 125 to 250 mg. three or four times daily.

*CHOLEDYL (oxtriphylline, choline theophyllinate tablets)  See oxtriphylline and read Drugs Used to Treat Bronchial Asthma, p. 138.

*cholestyramine (CUEMID, QUESTRAN)  Used to lower blood fat levels. Read Drugs Used to Treat Atherosclerosis, p. 98. *Adverse effects* May cause constipation, nausea, and diarrhea. Large doses may interfere with the absorption of fat and vitamins A, D, and K from the diet. Other drugs should be taken at least one hour before or four hours after taking cholestyramine. *Dose* By mouth, 4 G. three times daily. Maximum 24 G. daily.

*choline theophyllinate  See oxtriphylline (Choledyl).

*CHOLOXIN  See dextrothyroxine.

CHOOZ  A peppermint-oil chewing gum. See Antacids, p. 76.

*CHRONOTAB  See dexbrompheniramine.

*chymotrypsin  An enzyme which dissolves protein. It is obtained from beef pancreas and used in cough medicines to dissolve sputum. Read Drugs Used to Treat Coughs, p. 135. It is also taken by mouth to relieve swellings associated with abscesses or injury. *Adverse effects* May produce allergic reactions. Where allergy is suspected, a skin test should be carried out before use. It may produce irritation after swallowing and pain and swelling at the site of injection. *Dose* 50,000 to 100,000 units by mouth four times daily, or by intramuscular injection 2500 to 5000 units one to three times daily.

cimetidine  An antihistamine. Read Drugs Used to Treat Indigestion and Peptic Ulcers, p. 74.

cinnamedrine  Used to relieve painful spasms of the uterus, it is included in preparations for treating painful menstrual periods.

*CINNASIL  See rescinnamine.

*CITANEST  See prilocaine.

citric acid  Obtained from lemons and other citric fruits. It is used as a flavoring agent.

CLEARASIL  Regular tinted cream contains bentonite 11 5%, sulfur 8%, resorcinol 2%, and alcohol 10%. See bentonite, sulfur, and resorcinol. It is used to treat acne. Read Drugs Used to Treat Skin Disorders, p. 193.

*CLEOCIN  See clindamycin.

*clindamycin (CLEOCIN)  Similar effects and uses to those described under lincomycin. *Adverse effects* May occasionally cause nausea, vomiting, and diarrhea (although less than with lincomycin). Skin rashes and blood disorders have been reported. *Dose* By mouth, 150 to 450 mg. every six hours.

*clindinium (clindinium bromide)  An atropinelike drug used to treat peptic ulcers. See atropine, and read drugs Used to Treat Indigestion and Peptic Ulcers, p. 74. *Dose* By mouth, 2.5 to 5 mg. three or four times daily before meals and at bedtime.

*CLISTIN-D  Each tablet contains acetaminophen 300 mg., carbinoxamine maleate 2 mg., and phenylephrine hydrochloride 10 mg. See acetaminophen, carbinoxamine, and phenylephrine, and read Drugs Used to Treat Common Colds, p. 132.

*clofibrate (ATROMID-S)  Used to reduce high blood fat levels. Read Drugs Used to Treat Atherosclerosis, p. 98. *Adverse effects* May cause nausea, drowsiness, diarrhea, and weight gain. Itching, skin rashes, loss of hair (alopecia), and blood disorders have been reported. *Precautions* Should not be used by patients with impaired liver or kidney function. It should not be used during pregnancy. It may enhance the effects of anticoagulant drugs. *Dose* By mouth, 1.5 to 2 G. daily in divided doses.

\*CLOMID  See clomiphene.

\*clomiphene (CLOMID; clomiphene citrate)  Stimulates ovulation (see p. 178). It is used for the treatment of infertility in women. *Adverse effects* Include gastric upset, skin rashes, and visual disturbances. *Dose* By mouth, 50 mg. for five days beginning on fifth day of menstrual cycle, except in patients who have not menstruated recently.

\*clonidine (CATAPRES; clonidine hydrochloride)  Used to treat raised blood pressure (see p. 112). *Adverse effects* Dry mouth, drowsiness, constipation, and slowing of the heart rate may occur in the first few weeks of treatment. It may produce impotence, itching, swelling of the throat and face (angioneurotic edema), nausea, and drowsiness. *Precautions* In patients on clonidine a general anesthetic may cause a severe fall in blood pressure. A dangerous rebound increase in blood pressure may occur if use is stopped suddenly. *Dose* By mouth, 0.4 to 2 mg. daily in divided doses.

\*clopamide (AQUEX)  A diuretic drug with effects and uses similar to those described under chlorothiazide. Read Diuretics, p. 103.

\*CLOPANE  See cyclopentamine.

\*clorazepate (TRANXENE)  A benzodiazepine minor tranquilizer. See chlordiazepoxide, and read Minor Tranquilizers, p. 51. *Dose* By mouth, 15 to 60 mg. daily in divided doses.

\*clorexolone (NEFROLAN)  A diuretic drug. Read Diuretics, p. 103. It has actions, effects, and uses similar to those described under chlorothiazide. *Dose* By mouth, 10 to 50 mg. daily.

\*clorindione (INDALITAN)  Has effects and uses similar to those described under phenindione. Read Drugs Used to Prevent Blood from Clotting, p. 90. *Dose* By mouth, maintenance 2 to 4 mg. daily.

\*clotrimazole (LOTRIMIN, GYNE-LOTRIMIN)  An antifungal drug. Read Drugs Used to Treat Skin Disorders, p. 193. *Dose* Vaginal tablets (100 mg.) 1 at night for six nights. Also available as a cream for skin infections.

\*cloxacillin sodium (TEGOPEN)  A semisynthetic penicillin mainly of use in treating infections produced by one particular group of bacteria resistant to penicillin (penicillinase-producing staphylococci). Otherwise it is not as potent as penicillin G. Read Penicillins, p. 213. *Adverse effects and precautions* Similar to those described under penicillin G. It should not be used on the skin. *Dose* By mouth, 500 mg. before meals every six hours.

coal tar  Used in ointments to treat psoriasis and eczema. It may irritate the skin and cause acnelike eruptions.

\*cocaine  The oldest local anesthetic (see p. 191) but because of adverse effects and risks of drug dependence it is now seldom used except for local application to the eyes, ears, or nose. Unlike all other local anesthetics, it constricts small blood vessels and need not be given with epinephrine. *Adverse effects* Some people have an idiosyncrasy to cocaine and may become seriously ill, even after a small dose. They develop headaches and faintness, and may suddenly collapse and die. In other patients, it may cause the general adverse effects of any local anesthetic: excitation, restlessness, nausea, yawning, and vomiting, which may be followed by pallor, sweating, fall in blood pressure, twitching, convulsions, and unconsciousness. *Precautions* Should not be given to patients with myasthenia gravis. It should be given with caution to patients with disordered heart rhythm or impaired liver function. *Drug dependence* When taken by mouth, cocaine causes stimulation and a lift in mood. Large doses cause restlessness, trembling, and hallucinations. Cocaine addicts inject it under the skin or use it in the form of snuff. Its repeated use leads to drug dependence. The characteristics of cocaine dependence, described on p. 30, include a strong psychological dependence but no physical dependence. Persons dependent on cocaine develop an unbearable craving for the drug, loss of weight and memory, and mental deterioration.

**cocoa butter** A solid fat pressed from the roasted seeds of the cacao tree, *Theobroma cacao*. It is used as a basis for suppositories and vaginal insert tablets.

**codeine (methylmorphine)** A useful mild pain reliever. A weak cough suppressant, it is also of value in treating diarrhea. Read Morphine and Narcotic Pain Relievers, p. 115, Drugs Used to Treat Coughs, p. 135, and Drugs Used to Treat Diarrhea, p. 80. *Adverse effects* The most common adverse effects are constipation, nausea, vomiting, dizziness, and drowsiness. Very rarely, skin rashes occur in patients allergic to codeine. *Precautions* Should be given with caution to patients suffering from severe respiratory disorders (e.g., chronic bronchitis). It may increase the effects of other drugs which depress brain function (e.g., sedatives, tranquilizers, hypnotics). *Drug dependence* Prolonged use of high doses may rarely produce dependence of the morphine type. *Dose* By mouth, 10 to 60 mg. Not more than 200 mg. in 24 hours. Codeine, codeine phosphate, or codeine sulfate appear in many pain-relieving mixtures, cough mixtures, and antidiarrheal mixtures.

**\*COGENTIN** See benztropine.

**COLACE** See dioctyl sodium sulfosuccinate.

**\*colaspase** See l-asparaginase.

**\*colchicine** Used for the relief of pain in acute gout. Read Drugs Used to Treat Gout, p. 124. *Adverse effects* Large doses quickly produce diarrhea. Colchicine may also produce nausea, vomiting, and abdominal pains. Kidney and liver damage, dehydration, and loss of hair (after prolonged use) may rarely occur. *Precautions* Should be given with caution to the elderly and debilitated and to patients who suffer from impaired heart, liver, or kidney function. It should probably not be given to patients who suffer from disorders of the stomach or gut (e.g., colitis). *Dose* By mouth for acute attack of gout, 1 mg. initially followed by 0.5 mg. every two hours until relief is obtained or diarrhea develops. The total amount in a course of treatment should not exceed 10 mg.; maintenance dose, 0.5 to 2 mg. at night.

**cold cream** Contains rosewater 20 ml., white beeswax 18 G., borax 1 G., almond oil 61 G., and rose oil 0.1 ml.

*__colistimethate sodium__ See colistin.

*__colistin (COLY-MYCIN; colistin sulfate)__ An antibiotic with a range of activity similar to polymyxin B. Read Antibiotics, p. 210. It is poorly absorbed from the gut and is therefore used for treating gastroenteritis. *Adverse effects* May produce allergy and skin rashes, and in high dose it may cause kidney damage, dizziness, and migraine. *Dose* By mouth, 3 to 5 mg. per kg. of body weight daily in divided doses. Colistimethate sodium is a compound of colistin suitable for injections. *Dose* By mouth, 2.5 to 5 mg. per kg. of body weight daily in divided doses.

**collodion** A cellulose product used to protect cuts and abrasions by forming a film over the injured surface.

**COLOGEL** See methylcellulose, and read Drugs Used to Treat Constipation, p. 82.

*__COLY-MYCIN__ See colistin.

*__COMBID__ Contains isopropamide 5 mg. and prochlorperazine 10 mg. in each spansule. See isopropamide and prochlorperazine. *Dose* By mouth, 1 capsule every twelve hours.

*__COMPAZINE__ See prochlorperazine.

*__COMPOCILLIN V__ See phenoxymethylpenicillin.

**COMPOZ TABLETS** Contain methapyrilene hydrochloride 15 mg., pyrilamine maleate 10 mg., scopolamine aminoxide hydrobromide 0.15 mg. See methapyrilene, pyrilamine, and scopolamine. Read Sleeping Drugs and Sedatives, p. 43, and Antihistamine Drugs, p. 127.

**CONAR-A** Each tablet contains noscapine 15 mg., phenylephrine hydrochloride 10 mg., acetaminophen 300 mg., and guaifenesin 100 mg. Half of these doses are in each 5 ml. of suspension. See noscapine, phenylephrine, acetaminophen, and guaifenesin. Read Drugs Used to Treat Common Colds, p. 132, and Drugs Used to Treat Coughs, p. 135.

*conjugated estrogens  A mixture of two salts of estrogens—estrone and equilin. Read Female Sex Hormones, p. 166.

CONTAC  Each capsule contains belladonna alkaloids 0.25 mg., phenylpropanolamine hydrochloride 50 mg., and chlorpheniramine maleate 4.0 mg. See belladonna, phenylpropanolamine, and chlorpheniramine, and read Drugs Used to Treat Common Colds, p. 132, and Antihistamine Drugs, p. 127.

*COPAVIN  Each tablet or capsule contains codeine sulfate 15 mg. and papaverine hydrochloride 15 mg. See codeine and papaverine, and read Drugs Used to Treat Coughs, p. 135. Dose By mouth, 1 capsule or tablet after each meal and 2 capsules or tablets at bedtime.

COPE  Each tablet contains aspirin 421.2 mg., methapyrilene fumarate 15 mg., caffeine 32 mg. with antacids: dried aluminum hydroxide 25 mg. and magnesium hydroxide 50 mg. See aspirin, methapyrilene, caffeine, aluminum hydroxide, and magnesium hydroxide. Read Drugs Used to Treat Common Colds, p. 132.

CO-PYRONIL  Each capsule contains pyrrobutamine phosphate 15 mg., methapyrilene hydrochloride 25 mg., and cyclopentamine hydrochloride 15 mg. For pyrrobutamine and methapyrilene read Antihistamine Drugs, p. 127. For cyclopentamine see ephedrine and read Drugs Used to Treat Common Colds, p. 132. Dose By mouth, up to 2 capsules every eight hours.

*CORDRAN  See flurandrenolide.

CORICIDIN  Each tablet contains aspirin 390 mg., chlorpheniramine maleate 2 mg., and caffeine 30 mg. See aspirin, chlorpheniramine, and caffeine. Read Drugs Used to Treat Common Colds, p. 132.

CORICIDIN DEMILETS  Each children's chewable tablet contains phenylephrine 2.5 mg., chlorpheniramine maleate 0.5 mg., and aspirin 80 mg. See phenylephrine, chlorpheniramine, and aspirin, and read Drugs Used to Treat Common Colds, p. 132.

CORRECTOL  Each tablet contains yellow phenolphthalein 64.8 mg. and dioctyl sodium sulfosuccinate 100 mg. See phenolphthalein and dioctyl sodium sulfosuccinate, and read Drugs Used to Treat Constipation, p. 82.

*CORTEF  See hydrocortisone.

*corticotropin (ACTHAR; CORTIGEL; CORTROPHIN; ACTH; adrenocorticotropic hormone)  Stimulates the cortex of the adrenal glands and produces an increased output of hormones. The effects produced are similar to, but not identical with, those of cortisone. Read Corticosteroids, p. 160. Adverse effects Similar to those described under cortisone. Adverse effects upon the stomach and gut are less common. Acne and increased blood pressure are more common. Patients may sometimes become allergic to it. Precautions Should not be given to patients with peptic ulcers, active tuberculosis, signs of mental instability, or high blood pressure. It may make diabetic patients worse and increase their insulin needs. It may also mask the signs and symptoms of underlying infections. Patients should be seen and examined regularly by their doctor. *Withdrawal symptoms* May depress the natural ACTH produced by the master gland, the pituitary. This leads to changes in the gland caused by its underworking, so that if the drug is stopped, the pituitary gland cannot take over right away. The patient may then experience severe symptoms (see p. 162). Treatment should therefore be stopped very gradually in order to give the pituitary gland time to become active again. *Dose* Corticotropin is available for injection as corticotropin gelatin injection (ACTH gel, Acthar gel, Cortigel) and corticotropin zinc injection (Cortrophin zinc). These are long-acting and not suitable for injection into a vein. A preparation of corticotropin in sterile solution is available for intravenous injection. The dose needs careful calculation and control.

*CORTIGEL   See corticotropin.

*cortisone (CORTONE)   A corticosteroid (see p. 160). It has the effects of the naturally occurring adrenocortical hormone hydrocortisone. It is used in disorders of the adrenal glands which result in underproduction of hydrocortisone (Addison's disease), and it is used to treat inflammatory, allergic, and rheumatic disorders. Its effects are transitory, and relapse of the underlying condition soon occurs when the cortisone is stopped. With continued use of cortisone the master gland (the pituitary) stops producing the hormone which stimulates the adrenal glands to produce hydrocortisone. This results in disuse changes in the adrenal glands, so that if the cortisone is stopped the adrenal glands are not in a position to produce even the body's normal requirements of hydrocortisone. This produces serious consequences (see p. 162). Prolonged use of cortisone also leads to changes in salt, sugar, and protein used by the body. It reduces resistance to infection as well as the inflammatory response to infection; underlying infection may therefore go unnoticed. Cortisone should be used only for certain inflammatory disorders and when inflammation may be harmful, as in the eyes. It is better to use prednisone or prednisolone to treat asthma, rheumatoid arthritis, certain blood disorders, and other inflammatory or allergic disorders because it has less effect on body salts. In the case of asthma, the recently developed beclamethasone inhaler substantially reduces the adverse systemic effects of steroid therapy (see beclamethasone). *Adverse effects* Cortisone affects salt, sugar, and protein metabolism; healing and inflammation; and the pituitary and adrenal glands, resulting in salt and water retention, producing edema (a sign of which is ankle swelling), raised blood pressure, and alterations in blood potassium which may cause heart failure. Calcium and phosphorus metabolism are affected, which may result in bone softening and fractures. The blood sugar level increases. Cortisone may cause peptic ulcers with bleeding and perforation, delayed wound healing, and increased liability to infection. Prolonged application to the eyes may result in damage to the cornea and to sight; skin applications may cause wasting of skin tissues. Sudden collapse may occur if the drug is stopped (due to the adrenal glands not functioning), and growth may be slowed down in children. Large doses lead to development of "moon face," hairiness (hirsutism), swelling of the tissues over the lower part of the back of the neck and shoulders (called a buffalo hump), flushing, increased bruising, acne, and stripes (striae) on the skin, particularly around the lower abdomen and buttocks. Other adverse effects include disorders of the nervous system, mental disturbances, loss of periods (amenorrhea), and muscle weakness. *Precautions* Should not be given to patients with peptic ulcers, softening of bones (osteoporosis), or severe psychological disorders. It should be used with caution in patients who are elderly or have congestive heart failure, diabetes, infectious diseases, longstanding impairment of kidney function, or kidney failure. Patients with active or doubtfully active tuberculosis should not be given cortisone (unless it is part of the treatment and given along with antituberculous drugs). Normally the body produces more hydrocortisone in response to infection, anesthetics, surgery, shock, and injury. Patients who are receiving cortisone or who have been on cortisone in the previous two years may not be able to produce sufficient hydrocortisone themselves during anesthesia, surgery, or injury. They will therefore need to be given a supplementary dose of hydrocortisone. Cortisone's effects may be reduced by barbiturates and phenytoin. It may also affect the response to anticoagulant drugs. Applications to the skin, eyes, or ears should not be used in the presence of infection. When applied to large areas of the body surface under plastic occlusive dressings it is absorbed and may cause adverse effects. In certain cases it may be used combined with an antibacterial drug for lesions of the eyes, ears, or skin, but such a mixture should never be used to treat viral inflammation of the eyes, since there is a risk of causing blindness. *Dose* By mouth or intramuscular injection, 50 to 400 mg. daily in divided doses.

*CORTISPORIN Creams, ointments, ear drops, and eye drops contain various mixtures of polymyxin B, neomycin, gramicidin, bacitracin, and hydrocortisone. Read Antibiotics, p. 210, and Drugs Used to Treat Skin Disorders, p. 193.

*CORTONE ACETATE   See cortisone.

*CORTRIL   Hydrocortisone sprays, lotions, and ointments. See hydrocortisone, and read Corticosteroids, p. 160, and Drugs Used to Treat Skin Disorders, p. 193.

*CORTROPHIN   See corticotropin.

CORYBAN D   Contains phenylpropanolamine 25 mg., chlorpheniramine maleate 2 mg., ascorbic acid 25 mg., salicylamide 365 mg., and caffeine 30 mg. See phenylpropanolamine, chlorpheniramine, ascorbic acid, and salicylamide, and read Drugs Used to Treat Common Colds, p. 132.

*COSMEGEN   See dactinomycin.

*COTAZYM   See pancrelipase.

CO-TYLENOL   Each tablet contains phenylephrine hydrochloride 5 mg., chlorpheniramine maleate 1 mg., and acetaminophen 325 mg. See phenylephrine, chlorpheniramine, and acetaminophen. Read Drugs Used to Treat Common Colds, p. 132.

*COUMADIN   See warfarin.

*CRASNITIN   See l-asparaginase.

cream of tartar (potassium acid tartrate)   Used as a saline laxative. Read Drugs Used to Treat Constipation, p. 82.

creosote   A disinfectant. It is used in small doses in some cough mixtures, but is an irritant.

cresol   Used as an antiseptic and disinfectant (see p. 201). It has effects similar to those of phenol. It is also used in irritant skin applications (p. 202).

*cromolyn sodium (AARANE; INTAL; sodium cromoglycate)   Used to prevent attacks of asthma due to allergy. It appears to block certain processes in the allergic reaction. It is taken only by inhalation into the lungs or up the nose. It may be taken alone or with isoprenaline to prevent bronchospasm due to inhalation of the powder. Read Drugs Used to Treat Bronchial Asthma, p. 138. *Adverse effects* May cause irritation of the throat and bronchi, especially during infective illnesses. Sudden withdrawal may trigger an attack of asthma, particularly in those patients for whom it has permitted a reduction in corticosteroid dose. *Precautions* Should not be used in pregnancy. *Dose* By inhalation, 20 mg. every three to twelve hours.

*crotamiton   Used in skin applications to kill scabies and to prevent itching (see p. 200).

crystal violet   See gentian violet.

*crystalline IZS   Read Drugs Used to Treat Diabetes, p. 182.

*CRYSTICILLIN A.S. (procaine penicillin G suspension)   See procaine penicillin.

*CRYSTODIGIN   See digitoxin.

*CUEMID  See cholestyramine.

*CUPRIMINE  See penicillamine.

*curare  An extract from the bark of trees which grow in South America, used for making poisoned arrows by South American Indians. It paralyzes muscles and was formerly used in surgery. Tubocurarine has taken its place.

*cyanocobalamin (vitamin B$_{12}$)  A cobalt-containing substance used to treat anemias caused by vitamin B$_{12}$ deficiency. Read Vitamins, p. 155.

cyclamate (calcium cyclamate)  Formerly used as a sweetening agent. It may produce diarrhea when taken in high dosage. It may also sensitize the skin to sunlight.

*cyclandelate (CYCLOSPASMOL)  A vasodilator drug. Read Drugs Used to Treat Disorders of Circulation, p. 94. *Adverse effects* May produce dizziness, flushing, headache, nausea, and sweating in high dosage. *Dose:* By mouth, 100 to 200 mg. four to five times daily.

cyclizine (MAREZINE; cyclizine hydrochloride)  An antihistamine used to treat motion sickness, sickness of pregnancy, and other disorders associated with nausea and vomiting. Read Antihistamine Drugs, p. 127, and Drugs Used to Treat Nausea, Vomiting, and Motion Sickness, p. 71. *Adverse effects* Drowsiness and dizziness are the main adverse effects. *Dose* By mouth, 50 mg. 20 minutes before traveling. Dose should *not* be repeated more than twice in 24 hours.

*CYCLOGYL  See cyclopentolate.

cyclomethycaine (SURFACAINE; cyclomethycaine sulfate)  A sparingly soluble local anesthetic applied to cuts, abrasions, piles, and irritated skin. It may cause irritation and rashes. Read Drugs Used to Treat Skin Disorders, p. 193, and Local Anesthetics, p. 191.

cyclopentamine (CLOPANE)  An ephedrinelike drug used in nasal congestion. See ephedrine and Read Drugs Used to Treat Common Colds, p. 132.

*cyclopenthiazide (NAVIDREX)  A diuretic. It has actions, effects, and uses similar to those described under chlorothiazide. *Dose* 250 to 500 mcg. daily.

*cyclopentolate (cyclopentolate chloride)  Has effects similar to those described under atropine. Read Drugs Which Act on the Autonomic Nervous System, p. 145. It is used in eye drops.

*cyclophosphamide (CYTOXAN)  An anticancer drug (see p. 225). Also used as an immunosuppressant. *Adverse effects* May cause nausea, vomiting, and diarrhea, and sometimes bleeding colitis. Bleeding cystitis may be produced. It may cause bone marrow damage, producing blood disorders. Loss of hair is common at a dose of more than 35 mg. per kg. of body weight in eight days, but it regrows in two to three months, even if the drug is continued. *Precautions* Should not be given in pregnancy, to patients with any infection, or to patients whose bone marrow function may be reduced. *Dose* By mouth or injection, 100 to 150 mg. daily.

\*cycloserine (SEROMYCIN) An antibiotic drug active against many bacteria, including tuberculosis. Read Drugs Used to Treat Tuberculosis, p. 224. Its antibacterial activity is, however, lower than other antibiotics used to treat these infections; it is therefore used only as a reserve drug against bacteria resistant to other antibiotics or if the patient has become allergic to them. It is used principally to treat pulmonary tuberculosis and should be given in combination with antituberculous drugs in order to prevent development of resistance. *Adverse effects* The incidence of adverse effects is high, including headache, dizziness, drowsiness, twitching, speech difficulties, convulsions, and even unconsciousness. Abdominal symptoms may occur. With daily doses of less than 500 mg., adverse effects are rare. Allergic skin rashes occasionally occur; blood sugar levels may be reduced and certain tests for liver function altered. *Precautions* Should not be given to patients with epilepsy, mental disturbance, or impaired liver function. It should be given with caution to alcoholics and patients with impaired kidney function. Blood levels of the drug should be checked frequently. *Dose* By mouth, 250 to 750 mg. daily in divided doses.

\*CYCLOSPASMOL See cyclandelate.

\*cycrimine (PAGITANE HYDROCHLORIDE) Produces atropinelike effects. See atropine. Read Drugs Used to Treat Parkinsonism, p. 149. *Dose* By mouth, 5 to 45 mg. daily in divided doses.

\*cyproheptadine (PERIACTIN; cyproheptadine hydrochloride) An antihistamine drug. Read Antihistamine Drugs, p. 127. It is effective in small doses but is short-acting. It is also promoted as an appetite stimulant. *Dose* By mouth, 4 to 20 mg. daily in divided doses.

\*CYSTODIGIN See digitoxin.

\*cytarabine (CYTOSAR; cytarabine hydrochloride) An anticancer drug (see p. 225). *Adverse effects* May produce ulcers of the mouth, nausea, and vomiting. It may affect the eye (conjunctivitis and keratitis) and damage the bone marrow. *Precautions* Should not be used in pregnancy or in patients with depressed bone marrow function. *Dose* Depends upon the disorder being treated.

\*CYTOMEL See liothyronine.

\*CYTOSAR See cytarabine.

\*CYTOXAN See cyclophosphamide.

\*DACTIL See piperidolate.

\*dactinomycin (ACTINOMYCIN D; COSMEGEN) An anticancer drug (see

p. 225). Also used as an immunosuppressant. *Adverse effects* Nausea, vomiting, abdominal pain, and diarrhea may occur during treatment. Injections may be painful and produce local irritation. The skin marks of X-ray therapy may be made worse by dactinomycin. Days or weeks after treatment has stopped, the patient may develop blood disorders (due to bone marrow damage), nausea, vomiting, and diarrhea. *Precautions* Should probably be avoided during pregnancy. *Dose* 15 mcg. per kg. of body weight intravenously daily for five days.

**Dakin's solution** A solution of chlorinated lime used as a disinfectant.

\*DALIMYCIN See oxytetracycline.

\*DALMANE See flurazepam.

\*DANILONE See phenindione.

\*DANIVAC See danthron.

\*danthron (DANIVAC, DORBANE) An irritant laxative which may color the urine pink or red. Read Drugs Used to Treat Constipation, p. 82.

\*DANTRIUM See dantrolene.

\*dantrolene (DANTRIUM) A muscle relaxant. *Adverse effects* Include weakness, euphoria, light-headedness, dizziness, diarrhea, liver damage, and blood disorders. *Precautions* Effects on the brain may be enhanced by sedative-antianxiety drugs. Use with caution in patients with either lung or heart disease. *Dose* By mouth, 25 mg. twice daily, increasing to a maximum of 400 mg. per day.

\*DARANIDE See dichlorphenamide.

\*DARAPRIM See pyrimethamine.

\*DARBID See isopropamide.

\*DARCIL See phenethicillin.

\*DARICON See oxyphencyclimine.

\*DARVOCET-N Contains propoxyphene napsylate 50 mg. and acetaminophen 325 mg. See acetaminophen and propoxyphene, and read Aspirin, Nonnarcotic Pain Relievers, and Drugs Used to Treat Rheumatism and Arthritis, p. 118. *Dose* By mouth, 1 tablet every four hours as needed for pain.

\*DARVOCET-N 100 Contains propoxyphene napsylate 100 mg. and acetaminophen 650 mg. in each tablet. See acetaminophen and propoxyphene, and read Aspirin, Nonnarcotic Pain Relievers, and Drugs Used to Treat Rheumatism and Arthritis, p. 118. *Dose* By mouth, 1 tablet every four hours as needed for pain.

\*DARVON See propoxyphene.

\*DARVON COMPOUND-65 See propoxyphene compound 65.

\*DARVON-N Propoxyphene napsylate. See propoxyphene.

\*DARVON-N WITH A.S.A. Each pulvule contains propoxyphene hydrochloride 65 mg. and acetylsalicylic acid (aspirin) 325 mg. See propoxyphene and aspirin, and read Aspirin, Nonnarcotic Pain Relievers, and Drugs Used to Treat Rheumatism and Arthritis, p. 118. *Dose* By mouth, 1 capsule every four hours as needed for pain.

*daunorubicin (CERUBIDIN; daunorubicin hydrochloride)** An anticancer drug (see p. 225). *Adverse effects* May produce fever, nausea, vomiting, diarrhea, abdominal pain, sore mouth, skin rash, and loss of hair. Damage to the bone marrow may produce severe blood disorders. It may also damage the heart. Injections may produce pain and irritation. *Precautions* Should not be used in patients with heart disease or an infection. It should be used with utmost caution in pregnancy. *Dose* Varies according to the disorder being treated.

*DBI-TD** See phenformin.

DDT See chlorophenothane.

*DECADRON** See dexamethasone.

*DECA-DURABOLIN** See nandrolone.

DECAPRYN See doxylamine.

*DECLOMYCIN** See demeclocycline.

*dehydroemetine** Used to treat amebiasis (see p. 230). *Adverse effects and precautions* See emetine. *Dose* By intramuscular injection, 60 to 100 mg. daily.

*DELALUTIN** See hydroxyprogesterone.

*DELTA-CORTEF** See prednisolone.

*deltacortone** See prednisone.

*DELTALIN** See calciferol.

*delta methyl hydrocortisone (MEDROL)** See methylprednisolone.

*delta-1-cortisone** See prednisone.

*delta-1-hydrocortisone** See prednisone.

*DELTASONE** See prednisone.

*demeclocycline (DECLOMYCIN; demeclocycline hydrochloride; demethylchlortetracycline hydrochloride)** A tetracycline antibiotic (see p. 217). It is long-acting. *Adverse effects and precautions* Similar to those described under tetracycline, but in addition demeclocycline may cause skin sensitivity to sunlight. Patients should therefore avoid exposure to sunlight when receiving treatment with this drug. Salts of aluminum, calcium, and magnesium (e.g., antacid mixtures) and iron may decrease the absorption of demeclocycline from the gut and should not be given to patients receiving treatment with this drug. Milk, because it contains calcium, may also interfere with absorption. *Dose* By mouth, 300 to 900 mg. daily in divided doses.

*DEMEROL** See meperidine.

*demethylchlortetracycline** See demeclocycline.

*DEMULEN-21** Contains ethynodiol diacetate 1 mg. and ethinylestradiol 50 mcg. in each tablet. See ethynodiol and ethinylestradiol, and read Female Sex Hormones, p. 166, and Oral Contraceptives, p. 173.

**DEMURE** See benzethonium. It is used as an antiseptic douche.

*__DENDRID__ See idoxuridine.

*__deoxycortone__ See desoxycorticosterone.

*__DEPO-MEDROL__ Methylprednisolone acetate, a long-acting injection. For methylprednisolone see prednisolone, and read Corticosteroids, p. 160.

*__DEPO-PROVERA__ The injectable form of medroxyprogesterone. See medroxyprogesterone.

*__DERONIL__ See dexamethasone.

*__DES__ See diethylstilbestrol.

**DESENEX** Contains various amounts of undecylenic acid and zinc undecylenate. Used in antifungal skin applications. Read Drugs Used to Treat Skin Disorders, p. 193.

*__deserpidine__ (**HARMONYL**) Used to treat raised blood pressure. Read Drugs Used to Treat Raised Blood Pressure, p. 108. It has uses and effects similar to those described under reserpine. *Dose* By mouth, 250 mcg. three to four times daily for about two weeks, then a reduced daily dose of not more than 250 mcg.

*__desipramine__ (**NORPRAMIN; PERTOFRANE**; desipramine hydrochloride) A tricyclic antidepressant drug. Read Antidepressants, p. 56. *Adverse effects and precautions* Similar to those described under imipramine. *Dose* By mouth, initially 50 to 200 mg. daily in divided doses, changing to a maintenance dose of 75 to 150 mg. daily.

*__desoxycorticosterone__ (deoxycortone) A corticosteroid. Read Corticosteroids, p. 160.

*__desoxyephedrine__ See methamphetamine.

*__DESOXYN__ See methamphetamine.

*__dexamethasone__ (**DECADRON**) Effects, uses, and adverse effects similar to those of prednisone, but it is effective in lower doses. See prednisone, and read Corticosteroids, p. 160. *Dose* By mouth, 0.5 to 2 mg. daily in divided doses.

*__dexamphetamine__ See dextroamphetamine.

**dexbrompheniramine** (**DISOMER, CHRONOTAB**; dexbrompheniramine maleate) An antihistamine drug. Read Antihistamine Drugs, p. 127. *Dose* By mouth, 2 to 12 mg. daily in divided doses.

*__dexchlorpheniramine__ (**POLARAMINE**) An antihistamine drug. Read Antihistamine Drugs, p. 127. *Dose* By mouth, 2 mg. three or four times daily.

*__DEXEDRINE__ See dextroamphetamine.

*__dextroamphetamine__ (**DEXEDRINE**; dexamphetamine sulfate; dextroamphetamine sulfate) Produces effects similar to those described under amphetamine sulfate. Read Stimulants: Amphetamines, p. 64. *Dose* By mouth, 10 mg. three times a day.

**dextromethorphan (SILENCE IS GOLDEN; dextromethorphan hydrobromide)** A cough suppressant. Read Drugs Used to Treat Coughs, p. 135. *Adverse effects* May occasionally cause drowsiness and dizziness. No case of drug dependence has so far been reported. *Dose* By mouth, 15 to 30 mg. once to four times daily.

*dextropropoxyphene See propoxyphene.

dextrose A readily absorbable carbohydrate which acts as a source of energy. It may be given by mouth or by injection.

*dextrothyroxine (CHOLOXIN; dextrothyroxine sodium) Used to treat underworking of the thyroid gland. Read Drugs Used to Treat Thyroid Disorders, p. 187. *Adverse effects* May trigger angina, in which case the daily dose should be reduced. *Precautions* May increase the effects of anticoagulant drugs and upset the balance of treatment in patients suffering from diabetes. *Dose* By mouth, 1 to 8 mg. daily in divided doses.

*DIABINESE See chlorpropamide.

*DIAFEN See diphenylpyraline.

DIALOSE Each capsule contains dioctyl sodium sulfosuccinate 100 mg. and sodium carboxymethylcellulose 400 mg. See each constituent drug and read Drugs Used to Treat Constipation, p. 82.

DIALOSE PLUS Each capsule contains dioctyl sodium sulfosuccinate 100 mg., sodium carboxymethylcellulose 400 mg., and casanthranol 30 mg. See each constituent drug, and read Drugs Used to Treat Constipation, p. 82.

*DIAMOX See acetazolamide.

*DIANABOL See methandrostenolone.

*diazepam (VALIUM) A benzodiazepine minor tranquilizer. Read Minor Tranquilizers, p. 51. It has effects and uses similar to those of chlordiazepoxide and is used to relieve anxiety and tension. It also has muscle-relaxant properties, produces sedation, and is used to treat convulsions. Read Drugs Used to Treat Epilepsy, p. 142. *Adverse effects* Drowsiness, fatigue, and unsteady gait (ataxia), dryness of the mouth, and fall in blood pressure may occur. In some patients it may produce excitement and aggression instead of sedation (paradoxical reaction). It may produce changes in libido and cause constipation, incontinence, and trembling. Very rarely skin rashes and blood and liver disorders may occur. *Precautions* Should be used with caution in patients with impaired kidney or liver function and in the elderly and debilitated. "Normal" doses may make these patients unsteady on their feet, drowsy, and confused. Its effects are increased by alcohol, barbiturates, narcotics, or any other drug which depresses brain function. Diazepam may interfere with the ability to drive a motor vehicle or operate moving machinery. When given for prophylaxis along with other anticonvulsant drugs, diazepam may increase the frequency and severity of major convulsions, requiring an increased dosage of the other anticonvulsant. Also, abrupt withdrawal may be associated with a temporary increase in frequency and severity of convulsions. *Drug dependence* May very rarely cause dependence of the barbiturate/alcohol type. *Dose* By mouth, 5 to 30 mg. daily in divided doses.

*diazoxide (HYPERSTAT) Used in the emergency treatment of raised blood pressure. Read Drugs Used to Treat Raised Blood Pressure, p. 108. *Adverse effects* Causes water and salt retention, and a diuretic may be given with it. Diazoxide injected into a vein produces a rapid fall in blood pressure lasting up to 24 hours. It is used in emergencies in a dose of 300 mg.

*DIBENZYLINE See phenoxybenzamine.

*dibucaine (NUPERCAINE; dibucaine hydrochloride) A local anesthetic. See p. 191.

*dichlorophen Used to treat tapeworm. Read Drugs Used to Treat Worm Infections, p. 229. *Adverse effects* Include nausea, vomiting, colic, and diarrhea. It may also produce jaundice and skin rashes. *Precautions* Should not be used when fluid loss could be harmful, e.g., pregnancy, fever, heart disease. It should not be used in patients with liver impairment, and alcohol should be avoided. *Dose* By mouth, 6 G. daily for two days in divided doses.

*dichlorphenamide (DARANIDE; ORATROL) A diuretic drug used to reduce pressure inside the eyes in the treatment of glaucoma. Read Diuretics, p. 103. *Adverse effects* May cause loss of appetite, nausea, vomiting, numbness and tingling in the hands and feet, confusion, trembling, unsteadiness on the feet, and noises in the ears. Its use over prolonged periods may cause disturbances of salt and water balance. *Dose* By mouth, 50 to 300 mg. daily in divided doses.

*dicloxacillin (DYNAPEN, PATHOCIL, VERACILLIN; dicloxacillin sodium) Very similar to cloxacillin. Read Penicillins, p. 213. *Dose* By mouth, 125 to 500 mg. every six hours.

*dicloxacillin sodium See dicloxacillin.

dicophane See chlorophenothane.

*dicoumarol (DICUMAROL; bishydroxycoumarin) Effects and uses similar to those described under warfarin sodium. It may cause nausea, vomiting, and diarrhea. Read Drugs Used to Prevent Blood from Clotting, p. 90.

*DICUMAROL See dicoumarol.

*dicyclomine (BENTYL; dicyclomine hydrochloride) Weak atropine-like effects, but it does not act upon the brain. See atropine, and read Drugs Used to Treat Indigestion and Peptic Ulcers, p. 74. *Dose* By mouth, 30 to 60 mg. daily in divided doses.

*DIDREX See benzphetamine.

*dienestrol Effects and uses similar to the female sex hormone stilbestrol, but it is less potent. Read Female Sex Hormones, p. 166. *Dose* By mouth for menopausal symptoms, 0.1 to 1.5 mg. daily. To stop milk production, 1.5 mg. three times daily for three days, then 0.5 mg. daily for seven days.

*diethycarbamazine Used to treat worm infections (see p. 229). It is principally used to treat filariasis. *Adverse effects* Include loss of appetite, nausea and vomiting, headache, drowsiness, and allergic reactions (fever, muscle pains, skin rashes). *Precautions* Should not be used to treat patients with onchocerciasis because allergic reactions may affect the eyes. *Dose* By mouth, 2 mg. per kg. of body weight three times daily for one to three weeks.

*diethylpropion (TENUATE; TEPANIL) Used as an appetite depressant. Read Reducing Drugs, p. 68. *Adverse effects* Similar to those described under amphetamine sulfate, but diethylpropion produces less effects on the heart and circulation. It may produce drug dependence of the amphetamine type. *Dose* By mouth, 25 mg. three times daily one hour before meals, or 75 mg. of the sustained-release form in the morning (25 mg. may be taken in mid-evening if insomnia is not a problem).

*diethylstilbestrol (PABESTROL; stilbestrol, DES) A synthetic estrogen. Read Female Sex Hormones, p. 166.

diethyltoluamide Used as an insect repellent.

DI-GEL Tablets and liquids contain magnesium carbonate (strength not available) and simethicone 25 mg. in each tablet or 5 ml. See magnesium carbonate and simethicone, and read Drugs Used to Treat Indigestion and Peptic Ulcers, p. 74.

*digitalis (digitalis lanata leaf; digitalis leaf; prepared digitalis; powdered digitalis); digitoxin; digoxin (LANOXIN) These are cardiac glycosides. Read Drugs Used to Treat Heart Failure and Heart Rhythm Disorders, p. 86.

*digitoxin (CYSTODIGIN, PURODIGIN) Read Drugs Used to Treat Heart Failure and Heart Rhythm Disorders, p. 86.

*digoxin (LANOXIN) Read Drugs Used to Treat Heart Failure and Heart Rhythm Disorders, p. 86. *Precautions* Do not take with antacids or with antidiarrheal preparations containing kaolin and pectin.

*dihydrocodeine (DROCODE, PARACODIN; dihydrocodeine tartrate, dihydrocodeine acid tartrate) A mild-to-moderate pain reliever, also used as a cough suppressant. Read Morphine and Narcotic Pain Relievers, p. 115, and also Drugs Used to Treat Coughs, p. 135. *Adverse effects* These are similar to those described under morphine, but less pronounced. *Precautions* Dihydrocodeine should be given with caution to patients with impaired liver function and severe respiratory disorders such as asthma. *Drug dependence* It may produce dependence of the morphine type. *Dose* By mouth, 30 to 60 mg. when necessary, up to a maximum of 150 mg. in twenty-four hours.

*dihydroergocornine  See dihydroergotoxine.

*dihydroergocristine  See dihydroergotoxine.

*dihydroergokryptine  See dihydroergotoxine.

*dihydroergotamine (dihydroergotamine mesylate)  Used to treat migraine. Read Drugs Used to Treat Migraine, p. 125. It has effects and uses similar to those described under ergotamine, but it produces less vomiting and there is less risk of gangrene. *Dose* By intramuscular injection, 1 mg. at the first sign of impending headache, then 1 mg. at the end of the first hour and again at the end of the second hour, making a total of 3 mg. Once the minimum effective dose is determined, it may be given as a single dose at the beginning of an attack.

*dihydroergotoxine (HYDERGINE; dihydroergotoxine mesylate)  A mixture of three compounds—dihydroergocristine, dihydroergocornine, and dihydroergokryptine—used to treat migraine (see p. 127). It may produce nausea, but there is less risk of gangrene than with ergotamine. *Dose* Sucked under the tongue, 2 tablets (0.5 mg.) three times daily.

*dihydrostreptomycin  See streptomycin.

dihydroxyaluminum aminoacetate  Used as an antacid. Read Drugs Used to Treat Indigestion and Peptic Ulcers, p. 74.

dihydroxyaluminum sodium carbonate (ROLAIDS)  Used as an antacid. Read Drugs Used to Treat Indigestion and Peptic Ulcers, p. 74.

*diiodohydroxyquin (DIIODOQUIN)  Used to treat amebiasis of the gut. It has been used to treat *Trichomonas* vaginitis.

*DIIODOQUIN  See diiodohydroxyquin.

*dilabron  See isoetharine.

*DILANTIN SODIUM  See phenytoin.

*DILAUDID  See hydromorphone.

dimenhydrinate (DRAMAMINE; diphenhydramine theoclate)  An antihistamine drug. It is used to prevent and relieve motion sickness. Read Antihistamine Drugs, p. 127, and Drugs Used to Treat Nausea, Vomiting, and Motion Sickness, p. 71. *Adverse effects* One of its main adverse effects is drowsiness. *Dose* By mouth, 25 to 50 mg. half an hour before traveling and up to four times daily.

*DIMETANE  See brompheniramine.

*DIMETAPP elixir  5 ml. contains brompheniramine maleate 4 mg., phenylephrine hydrochloride 5 mg., and phenylpropanolamine hydrochloride 5 mg. For brompheniramine read Antihistamine Drugs, p. 127. For phenylephrine and phenylpropanolamine see ephedrine and read Drugs Used to Treat Common Colds, p. 132. Also read Drugs Used to Treat Coughs, p. 135. *Dose* By mouth, 1 to 2 teaspoonfuls (5 to 10 ml.) three to four times daily.

*DIMETAPP EXTENTABS  Same as Dimetapp, but each tablet contains 12 mg., 15 mg., and 15 mg. respectively. For brompheniramine read Antihistamine Drugs, p. 127. For phenylephrine and phenylpropanolamine see ephedrine and read Drugs Used to Treat Common Colds, p. 132. Also read Drugs Used to Treat Coughs, p. 135. *Dose* By mouth, 1 tablet every eight to twelve hours.

dimethicone (silicone)  Used as a water-repellent in skin applications.

*dimethisterone  Effects and uses similar to progesterone. In large doses it may cause pain in the lower abdomen, fullness of the breasts, and vertigo. See progesterone; and read Female Sex Hormones, p. 166. *Dose* By mouth, 15 to 40 mg. daily in divided doses.

*dimethylamine  See diphenhydramine.

*dimethylaminobenzoate  See tetracaine.

dimethylcarbate  Used as an insect repellent.

dimethylphthalate  Used as an insect repellent.

dioctyl calcium sulfosuccinate  Read entry under dioctyl sodium sulfosuccinate.

dioctyl sodium sulfosuccinate (COLACE)  Lowers surface tension and has detergent properties. It is used as a laxative, to soften wax in the ears, and is included in some tablets in order to make them dissolve more quickly in the stomach. Read Drugs Used to Treat Constipation, p. 82. *Dose* By mouth, 50 to 100 mg. on alternate days.

*DIODOQUIN  See diiodohydroxyquin.

*DIPAXIN  See diphenadione.

*diphenadione (DIPAXIN)  An anticoagulant drug. Read Drugs Used to Prevent Blood from Clotting, p. 90. *Adverse effects* May produce nausea and overdosage causes bleeding. *Dose* By mouth, 2.5 to 30 mg. daily.

*diphenhydramine (BENADRYL; diphenhydramine hydrochloride; dimethylamine hydrochloride)  An antihistamine drug. Read Antihistamine Drugs, p. 127. It is one of the least effective antihistamines, but produces more drowsiness. For this reason it is used to induce sleep, usually in combination with a hypnotic drug. *Dose* By mouth, 50 to 200 mg. daily in divided doses or by injection as a single dose.

*diphenoxylate (present in LOMOTIL) Reduces the mobility of the gut and is used to treat diarrhea. See Drugs Used to Treat Diarrhea, p. 80. *Adverse effects* Include itching, skin rash, drowsiness, insomnia, dizziness, restlessness, changes in mood, abdominal distention, and nausea. *Precautions* Should not be used in patients with impaired liver function. It may increase the effects of barbiturates and other depressant drugs. Adverse effects may be exaggerated in infants and children, and it should therefore be used with caution. *Drug dependence* May produce drug dependence of the morphine type, which is said to be discouraged by the addition of atropine (as in Lomotil). *Dose* By mouth, 5 to 40 mg. daily in divided doses.

*diphenylhydantoin See phenytoin.

*diphenylpyraline (DIAFEN; HISPRIL; diphenylpyraline hydrochloride) An antihistamine drug. Read Antihistamine Drugs, p. 127.

*dipyridamole (PERSANTINE) Used to treat angina. Read Drugs Used to Treat Heart Failure and Heart Rhythm Disorders, p. 86. *Adverse effects* May cause headache, dizziness, faintness, and gastric upsets. *Dose* By mouth, 25 to 50 mg. two or three times daily.

*DISIPAL See orphenadrine.

*DISOMER See dexbrompheniramine.

*disulfiram (ANTABUSE) Used to treat alcoholism. It is not a cure, and it is used because it produces unpleasant effects when alcohol is taken. These unpleasant effects are caused by an accumulation in the blood of a breakdown product of alcohol called acetaldehyde. Within 15 minutes of taking alcohol, disulfiram may produce red eyes, flushed face, throbbing headache, rapid heartbeat, dizziness, nausea, sweating, and vomiting. An irritation in the throat, deep breathing, and a fall in blood pressure may occur. The effects last from 30 minutes to an hour in mild cases and up to several hours in severe attacks. The intensity and duration vary greatly among individuals; initial treatment should therefore be carried out only in a hospital. A careful dosage regimen needs to be worked out, starting with a high dose and slowly working down to a maintenance dose. *Adverse effects* May cause indigestion, bad breath, body odor, drowsiness, headache, impotence, allergic skin rashes, and nerve damage (peripheral neuritis). *Precautions* Even small quantities of alcohol may produce a severe reaction which may result in heart failure, unconsciousness, convulsions, and even death. It should not be used during pregnancy, or for patients with heart disease, severe psychological disorders, or drug dependence. It should be used with the utmost caution in patients with impaired liver or kidney function, epilepsy, chronic bronchitis, or diabetes. It increases the effects of coumarin anticoagulants and phenytoin. Acute confusion may occur when given with metronidazole (Flagyl). It should only be used if the patient has clear knowledge of the expected benefits and risks. *Dose* By mouth, 250 mg. daily for the first two or three weeks, then 125 to 500 mg. daily.

**dithranol (anthralin)** Used to treat psoriasis. Some patients are sensitive to it, and a small area of skin should be tested first. It stains the skin, causes a burning sensation, and irritates the eyes.

\*DIUCARDIN See hydroflumethiazide.

\*DIUPRES Each tablet contains chlorothiazide 250 mg. or 500 mg. and reserpine 0.125 mg. See chlorothiazide, and read Diuretics, p. 103. See reserpine, and read Drugs Used to Treat Raised Blood Pressure, p. 108. *Dose* By mouth, Diupres 250, one tablet one to four times daily. Diupres 500, one tablet one to two times daily.

\*DIURIL See chlorothiazide.

\*DOLENE See propoxyphene.

\*DOLENE COMPOUND 65 See propoxyphene compound 65.

DOMEBORO See aluminum acetate.

DOME-PASTE **bandage** See zinc gelatin.

**domiphen (domiphen hydrochloride)** An antiseptic with properties similar to those described under cetrimide. It is used in throat lozenges and antiseptic skin applications. In high concentrations it may be used as a disinfectant.

DONNAGEL Contains the same ingredients as Donnatal, except for the phenobarbital. It also contains kaolin and pectin. It is used to control diarrhea. See Donnatal, kaolin, and pectin. Read Drugs Used to Treat Diarrhea, p. 80.

\*DONNAGEL-PG Donnagel with added opium.

\*DONNATAL Each tablet or capsule and each 5 ml. contain hyoscyamine sulfate 0.1037 mg., atropine sulfate 0.0194 mg., hyoscine hydrobromide 0.0065 mg., and phenobarbital 16.2 mg. See atropine, and read Drugs Which Act on the Autonomic Nervous System, p. 145. See phenobarbital, and read Sleeping Drugs and Sedatives, p. 43. *Dose* By mouth, 1 or 2 tablets, capsules, or teaspoonfuls three to four times daily.

\*DOPAR See levodopa.

DORBANE See danthron.

\*DORIDEN See glutethimide.

DOXAN Contains dioctyl sodium sulfosuccinate 60 mg. and danthron 50 mg. See dioctyl sodium sulfosuccinate and danthron, and read Drugs Used to Treat Constipation, p. 82. *Dose* By mouth, 1 or 2 tablets at bedtime.

\*doxepin (SINEQUAN; **doxepin hydrochloride**) A tricyclic antidepressant drug. Read Antidepressants, p. 56. It has effects similar to imipramine but produces more drowsiness. *Dose* By mouth, 30 to 150 mg. daily in divided doses.

**DOXIDAN** Contains dioctyl calcium sulfosuccinate 60 mg. and danthron 50 mg. See dioctyl sodium sulfosuccinate and danthron, and read Drugs Used to Treat Constipation, p. 82. *Dose* By mouth, 1 or 2 capsules at bedtime.

*doxorubicin (ADRIAMYCIN) An anticancer antibiotic. Read Drugs Used to Treat Cancer, p. 225. *Adverse effects* Complete loss of hair often occurs, and in some cases nausea, vomiting, and diarrhea. In children, it causes darkening of the skin creases and nail beds. *Dose* 60–75 mg. per square meter of body surface by intravenous injection at 21-day intervals.

*doxycycline (VIBRAMYCIN; doxycycline hydrochloride) Effects, uses, and adverse effects similar to those described under tetracycline. See tetracycline, and read Antibiotics, p. 210. It is well absorbed, even when taken with food, and acts for a long time; its excretion is slow, and it is possible to get high blood levels with a once-daily dosage. *Dose* By mouth, 100 to 200 mg. daily.

*doxylamine (DECAPRYN; doxylamine succinate) An antihistamine drug. Read Antihistamine Drugs, p. 127. *Dose* By mouth, 25 mg. up to four times daily as necessary.

**DRAMAMINE** See dimenhydrinate.

*DRISDOL See calciferol.

**DRISTAN** Each capsule contains phenylephrine 5 mg. and chlorpheniramine 4 mg.; each tablet, phenylephrine 5 mg., phenindamine 10 mg. Both also contain aspirin, caffeine, aluminum hydroxide, and magnesium carbonate (strengths not available). See constituent drugs, and read Drugs Used to Treat Common Colds, p. 132, and Drugs Used to Treat Coughs, p. 135.

*DRIXORAL See dexbrompheniramine.

*DROCODE See dihydrocodeine.

*DROLBAN See dromostanolone.

*dromostanolone (DROLBAN, MASTERANE; dromostanolone propionate) A male sex hormone. Read Male Sex Hormones, p. 163, and Anabolic Steroids, p. 165. *Dose* 100 mg. three times weekly by intramuscular injection.

**DULCOLAX** See bisacodyl.

*DUPHASTON See dydrogesterone.

*DURABOLIN See nandrolone.

*DUVADILAN See isoxsuprine.

*DYAZIDE tablets Contains triamterene 50 mg. and hydrochlorothiazide 25 mg. See triamterene and hydrochlorothiazide, and read Diuretics, p. 103.

*dydrogesterone (DUPHASTON; GYNOREST) Effects similar to those described under progesterone. Read Female Sex Hormones, p. 166. It is used to treat disorders of menstruation along with estrogens, to treat painful periods, and to treat patients who have had repeated miscarriages. It is of no value as an oral contraceptive. *Adverse effects* May cause nausea, vomiting, and breakthrough bleeding (this usually responds to a reduction in dose and increased frequency of administration). *Dose* For treatment of painful periods, by mouth, 5 to 10 mg. daily in divided doses (from the 5th to 23rd day of the cycle).

\*DYMELOR   See acetohexamide.

\*DYNAPEN   See dicloxacillin.

\*DYRENIUM   See triamterene.

\*echothiophate   See pholine iodide.

ECOTRIN   See aspirin.

\*EDECRIN   See ethacrynic acid.

\*edrophonium (TENSILON)   Effects and uses similar to neostigmine. It is used to diagnose myasthenia gravis and has been used to treat disorders of heart rhythm. Read Drugs Which Act on the Autonomic Nervous System, p. 145.

EFFERSYLLIUM   Effervescent psyllium, a bulk laxative. See psyllium, and read Drugs Used to Treat Constipation, p. 82.

\*EFUDEX solution and cream   See fluorouracil.

\*ELAVIL   See amitriptyline.

\*ELIXOPHYLLIN   See theophylline.

EMETE-CON   See benzquinamide.

\*emetine   Used in the treatment of amoebic dysentery, amoebic hepatitis, and liver abscess. It irritates the stomach lining. In small doses it increases bronchial secretion and causes sweating and vomiting. Prolonged use may cause damage to the liver, kidneys, muscles, nerves, and heart muscle. *Dose* By subcutaneous or intramuscular injection 1 mg. per kg. of body weight, not to exceed 65 mg. daily, for three to ten days.

EMPIRIN COMPOUND   Each tablet contains aspirin 227 mg., phenacetin 162 mg., and caffeine 15 mg. See aspirin, phenacetin, and caffeine.

\*EMPIRIN COMPOUND with codeine   A compound preparation, each tablet containing aspirin 227 mg., phenacetin 162 mg., caffeine 15 mg., and codeine (in various strengths of 7.5 mg., 15 mg., 30 mg., or 60 mg.). See aspirin, phenacetin, caffeine, and codeine, and read Aspirin, Nonnarcotic Pain Relievers, and Drugs Used to Treat Rheumatism and Arthritis, p. 118. *Dose* By mouth, 1 or 2 tablets three times daily as needed.

\*E-MYCIN   See erythromycin.

\*ENDURON   See methyclothiazide.

\*ENDURONYL   Contains methyclothiazide 5 mg. and deserpidine 0.25 mg. See methyclothiazide, and read Diuretics, p. 103. See deserpidine, and read Drugs Used to Treat Raised Blood Pressure, p. 108. *Dose* By mouth, 1 tablet daily.

\*ENOVID Each tablet contains norethynodrel 5 mg. and mestranol 0.075 mg. Read Oral Contraceptive Drugs, p. 173.

\*ENOVID E Each tablet contains norethynodrel 2.5 mg. and mestranol 0.1 mg. Read Oral Contraceptive Drugs, p. 173.

\***ephedrine (ephedrine hydrochloride)** Has stimulating effects which resemble epinephrine and amphetamines. When given by mouth it constricts small blood vessels and raises the blood pressure, relaxes the muscles in the bronchi, slows down movements in the gut, and contracts the uterus. It also has effects on the bladder and the pupils, and it stimulates the central nervous system. It is used mainly to prevent attacks of asthma. Read Drugs Used to Treat Bronchial Asthma, p. 138. *Adverse effects* If given to patients sensitive to ephedrine, or if given in large doses, it may cause nausea, vomiting, giddiness, headache, sweating, thirst, palpitations, anxiety, restlessness, trembling, insomnia, and muscular weakness. *Precautions* Should not be used in patients with high blood pressure, coronary thrombosis, or overworking of the thyroid gland. It should be given with caution to patients with heart disease, and it may cause retention of urine in patients with enlarged prostate glands (who may already have difficulty urinating). Ephedrine should not be used in patients being treated with monoamine oxidase inhibitor antidepressant drugs or within two weeks of stopping such drugs. *Dose* By mouth, 30 mg. three times daily, up to a maximum daily dose of 150 mg.

EPI-CLEAR SCRUB CLEANSER See aluminum oxide.

\***epinephrine (adrenaline)** Acts on the nerve endings of the sympathetic nervous system. It produces the sort of effects caused by fear or emotion: blanched skin (caused by constriction of small arteries), dilation of the pupils, inhibition of the movements of the gut and bladder, and release of glucose by the liver. In addition it increases the blood supply to muscles, stimulates the heart, increases the heart rate, and relaxes the uterus and bronchial muscles. These are stress effects and prepare the body for what may be called "fight or flight." Epinephrine is used medically to treat asthma and to treat shock produced in severe allergic reactions. Because epinephrine constricts small blood vessels, it is often mixed with injections of a local anesthetic to prevent the anesthetic from getting washed away in the bloodstream too quickly, thereby prolonging its effects. *Adverse effects* Are common, and include anxiety, breathlessness, restlessness, palpitations, rapid heartbeat, trembling, weakness, dizziness, headache, and coldness of the hands and feet. Such reactions may occur even with small doses used by dentists in local anesthetic injections. Nervous and tense individuals easily develop these symptoms when given epinephrine, and so do patients with overworking of their thyroid glands. Gangrene of the fingers may occur after the injection of a combined solution of epinephrine and local anesthetic into a finger. *Precautions* Should not be used in patients who have overworking of their thyroid glands, coronary artery disease or a disorder of heart rhythm, high blood pressure, or hardening of the arteries (arteriosclerosis). It may cause a severe irregularity of heart rhythm in patients undergoing anesthesia with halothane, chloroform, or cyclopropane, and in patients being treated with quinidine or digitalis. Dentists should use caution when giving epinephrine to patients currently using other drugs such as antidepressants. *Dose* As a single dose by subcutaneous injection, 200 to 250 mcg.

*EPODYL   See ethoglucid.

EPSOM SALTS   See magnesium sulfate.

*EQUAGESIC   Each tablet contains aspirin 250 mg., ethoheptazine citrate 75 mg., and meprobamate 150 mg. See aspirin and ethoheptazine, and read Aspirin, Nonnarcotic Pain Relievers, and Drugs Used to Treat Rheumatism and Arthritis, p. 118. See meprobamate, and read Minor Tranquilizers, p. 51. *Dose* By mouth, 1 or 2 tablets three to four times daily, as needed.

*EQUANIL   See meprobamate.

*equilin   An estrogen. Read Female Sex Hormones, p. 166.

ergocalciferol   See calciferol.

*ERGOMAR   See ergotamine.

*ergometrine   See ergonovine.

*ergonovine (ERGOTRATE; ergometrine maleate; ergonovine maleate) Causes contractions of the uterus and is used to prevent bleeding from the uterus after childbirth. *Adverse effects* Are rare if the drug is used properly. Nausea and vomiting may occur. Intravenous injections may cause the blood pressure to increase. *Precautions* Should not be used during the first or second stages of labor, since this may cause death of the fetus and rupture of the uterus. *Dose* By mouth, 0.5 to 1 mg. By intravenous injection, 100 to 500 mcg.

*ergot   Obtained from a fungus which grows on rye, it contains several chemicals (ergot alkaloids). Some of these are used to treat migraine and to contract the uterus after childbirth.

*ergotamine (ERGOMAR, GYNERGEN; ergotamine tartrate)   Stimulates and, in large doses, paralyzes the endings of the sympathetic nerves. It constricts small blood vessels and the uterus. Its main use is in the treatment of migraine. Read Drugs Used to Treat Migraine, p. 125. *Adverse effects* Is isolated from ergot and is in fact a derivative of lysergic acid diethylamide (LSD). The dose used to treat migraine may cause headache, nausea, and vomiting, and occasionally muscle weakness and pain. In large repeated doses it can produce all the symptoms of ergot poisoning: coldness of the skin, severe muscle pains, gangrene of the hands and feet, thromboses, angina, alteration of heart rate and blood pressure, confusion, drowsiness, paralysis, and convulsions. *Precautions* Should not be used in pregnancy or in patients with circulatory diseases or impaired kidney or liver function. Its effects are increased by epinephrinelike drugs. *Dose* By mouth, 1 to 2 mg. (maximum in 24 hours—6 mg.). By subcutaneous or intramuscular injection, 250 to 500 mcg.

*ERGOTRATE   See ergonovine.

*ERYPAR   See erythromycin stearate.

*erythritol   See erythrityl.

*erythrityl (CARDILATE; erythrityl tetranitrate; erythritol)   Effects and uses similar to those described under nitroglycerin. Read Drugs Used to Treat Angina, p. 100.

*ERYTHROCIN   See erythromycin.

*erythromycin (E-MYCIN; ERYTHROCIN; ILOTYCIN)   An antibiotic. Read Antibiotics, p. 210. It is partly destroyed by acid in the stomach and has to be taken in specially coated tablets (enteric-coated). *Adverse effects* Rare and usually mild. They include abdominal pains and skin rashes. *Dose* By mouth, 1 to 4 G. daily in divided doses.

*erythromycin estolate (ILOSONE)   See erythromycin. This preparation is rapidly absorbed, producing high blood levels, *but* can cause jaundice when treatment is repeated or is continued for more than ten days.

*erythromycin stearate (BRISTAMYCIN; ERYPAR; SK-ERYTHROMYCIN)   See erythromycin. It is less bitter and is given in the same dosages as erythromycin.

*eserine   See physostigmine.

*ESIDRIX   See hydrochlorothiazide.

*esterified estrogens   Semisynthetic salts of estrogens—estrone and equilin. Read Female Sex Hormones, p. 166.

*ESTINYL   See ethinyl estradiol.

*estradiol (estradiol benzoate; estradiol cypionate)   The most active of the naturally occurring estrogens. Read Female Sex Hormones, p. 166. *Dose* 1 to 5 mg. daily by intramuscular injection.

*ESTRIN   See estrone.

*estrone   A naturally occurring estrogen. Read Female Sex Hormones, p. 166. *Dose* By mouth, 1.5 to 4.5 mg. daily.

ethacridine   An antiseptic and disinfectant. See p. 201.

*ethacrynic acid (EDECRIN)   A rapidly acting diuretic drug. Read Diuretics, p. 103. *Adverse effects* May cause loss of appetite, nausea, vomiting, and diarrhea in high doses. Single large doses or prolonged use may cause severe disturbances of the body's salt and water balance, resulting in weakness, muscle cramps, thirst, skin rashes, headaches, blurred vision, confusion, or low blood sugar. Increased blood uric acid levels may occur. Blood disorders, temporary or permanent deafness, and breast enlargement have been reported. *Precautions* See chlorothiazide. *Dose* By mouth, 50 to 200 mg. daily in divided doses.

*ethambutol (MYAMBUTOL) Used to treat tuberculosis. Read Drugs Used to Treat Tuberculosis, p. 224. *Adverse effects* Most serious adverse effect is progressive blindness with loss of copper and zinc from the body. This is reversible if the drug is stopped early enough. *Precautions* Should be used with caution in patients with impaired kidney function. Blood levels must be checked repeatedly and kept below a certain level (5 mcg. per ml.). The eyes should be examined at frequent intervals. *Dose* By mouth, 25 mg. per kg. of body weight daily for two months, followed by 15 mg. per kg. body weight daily.

*ethchlorvynol (PLACIDYL) A sleeping drug. Read Sleeping Drugs and Sedatives, p. 43. *Adverse effects* Include dizziness, nausea and vomiting, confusion, and ataxia. Long-term use may affect vision (amblyopia). *Precautions* Should not be used in patients with marked impairment of liver, kidney, or heart function. Its effects may be increased by alcohol (sometimes quite severely) and by other drugs such as sedatives. It interferes with the ability to drive motor vehicles and operate moving machinery. *Drug dependence* May produce drug dependence of the barbiturate/alcohol type. *Dose* By mouth, sleeping dose, 0.25 to 1 G.

*ethinamate (VALMID) A nonbarbiturate sleeping drug with effects similar to chloral hydrate. See chloral hydrate, and read Sleeping Drugs and Sedatives, p. 43.

*ethinylestradiol (ESTINYL, FEMINONE) Effects and uses of the estrogens. Read Female Sex Hormones, p. 166. It may cause headache, dizziness, nausea, and vomiting.

*ethionamide (TRECATOR) An antibacterial drug. Read Drugs Used to Treat Tuberculosis, p. 224. It should be given in combination with other antituberculosis drugs in order to prevent the development of drug-resistant bacteria. *Adverse effects* May cause a metallic taste in the mouth, soreness of the gums, excessive salivation, nausea, vomiting, diarrhea, and loss of appetite. Acne, alopecia (loss of hair), liver damage, fall in blood pressure, convulsions, headache, enlargement of the breasts, impotence, insomnia, damage to peripheral nerves, menstrual disturbances, slight deafness, and skin rashes have been reported. It may produce mental breakdown in alcoholics. *Precautions* Should be given with caution to patients with depression or other psychological disorders, to chronic alcoholics, and to patients with epilepsy. It may make the control of diabetes difficult, and it may increase the adverse effects of other antituberculous drugs. It should not be given in pregnancy, since it causes abnormality in the baby. *Dose* By mouth, 0.5 to 1 G. daily in divided doses.

\*ethisterone (anhydrohydroxyprogesterone; pregneninolone; ethinyltestosterone) Effects and uses similar to progesterone. Read Female Sex Hormones, p. 166.

\*ethoglucid (EPODYL) An anti-cancer drug. Read Drugs Used to Treat Cancer, p. 225. *Adverse effects* These include nausea, vomiting, loss of hair, fluid retention, pain and irritation at site of injection and bone-marrow damage leading to blood disorders. *Precautions* It should be given with caution to patients whose bone-marrow function may be depressed. *Dose* Varies according to the treatment program being followed.

\*ethoheptazine (ZACTANE) A mild pain reliever. It may produce stomach discomfort, nausea, dizziness, drowsiness, and itching. *Dose* By mouth, 75 to 150 mg. three or four times daily.

ethohexadiol Used as an insect repellent.

\*ethopropazine (PARSIDOL; ethopropazine hydrochloride) Produces effects similar to those described under atropine. It is used to treat Parkinsonism. See atropine, and read Drugs Used to Treat Parkinsonism, p. 149. *Dose* By mouth, 10 mg. two to four times daily, increasing by 5 mg. per dose every three to four days until symptoms are controlled or side effects become serious. In elderly or sensitive patients the dose should not exceed 25 mg. three to four times daily. Maximum dose is 250 mg. four times daily in persons with exceptional tolerance.

\*ethosuximide (ZARONTIN) An anticonvulsant drug used to treat petit mal epilepsy. Read Drugs Used to Treat Epilepsy, p. 142. *Adverse effects* Mild transient effects include headache, nausea, drowsiness, apathy, mood changes, unsteadiness on the feet (ataxia), and loss of appetite. It may cause skin rashes, blood disorders, Parkinsonism, and oversensitivity to bright light. If given to patients with temporal lobe epilepsy, it may cause mental breakdown. *Precautions* Should be given with extreme caution to patients with impaired liver or kidney function. *Dose* By mouth, 500 to 2000 mg. daily in divided doses.

\*ethotoin (PEGANONE) An anticonvulsant drug used to treat epilepsy. Read Drugs Used to Treat Epilepsy, p. 142. It has effects similar to phenytoin, but it is much less effective, and is also less liable to produce adverse effects. It is usually given in combination with other anticonvulsant drugs in the treatment of grand mal epilepsy. *Adverse effects* Seldom produces visual disturbances or thickening of the gums (see phenytoin), but it occasionally causes skin rashes, nausea, vomiting, dizziness, headache, and drowsiness. It may occasionally cause paranoid symptoms when given with phenacemide. *Dose* By mouth, 1 to 3 G. daily in divided doses.

\*ETHRIL   See erythromycin.

ethyl alcohol   See alcohol.

\*ethyl aminobenzoate   See benzocaine.

\*ethylenediamine   Used in combination with theophylline. See aminophylline.

\*ethylestrenol (MAXIBOLIN)   An anabolic (body-building) steroid with effects, uses, and adverse effects similar to those described under methandrostenolone. Read Anabolic Steroids, p. 165. *Dose* By mouth, 4 to 16 mg. once daily for up to six weeks.

\*ethynodiol (ethynodiol diacetate)   A synthetic female sex hormone. Read Female Sex Hormones, p. 166. Its effects and uses are similar to those described under norethisterone. It is used in conjunction with estrogens as an oral contraceptive agent and in the treatment of disorders of menstruation.

\*ETRAFON   Tablets contain combinations of amitriptyline and perphenazine in various doses. See amitriptyline and perphenazine, and read Major Tranquilizers, p. 53, and Antidepressants, p. 56. *Dose* By mouth; varies according to the strengths of combinations being used and the patient's response.

eucalyptol   Has the actions and uses of eucalyptus oil but is less irritating. It is used in irritant skin applications (see p. 202). It has some antiseptic properties and is used in some temporary dental fillings.

eucalyptus   Used in inhalations, throat pastilles, and liniments.

eucalyptus oil   Used in inhalations, throat pastilles, and liniments.

eusol   A chlorinated lime and boric acid solution used as an antiseptic. See chlorinated lime and borax, taking note of the warnings under borax.

\*EUTHYROID   See liotrix.

EXCEDRIN   Each tablet contains aspirin 200 mg., salicylamide 130 mg., acetaminophen 100 mg., and caffeine 65 mg. See aspirin, salicylamide, acetaminophen, and caffeine, and read Aspirin, Nonnarcotic Pain Relievers, and Drugs Used to Treat Rheumatism and Arthritis, p. 118.

EXCEDRIN P.M.   Each tablet contains aspirin 195 mg., salicylamide 150 mg., acetaminophen 162 mg., and methapyrilene fumarate 25 mg. See aspirin, salicylamide, acetaminophen, and methapyrilene. Read Drugs Used to Treat Common Colds, p. 132, and read Aspirin, Nonnarcotic Pain Relievers, and Drugs Used to Treat Rheumatism and Arthritis, p. 118.

EX-LAX   Contains phenolphthalein. See phenolphthalein, and read Drugs Used to Treat Constipation, p. 82.

*FANSIL See sulfadoxine.

FDS A vaginal deodorant spray (see p. 206).

*FEEN-A-MINT chewing gum See phenolphthalein.

FEMINIQUE A vaginal douche liquid containing benzethonium chloride 0.5%, alcohol 14%, lactic acid, and perfume. See benzethonium and lactic acid.

*FEMINONE See ethinylestradiol.

*fenfluramine (PONDIMIN) A weight-reducing drug. Read Reducing Drugs, p. 68. *Adverse effects* May cause drowsiness, dry mouth, dizziness, nausea, diarrhea, fatigue, and aching pains. Rarely, it causes itching of the skin and disturbed sleep. High doses may cause vivid and bad dreams. *Precautions* May increase the effects of certain drugs used to treat blood pressure: bethanidine, guanethidine, methyldopa, and reserpine. It should not be given to patients on monoamine oxidase inhibitor antidepressant drugs, and probably not to patients who are depressed or in the first three months of pregnancy. *Dose* By mouth, 20 to 120 mg. daily in divided doses.

FEOSOL See ferrous sulfate.

FERGON Is ferrous gluconate, an oral iron preparation. Read Iron, p. 152.

FER-IN-SOL Is ferrous sulfate, an oral iron preparation. Read Iron, p. 152.

FERRO-SEQUELS Each capsule contains ferrous fumarate 150 mg. and dioctyl sodium sulfosuccinate 100 mg. See ferrous fumarate and dioctyl sodium sulfosuccinate. Read Iron, p. 152.

ferrous fumarate An iron salt taken by mouth for iron deficiency. Read Iron, p. 152.

ferrous gluconate An iron salt taken by mouth for iron deficiency. Read Iron, p. 152.

ferrous succinate An iron salt taken by mouth for iron deficiency. See Iron, p. 152.

ferrous sulfate and other iron preparations Read Iron, p. 152.

*FIORINAL Each capsule or tablet contains butalbital 50 mg., caffeine 40 mg., aspirin 200 mg., and phenacetin 130 mg. See butalbital, and read Sleeping Drugs and Sedatives, p. 43. See aspirin, phenacetin, and caffeine, and read Aspirin, Nonnarcotic Pain Relievers, and Drugs Used to Treat Rheumatism and Arthritis, p. 118. *Dose* By mouth, 1 to 2 tablets or capsules repeated if necessary up to six times daily.

*FIORINAL with codeine Contains the ingredients of Fiorinal plus codeine in varying amounts (8, 16, or 32 mg.). See Fiorinal and codeine. *Dose* By mouth, 1 to 2 tablets or capsules repeated if necessary up to six times daily.

FIZRIN powder Contains aspirin 324 mg., sodium bicarbonate 1.82

G., sodium carbonate 400 mg., and citric acid 1.5 G. See aspirin and sodium bicarbonate.

*FLAGYL See metronidazole.

FLEET enema Contains sodium phosphate 6 G. and sodium biphosphate 16 G. in each 100 ml. These salts cause an increase in the bulk of the feces by causing osmosis of water into the lower bowel, thus stimulating the muscles to contract and evacuate the bowel. See Drugs Used to Treat Constipation, p. 82.

FLETCHER'S CASTORIA A liquid senna laxative. See senna.

*FLORINEF See fludrocortisone.

*floxuridine (FUDR) An anticancer drug (see p. 227). *Adverse effects* These include nausea, vomiting, loss of appetite, skin rash, loss of hair, nail damage, and pigmentation of the skin. It may produce damage to the lining membrane of the mouth, stomach and gut, fever, hemorrhage, and bone-marrow damage leading to blood disorders. *Precautions* It should not be given to patients whose bone-marrow function may be depressed, and it should be given with caution to patients whose liver function is impaired. *Dose* Varies according to treatment program being followed.

*flucytosine (ANCOBON) An antifungal drug (see pp. 212–13). Also used in antifungal skin applications (p. 200). *Dose* By mouth, 100 mg. per kg. of body weight daily in four divided doses.

*fludrocortisone (FLORINEF; fludrocortisone acetate) A corticosteroid. Read Corticosteroids, p. 160.

*flumethasone A corticosteroid. Read Corticosteroids, p. 160. Used in skin applications. Read Drugs Used to Treat Skin Disorders, p. 193.

*fluocinolone (SYNALAR; FLUONID; fluocinolone acetonide) A corticosteroid used in skin applications. Read Drugs Used to Treat Skin Disorders, p. 193, and Corticosteroids, p. 160.

*fluocinonide A corticosteroid. Read Corticosteroids, p. 160. Used in skin applications. Read Drugs Used to Treat Skin Disorders, p. 193.

*FLUONID See fluocinolone.

*fluorometholone A corticosteroid. Read Corticosteroids, p. 160. Used in skin applications. Read Drugs Used to Treat Skin Disorders, p. 193.

*FLUOROPLEX See fluorouracil.

*fluorouracil (EFUDEX, FLUOROPLEX) An anticancer drug. Read Drugs Used to Treat Cancer, p. 225. *Adverse effects* Include nausea, vomiting, loss of appetite, skin rash, loss of hair, nail damage, and pigmentation of the skin. It may produce damage to the lining membrane of the mouth, stomach, and gut, fever, hemorrhage, and bone-marrow damage leading to blood disorders. *Precautions* Should not be given to patients whose bone-marrow function may be depressed, and should be given with caution to patients whose liver function is impaired. *Dose* 6 to 15 mg. per kg. of body weight by intravenous injection.

\*fluoxymesterone (ULTANDREN, HALOTESTIN, ORA-TESTRYL) A male sex hormone with effects similar to those described under testosterone. Read Male Sex Hormones, p. 163. *Dose* By mouth, 2 to 30 mg. daily.

\*fluphenazine (PERMITIL; PROLIXIN; fluphenazine hydrochloride) A major tranquilizer. Read Major Tranquilizers, p. 53. It also has anti-vomiting properties. Read Drugs Used to Treat Nausea, Vomiting, and Motion Sickness, p. 71. *Adverse effects* May produce Parkinsonism and other disorders of movement and coordination. Some of these effects are irreversible. Occasionally fluphenazine may cause milk to come from the breasts (galactorrhea), abdominal pain, and jaundice. For other adverse effects and precautions refer to chlorpromazine. *Dose* By mouth, for anxiety states, 1 to 2 mg. daily in divided doses. As a major tranquilizer for psychotic disorders, up to 15 mg. daily in divided doses.

\*fluprednisolone (ALPHADROL) A corticosteroid. See prednisone, and read Corticosteroids, p. 160.

\*flurandrenolide (CORDRAN; flurandrenolone) A corticosteroid. Read Corticosteroids, p. 160. Used in skin applications. Read Drugs Used to Treat Skin Disorders, p. 193.

\*flurandrenolone See flurandrenolide.

\*flurazepam (DALMANE) A benzodiazepine drug used to treat insomnia. See chlordiazepoxide, and Read Sleeping Drugs and Sedatives, p. 43. *Dose* By mouth, 15 to 30 mg. before bedtime.

\*folic acid (FOLVITE; pteroylglutamic acid) Present in many foods; it is necessary for cell division and for the normal production of red blood cells. Read Vitamins, p. 155. Symptoms of folic acid deficiency include sore tongue, anemia, diarrhea, and loss of weight. Folic acid deficiency may occur in pregnancy, in patients with certain disorders of the stomach and bowels which interfere with absorption (e.g., sprue, coeliac disease, after gastrectomy), after prolonged use of large doses of pyrimethamine (used to prevent malaria), and in patients with epilepsy treated with anticonvulsant drugs (particularly primidone and phenytoin, but also phenobarbital). In this last disorder, folic acid deficiency can lead to mental deterioration, which can be prevented by giving folic acid and vitamin $B_{12}$. Folic acid deficiency may also occur in pregnancy, and it is now often given routinely along with iron during the prenatal period. *Adverse effects* Appears to be nontoxic in human beings. *Precautions* Should not be used to treat pernicious anemia, since, unlike vitamin $B_{12}$, it does not prevent the nerve damage complications of pernicious anemia. *Dose* By mouth, initially, 0.1 to 1 mg. daily. Maintenance, 0.2 to 0.5 mg. daily.

**FOLVITE** See folic acid.

**formaldehyde in solution (formalin)** Used in varying strengths as an antiseptic and disinfectant. It is also used to treat warts and foot perspiration, and in throat lozenges.

**formalin** See formaldehyde.

**4-WAY COLD TABLETS** Each tablet contains phenylephrine hydrochloride 5 mg., aspirin 324 mg., yellow phenolphthalein 15 mg., and magnesium hydroxide 125 mg. See phenylephrine, aspirin, phenolphthalein, and magnesium hydroxide. Read Drugs Used to Treat Common Colds, p. 132.

**frangula** A liquid extract of dried bark of *Rhamnus frangula.* It has properties similar to those of cascara sagrada and is used in laxative preparations. Read Drugs Used to Treat Constipation, p. 82.

**\*FUDR** See floxuridine.

**\*FULVICIN** See griseofulvin.

**\*FUNGIZONE** See amphotericin B

**\*FURACIN** See nitrofurazone.

**\*FURADANTIN** See nitrofurantoin.

**\*furosemide (LASIX)** A diuretic. Read Diuretics, p. 103. It works quickly when taken by mouth and lasts for about four to six hours. *Adverse effects* May produce nausea and diarrhea. Continued use may cause salt and water loss, resulting in weakness, muscle cramps, pins and needles, thirst, and loss of appetite. It may trigger an attack of gout in someone prone to that disease. It may also produce blood disorders and cause the blood sugar to increase and sugar to appear in the urine. Prolonged use may cause a fall in blood sodium, calcium, and potassium; a fall in potassium sensitizes heart muscle to digitalis. *Precautions* Should not be used in patients with acute impairment of kidney function. When the blood potassium is low, it should be used with caution in patients with impaired liver function. For general precautions read Diuretics, p. 103. *Dose* By mouth, 40 to 200 mg. daily in divided doses, reducing to a maintenance dose every other day or on three successive days each week.

**\*gallamine (gallamine triethiodide)** A muscle relaxant which is used along with general anesthetics in surgical operations. Read Drugs Which Act on the Autonomic Nervous System, p. 145. It may produce rapid beating of the heart. For precautions see tubocurarine.

**gamma benzene hexachloride** Used to treat scabies and lice.

**\*GANTANOL** See sulfamethoxazole.

**\*GANTRISIN** See sulfisoxazole.

*GARAMYCIN See gentamicin.

GAVISCON Each tablet contains alginic acid 200 mg., magnesium trisilicate 20 mg., dried aluminum hydroxide gel 80 mg., and sodium bicarbonate 70 mg. See magnesium trisilicate and aluminum hydroxide, and read Drugs Used to Treat Indigestion and Peptic Ulcers, p. 74. *Dose* By mouth, 2 to 4 tablets chewed after meals and at bedtime followed by half a glass of water. Do not swallow whole.

GELUSIL Each tablet contains magnesium trisilicate 500 mg. and dried aluminum hydroxide 250 mg. Also available as a suspension. See magnesium trisilicate and aluminum hydroxide, and read Drugs Used to Treat Indigestion and Peptic Ulcers, p. 74.

GELUSIL M 5 ml. contains magnesium trisilicate 500 mg., aluminum hydroxide 250 mg., and magnesium hydroxide 100 mg. See aluminum hydroxide, magnesium hydroxide, and trisilicate. Read Drugs Used to Treat Indigestion and Peptic Ulcers, p. 74.

*gentamicin (GARAMYCIN; gentamicin sulfate) An antibiotic. Read Antibiotics, p. 210. It is not absorbed by mouth and has to be given by injections and used in ointments. *Adverse effects* By injection may produce deafness and disorders of balance, which may be permanent. It may also produce kidney damage, skin rashes, and fevers. *Precautions* Should be used in pregnancy or infancy only if no safer treatment is available. *Dose* Varies according to age, weight, disease, kidney function, and route of administration.

gentian violet (crystal violet) Used in antiseptic skin applications against bacteria, worms, and fungi.

*GEOCILLIN See carbenicillin.

*GEOPEN See carbenicillin.

GERITOL Read Iron, p. 152.

GLAUBER'S SALTS Sodium sulfate, used as a laxative. Read Drugs Used to Treat Constipation, p. 82.

*GLAUCON See epinephrine.

*globin zinc suspension An insulin preparation. Read Drugs Used to Treat Diabetes, p. 182.

*glucagon Used to treat low blood sugar caused by too much insulin or other drugs. Read Drugs Used to Treat Diabetes, p. 182. *Dose* By subcutaneous injection, 1 mg.

glucose A readily absorbable carbohydrate which acts as a source of energy. It may be given either by mouth or by injection.

glutaraldehyde Used as an antiseptic (see p. 202).

*glutethimide (DORIDEN) Used as a sedative and sleeping drug. Read Sleeping Drugs and Sedatives, p. 43. *Adverse effects* May produce nausea, dizziness, excitement, and skin rashes. Blood disorders and nerve damage have been reported, rarely, in patients allergic to glutethimide. Very rarely, long-term use may produce toxic psychoses, convulsions, and fever. *Precautions* Can markedly increase the effects of alcohol. *Drug dependence* Produces dependence of the barbiturate/alcohol type. *Dose* By mouth, 250 to 500 mg. at night.

**glycerin** See glycerol.

**glycerol (glycerin)** Used as a lubricant, and as a sweetening agent in mixtures and pastilles. It has been used as a diuretic. Glycerol suppositories are used to treat constipation. Glycerol is included in creams and jellies and in ear drops to soften wax. *Adverse effects* Large doses by mouth may cause headache, thirst, and nausea.

**glyceryl guaiacolate** See guaifenesin.

**glyceryl triacetate** Used in skin applications to treat fungal infections. Read Drugs Used to Treat Skin Disorders, p. 193.

\*glyceryl trinitrate See nitroglycerin.

**glycine** Included in some preparations to reduce irritation of the stomach produced by certain drugs.

**glycirrhiza (licorice root)** Used as a flavoring agent in cough medicines.

**glycocoll** See aminoacetic acid.

\*glycopyrrolate (ROBINUL) Produces atropinelike effects and is used to treat peptic ulcers. See atropine, and read Drugs Used to Treat Indigestion and Peptic Ulcers, p. 74. *Adverse effects* See atropine. *Dose* By mouth, 1 to 2 mg. three times daily.

\*gold (MYOCHRYSINE; gold sodium thiomalate; sodium aurothiomalate; sodium aurothiosuccinate) Used to treat rheumatoid arthritis. A compound of gold is given in a water or oil solution by deep intramuscular injection. It is slowly absorbed, stored in the body, and slowly excreted in the urine. It is not known how it works. Read Aspirin, Nonnarcotic Pain Relievers, and Drugs Used to Treat Rheumatism and Arthritis, p. 118. *Adverse effects* Up to half the patients receiving gold treatment develop adverse effects. These may be severe, occasionally resulting in death if not discontinued. Skin rashes, itching, blood disorders, liver damage, kidney damage, colitis, stomatitis, sensitivity of the skin to sunlight, and occasionally neuritis and encephalitis may occur. An injection may trigger an attack of acute rheumatoid arthritis. *Precautions* Should not be given to patients with impaired kidney or liver function, blood disorders, dermatitis, or other skin disorders. It should be given with caution in pregnancy and to patients with high blood pressure. Before each injection patients should be carefully examined, particularly for stomatitis, fever, debility, bleeding disorders, sore throats, and skin rashes. The urine should be examined, and repeated blood tests should be carried out. Any sign of intolerance to gold is an indication to stop the drug immediately, and in certain cases to start the patient off on an antidote—dimercaprol or penicillamine. Patients should report any untoward symptoms such as fever, debility, sore throat, sore mouth, skin rash, or diarrhea as soon as they occur. *Dose* By deep intramuscular injection, 10 to 50 mg. weekly. No more than 750 mg. in one course.

*gold sodium thiomalate  See gold.

*gramicidin  An antibiotic used in skin applications. Read Drugs Used to Treat Skin Disorders, p. 193.

*GRIFULVIN  See griseofulvin.

*GRISACTIN  See griseofulvin.

*griseofulvin (FULVICIN, GRIFULVIN, GRISACTIN, GRIS PEG)  An antibiotic used to treat fungus infections of the nails, hair, and skin. Read Antibiotics, p. 210. *Adverse effects* May cause headache, stomach upsets, and skin rashes, which are usually mild and short-lasting. Rarely, severe allergic reactions to griseofulvin may produce dermatitis, swelling of the throat, blood disorders, skin sensitivity to sunlight, and bad headaches. Swelling of the breasts and brown coloration of the area around the nipples have occurred in children. *Precautions* Should not be used in patients suffering from porphyria. It may increase the effects of alcohol and decrease the effects of anticoagulant drugs. Barbiturates can reduce the effectiveness of griseofulvin. *Dose* By mouth, 0.5 to 1 G. daily in four equally divided doses given at six-hour intervals.

*GRIS PEG  See griseofulvin.

guaifenesin (glyceryl guaiacolate)  Included in many cough mixtures as a cough expectorant. Read Drugs Used to Treat Coughs, p. 135. *Dose* By mouth, 100 mg. every three to four hours.

*guanethidine (ISMELIN; guanethidine sulfate)  Lowers the blood pressure. Read Drugs Used to Treat Raised Blood Pressure, p. 108. *Adverse effects* Commonest adverse effects at the start of treatment are diarrhea and a drop in blood pressure on exertion, producing dizziness, faintness, weakness, and lassitude (particularly in the mornings). These decrease in severity as treatment is continued. Other frequent adverse effects are slowing of the heart rate, breathlessness, and edema (the last often recognized by swelling of the ankles). Nausea, vomiting, pain in the cheeks (parotid glands), stuffy nose, blurred vision, muscle pains, trembling, dermatitis, failure to ejaculate, frequent urination, and depression of mood may occur. *Precautions* Should be used with caution in patients with defective blood supply to the brain, kidneys, or heart. The blood-pressure-lowering effects are decreased by antidepressant drugs. Patients may become very sensitive to the effects of amphetamines and other similar drugs. *Dose* By mouth, 10 to 75 mg. daily in divided doses until the desired reduction in blood pressure is obtained.

**gum arabic** See acacia.

**gum tragacanth** A gum used as a laxative. Read Drugs Used to Treat Constipation, p. 82.

*GYNE-LOTRIMIN See clotrimazole.

*GYNERGEN See ergotamine.

*GYNOREST See dydrogesterone.

*HALDOL See haloperidol.

HALEY'S M-O Contains mineral oil and milk of magnesia. For mineral oil, see petrolatum liquid, and for milk of magnesia, see magnesium hydroxide, and read Drugs Used to Treat Constipation, p. 82.

*haloperidol (HALDOL) A major tranquilizer. Read Major Tranquilizers, p. 53. It also has antivomiting effects. Read Drugs Used to Treat Nausea, Vomiting, and Motion Sickness, p. 71. *Adverse effects* Dose-related adverse effects commonly include muscle rigidity, trembling and incoordination (dystonias and dyskinesias), depression, blood disorders, and loss of weight. *Precautions* Should not be given to patients with Parkinsonism. It may reduce the effects of anticoagulant drugs. *Dose* By mouth, initial dose, 1 to 30 mg. daily. Maintenance dose, 2 to 6 mg. daily. For anxiety, 0.5 mg. daily.

*HALOTESTIN See fluoxymesterone.

**hamamelis water** See witch hazel.

*HARMONYL See deserpidine.

**hashish** Concentrate of marijuana. Read about marijuana in Dependence on Drugs, p. 23.

*HEDULIN See phenindione.

*heparin (heparin sodium) Prevents the blood from clotting. Read Drugs Used to Prevent Blood from Clotting, p. 90. Its main use is in the treatment of patients suffering from thrombosis in a vein or artery. It is ineffective by mouth and must be given by injection usually every four or six hours because it is short-acting. *Adverse effects* Main adverse effect is bleeding, from any site. Rarely, fever and allergic reactions may occur. Nose-bleeds, red blood cells in the urine, and bruising are the signs of overdosage. Transient loss of hair and diarrhea may occur. *Precautions* Should not be used in patients with jaundice, bleeding disorders (e.g., hemophilia), peptic ulcers, or impairment of kidney or liver function. *Dose* 5000 to 15,000 units by subcutaneous, intramuscular, or intravenous injection.

*HERPLEX See idoxuridine.

HEXA-BETALIN See pyridoxine.

**hexachlorophene** Used as an antiseptic (see p. 202). By mouth it may produce diarrhea, drowsiness, and dizziness. Repeated skin applications may, rarely, make the skin sensitive to sunlight. When applied repeatedly to the skin in premature babies, it may produce brain damage.

*hexamethylenamine  See methenamine mandelate.

HEXAVITAMIN  Each tablet contains vitamin A 5000 units, vitamin B₁ 2 mg.; vitamin B₂ 3 mg., ascorbic acid 75 mg., vitamin D 400 units, and nicotinamide 20 mg. Read Vitamins, p. 155. *Dose* By mouth, 1 tablet daily.

*hexestrol  A synthetic estrogen. Read Female Sex Hormones, p. 166.

*hexobarbital (SOMBULEX)  A barbiturate sleeping drug. Read Sleeping Drugs and Sedatives, p. 43. *Dose* By mouth, 250 to 500 mg. at bedtime.

*hexylresorcinol (SUCRETS)  Used to treat roundworms and dwarf tapeworms and other worm infections. See Drugs Used to Treat Worm Infections, p. 229. *Adverse effects* Crystals may produce ulcers of the mouth; it must therefore be given only in solution, in gelatin capsules, or as coated pills or tablets. It should be given with caution to patients with peptic ulcers. *Dose* By mouth, 1 G. as a single dose.

*HIPREX  See methenamine hippurate.

*HISPRIL  See diphenylpyraline.

*HISTADYL  See methapyriline.

*homatropine  Has uses and effects similar to those described under atropine.

*HUMATIN  See paromomycin.

*hycanthone  Used to treat worm infections. Read Drugs Used to Treat Worm Infections, p. 229. It is used to treat blood fluke. *Adverse effects* Include nausea, vomiting, muscle pains, diarrhea, and loss of weight. It may damage the liver and produce death. *Precautions* Should not be used in pregnancy or within one month after delivery. It should not be used in children under three years of age or weighing less than 15 kg. It should not be used in patients with impaired liver function or taken with a phenothiazine antivomiting drug (see p. 53). *Dose* By deep intramuscular injection in a single dose of 2.5 to 30 mg. per kg. of body weight up to a maximum of 200 mg.

*HYDERGINE  Contains dihydroergocristine 0.1 mg., dihydroergocornine 0.1 mg., and dihydroergokryptine 0.3 mg. in each ml. See ergot, and read Drugs Used to Treat Disorders of Circulation, p. 93, and Drugs Used to Treat Migraine, p. 125. *Dose* Two tablets, sucked under the tongue three times daily.

*hydralazine (APRESOLINE; hydralazine hydrochloride)  Used to treat raised blood pressure. Read Drugs Used to Treat Raised Blood Pressure, p. 108. *Adverse effects* Include nausea, vomiting, headache, a fall in blood pressure when the patient stands up, rapid beating of the heart, flushing, sweating, pins and needles, numbness in the hands and feet, trembling, breathlessness, skin rashes, difficult urination, and depressed mood. These usually occur in the first few weeks of treatment. Prolonged use may produce signs and symptoms of rheumatoid arthritis or acute lupus erythematosus. *Precautions* Should be used with caution in patients with coronary artery disease or rapid heartbeat. Should not be used alone in patients with angina. As with most of these drugs, a severe fall in blood pressure may occur in patients given a general anesthetic. *Dose* By mouth, 10 mg. four times daily, increasing to 50 mg. four times daily if necessary.

*HYDREA  See hydroxyurea.

*hydrochlorothiazide (HYDRODIURIL; ORETIC; ESIDRIX)  A diuretic. Read Diuretics, p. 103. It has effects and uses similar to those described under chlorothiazide, but it is effective in smaller doses. It works in about two hours, reaches a maximum in four, and lasts for about six to twelve hours. *Adverse effects and precautions* See chlorothiazide. *Dose* By mouth, 25 to 100 mg. daily or on alternate days.

*hydrocodone  Has actions and effects similar to those described under codeine. It is used principally to treat cough. Read Drugs Used to Treat Coughs, p. 135. *Adverse effects* See codeine. It is more likely than codeine to produce drug dependence of the morphine type. *Dose* By mouth, 5–10 mg. three or four times daily, maximum in 24 hours 60 mg.

*hydrocortisone (CORTEF)  Occurs naturally in the body and is produced by the adrenal glands. It has similar effects and uses to those described under cortisone. It is given by mouth or injection, and is applied externally in ointments, creams, and lotions. Read Corticosteroids, p. 160. *Adverse effects and precautions* Discussed in the section on corticosteroids and under cortisone. *Dose* By mouth, 10 to 300 mg. daily in divided doses.

*hydrocortisone acetate  Effects and uses similar to those described under cortisone. It is used in eye drops, creams, and ointments. Read Corticosteroids, p. 160, and Drugs Used to Treat Skin Disorders, p. 193. *Dose* By injection into a joint or painful lesion, 5 to 50 mg.

*hydrocortisone sodium succinate  Used in hydrocortisone preparations for injections, as is hydrocortisone sodium phosphate.

*HYDRODIURIL  See hydrochlorothiazide.

*hydroflumethiazide (SALURON; DIUCARDIN)  A diuretic. Read Diuretics, p. 103. It has effects and adverse effects similar to those described under chlorothiazide. *Dose* By mouth, 25 to 100 mg. daily.

hydrogen peroxide  Used to cleanse wounds. It is a very weak antiseptic, however, and probably should not be used. Its use as a mouthwash may cause "hairy tongue" due to increased growth of taste buds.

*hydromorphone (DILAUDID) A narcotic analgesic similar to morphine. See morphine, and read Morphine and Narcotic Pain Relievers, p. 115. It causes dependence of the morphine type. *Dose* By mouth or subcutaneous injection, 1 to 4 mg. four to six times daily.

*HYDROMOX See quinethazone.

*HYDROPRES 25 and 50 Each tablet contains hydrochlorothiazide 25 mg. or 50 mg. combined with reserpine 0.125 mg. See hydrochlorothiazide, and read Diuretics, p. 103. See reserpine, and read Drugs Used to Treat Raised Blood Pressure, p. 108. *Dose* By mouth, Hydropres 25, one tablet one to four times daily; Hydropres 50, one tablet once or twice daily.

*hydroxocobalamin Used to treat pernicious anemia. Read Vitamins, p. 155.

*hydroxychloroquine (PLAQUENIL; hydroxychloroquine sulfate) An antimalarial drug. Read Drugs Used to Treat Malaria, p. 227. It has effects and uses similar to those described under chloroquine. Its main use, however, has been in the treatment of rheumatoid arthritis and lupus erythematosus. Read Aspirin, Nonnarcotic Pain Relievers, and Drugs Used to Treat Rheumatism and Arthritis, p. 118. *Adverse effects and precautions* Similar to those listed under chloroquine. Prolonged use of hydroxychloroquine may cause nausea, diarrhea, and cramps in the abdomen. Its use for long periods exceeding one to two years may irreversibly damage the eyes (retinopathy). *Dose* By mouth, antimalarial suppression, 400 mg. weekly; malarial treatment, 400 to 1200 mg. daily in divided doses. Giardiasis, 200 to 400 mg. three times daily for five days. Rheumatoid arthritis etc., 200 to 1200 mg. daily in divided doses.

*hydroxyprogesterone (DELALUTIN; hydroxyprogesterone hexanoate; hydroxyprogesterone caproate) Effects and uses similar to progesterone. It is used in threatened and habitual miscarriage and to treat disorders of menstruation. Read Female Sex Hormones, p. 166. *Dose* 250 to 500 mg. once or twice weekly by intramuscular injection.

*hydroxyurea (HYDREA) An anticancer drug. Read Drugs Used to Treat Cancer, p. 225. *Adverse effects* Include nausea, vomiting, confusion, skin rashes, loss of hair, abdominal pain, diarrhea, blood in the stool, and convulsions. A common effect is reversible damage to the bone marrow, producing blood disorders. *Precautions* Should not be used in pregnancy. Because it may cause kidney damage, it should be used with caution in patients with impaired kidney function. *Dose* By mouth, 20 to 30 mg. per kg. of body weight daily as a single dose or 80 mg. per kg every third day.

*hydroxyzine (ATARAX; VISTARIL; hydroxyzine pamoate; hydroxyzine hydrochloride) Used to treat nausea and vomiting. It is also used as an antianxiety drug, and it has antihistamine properties. Read Antihistamine Drugs, p. 127, Minor Tranquilizers, p. 51, and Drugs Used to Treat Nausea, Vomiting, and Motion Sickness, p. 71. *Adverse effects* Include drowsiness, headache, dry mouth, and itching. High doses may produce trembling and convulsions. *Precautions* Increases the effects of alcohol and other depressant drugs. It should not be given during pregnancy, and it must be used with caution by those who drive motor vehicles or operate moving machinery. It increases the effects of coumarin anticoagulant drugs. *Dose* By mouth, 25 to 100 mg. three times daily.

*HYGROTON See chlorthalidone.

*hyoscine See scopolamine.

*hyoscyamine See atropine.

*HYPERSTAT See diazoxide.

IBERET 500 Each tablet contains ascorbic acid (vitamin C) 500 mg., ferrous sulfate 525 mg., and B vitamins. Read Iron, p. 152, and Vitamins, p. 155.

*ibuprofen (MOTRIN) An antirheumatic drug. Read Aspirin, Nonnarcotic Pain Relievers, and Drugs Used to Treat Rheumatism and Arthritis, p. 118. *Adverse effects* Like all antirheumatic drugs, it may produce irritation of the stomach, and it should be taken with or after meals. It may cause nausea, indigestion, and skin rash. *Precautions* Should probably not be used in patients with impaired liver function, and it should be used with caution in the first three months of pregnancy. *Dose* By mouth, 300 to 400 mg. three to four times daily.

ichthammol A slightly antibacterial substance that irritates the skin. It has been used in skin applications. Read Drugs Used to Treat Skin Disorders, p. 193.

*idoxuridine (DENDRID; HERPLEX; STOXIL) An antiviral agent. It is used as drops to treat virus ulcers on the eye and also cold sores (herpes simplex) and shingles (herpes zoster). *Dose* By mouth, up to 600 mg. per kg. of body weight daily for five days may be given for generalized virus infection. It should not be used during pregnancy.

*ILETIN See insulins.

*ILOSONE (erythromycin estolate) See erythromycin.

*ILOTYCIN See erythromycin.

*IMFERON See iron dextran solution. Read Iron, p. 152.

*imipramine (TOFRANIL; PRESAMINE; imipramine hydrochloride) A tricyclic antidepressant drug. Read Antidepressants, p. 56. The relief of symptoms is slow, and it may be up to two or three weeks before the patient feels any improvement. It has been used to treat bed-wetting in children. *Adverse effects* During the first few weeks of treatment, dose-related adverse effects occur. They usually disappear. They include dryness of the mouth, blurred vision, constipation, retention of urine, rapid beating of the heart, fall in blood pressure, and sweating. Nausea, vomiting, fatigue, trembling, unsteadiness when walking, excessive energy, and milk from the breasts (galactorrhea) may occur. *Precautions* Should be given with caution to patients with heart disease, glaucoma, epilepsy, enlarged prostate gland, or pyloric stenosis (a narrowing of the outlet from the stomach). Local anesthetic solutions containing adrenaline should be used with care in patients taking imipramine or any other tricyclic antidepressant drug. Caution is also necessary when giving imipramine to patients taking alcohol, barbiturates, and atropinelike drugs. It should not be given to patients who are taking monoamine oxidase inhibitor antidepressants and preferably not within two weeks of stopping such drugs. Imipramine may decrease the effectiveness of the blood-pressure-lowering drugs guanethidine and methyldopa *Dose* By mouth, 50 to 300 mg. daily in divided doses, using smaller doses (e.g., 10 to 50 mg. daily) in the elderly.

*IMURAN   See azathioprine.

*INDALITAN   See clorindione.

*INDERAL   See propranolol.

*INDOCIN   See indomethacin.

*indomethacin (INDOCIN)   Relieves inflammation, reduces high temperature, and relieves pain. It is used to treat gout, rheumatoid arthritis, and other rheumatic disorders. Read Aspirin, Nonnarcotic Pain Relievers, and Drugs Used to Treat Rheumatism and Arthritis, p. 118, and Drugs Used to Treat Gout, p. 124. *Adverse effects* Most common adverse effects are headache and dizziness. These are dose-related, and disappear if the dose is reduced. Loss of appetite, nausea, vomiting, dyspepsia, and diarrhea may occur and are not dose-related. Ulceration of the stomach with bleeding may sometimes occur without the warning symptoms of dyspepsia. Blood disorders, skin rashes, and edema may also occur. *Precautions* Should be given with caution to patients with impaired liver or kidney function. It should not be given to patients with a history of peptic ulcer, and probably not to pregnant women. *Dose* By mouth, 50 to 150 mg. daily in divided doses.

*INH   See isoniazid.

*INHISTON   See pheniramine.

*insulin lente   A type of insulin preparation. Read Drugs Used to Treat Diabetes, p. 182.

*insulins See general discussion of insulins in section on Drugs Used to Treat Diabetes, p. 182.

*insulin semilente A type of insulin preparation. Read Drugs Used to Treat Diabetes, p. 182.

*insulin semilente amorphous An insulin preparation. Read Drugs Used to Treat Diabetes, p. 182.

*insulin ultralente An insulin preparation. Read Drugs Used to Treat Diabetes, p. 182.

*insulin zinc suspension An insulin preparation. Read Drugs Used to Treat Diabetes, p. 182.

*insulin zinc suspension crystalline An insulin preparation. Read Drugs Used to Treat Diabetes, p. 182.

*INTAL See cromolyn sodium.

*INVERSINE See mecamylamine.

iodine Used as an antiseptic (see p. 202). 1% iodine tincture is used on unbroken skin, 2% iodine solution on wounds, because it is less irritating than the tincture.

*iodochlorhydroxyquin (VIOFORM) Similar in uses and adverse effects to diiodohydroxyquin, except that a rare but serious eye disease now precludes its once-popular use for "traveler's diarrhea." See diiodohydroxyquin. *Dose* By mouth, 500 to 750 mg. three times daily for ten days.

*IONAMIN See phentermine.

*iopanoic acid (TELEPAQUE) Used as a diagnostic agent in the detection of gallstones. It greatly increases the visibility of the gallstones on an X-ray.

ipecac Produces the effects of its principal alkaloids, emetine and cephaeline. In small doses it is used as a cough expectorant. Read Drugs Used to Treat Coughs, p. 135. It is also used to induce vomiting after poisoning. *Adverse effects* Has an irritant effect on the stomach and gut. Large doses produce vomiting and diarrhea. It may also produce irregular heartbeat and cause protein to appear in the urine (albuminuria). *Dose* By mouth, 15 to 20 ml. of ipecac syrup after two or three large (8 oz.) glasses of water, to induce vomiting. This may be repeated after 15 to 20 minutes if vomiting does not occur.

iron Read Iron, p. 152.

*iron dextran solution (IMFERON) Given by injection to treat iron-deficiency anemia. Read Iron, p. 152. *Adverse effects* May produce pain and brown staining at the site of injection. Fever, allergic reactions, and rapid heartbeat may occur. After intravenous injections an allergic reaction causing death may very rarely occur, and thrombosis may occur at the site of injection. *Precautions* Should be given with caution to anyone who has suffered from a previous adverse drug reaction. The patient should be kept under close observation for at least one hour after an intravenous injection. It should not be given to patients with severe impairment of liver function or with depression of blood cell production in the bone marrow.

*iron sorbitex (JECTOFER; iron sorbitol)  Used to treat iron-deficiency anemia. Read Iron, p. 152. *Adverse effects* Include flushing, nausea, vomiting, metallic taste in the mouth, loss of taste, dizziness, disorientation, blurred vision, headache, and painful muscles. It turns the urine black in some patients and may produce pain and staining at the site of injection. *Precautions* Should not be given to patients with kidney disease and not within 24 hours of taking iron by mouth.

*iron sorbitol  See iron sorbitex.

*ISMELIN  See guanethidine.

*isoamyl nitrite  See amyl nitrite.

*isocarboxazid  A monoamine oxidase inhibitor antidepressant drug. Read Antidepressants, p. 56. *Adverse effects and precautions* Similar to those discussed under phenelzine. *Dose* By mouth, 10 to 30 mg. daily in divided doses.

*isoetharine (DILABRON)  Effects and uses similar to those described under isoproterenol, except that the side effect on the heart is less pronounced. Read Drugs Used to Treat Bronchial Asthma, p. 138.

*isoniazid (INH)  An antibacterial drug used to treat tuberculosis. Read Drugs Used to Treat Tuberculosis, p. 224. It is used principally in the treatment of tuberculosis of the lungs, but it may also be used to treat tuberculous meningitis and tuberculosis of the kidneys and bladder. Bacterial resistance develops within a few weeks of use, so it should always be given with ethambutol, rifampin, and/or streptomycin, depending upon the severity of the disease. This greatly reduces the risk of resistance. *Adverse effects* May cause constipation, difficulty in starting urination, dryness of the mouth, and vertigo. In doses above 10 mg. per kg. of body weight per day patients may develop inflammation of nerves (peripheral neuritis), producing numbness, pins and needles, and weakness. This may be prevented by giving 100 mg. vitamin $B_6$ (pyridoxine) daily. Isoniazid usually lifts the mood, but it may also cause mental disturbances which are usually reversed on withdrawal of the drug. Hypersensitivity reactions include fever, skin rashes, swollen glands (lymphadenopathy), and, rarely, blood disorders and jaundice. Raised blood sugar and swollen breasts (gynecomastia) have been associated with isoniazid treatment. Withdrawal symptoms may occur on stopping the drug; these include headache, irritability, nervousness, insomnia, and excessive dreaming. *Precautions* Should be given with caution to patients suffering from convulsive disorders, chronic alcoholism, or impaired kidney or liver function. It should preferably not be used in pregnant women. Some patients inactivate it slowly, and therefore they may develop adverse effects on smaller doses. Tuberculosis bacteria rapidly become resistant to isoniazid, and therefore it should not be used alone except for prevention. *Dose* By mouth, 300 to 600 mg. daily in divided doses.

*isophane insulin   An insulin preparation. Read Drugs Used to Treat Diabetes, p. 182.

*isoprenaline   See isoproterenol.

*isopropamide (DARBIN)   Has atropinelike effects and is used to treat peptic ulcers and intestinal spasm. Read Drugs Used to Treat Diarrhea, p. 80. See atropine. *Dose* By mouth, 5–10 mg. every twelve hours.

*isoproterenol (isoproterenol hydrochloride; isoprenaline hydrochloride)   Acts like epinephrine on special nerve endings. It relaxes bronchial muscles, dilates peripheral blood vessels, causes a fall in blood pressure, increases the heart rate, and stimulates the heart muscle. It is used to treat bronchial asthma. Read Drugs Used to Treat Bronchial Asthma, p. 138. It may also be used to treat disordered heart rhythms (see p. 90). *Adverse effects* It may cause rapid beating of the heart, chest pain, faintness, dizziness, headache, nervousness, trembling, and weakness. Irregularities of the heartbeat may occur. *Precautions* Should not be used in patients with acute coronary heart disease or asthma due to heart disease. It should be used with caution in patients with overworking thyroid glands (hyperthyroidism). It should never be given at the same time as epinephrine, but may be used simultaneously with phenylephrine. Tolerance may develop to isoproterenol inhaled in an aerosol; in such cases the dose should not be increased but the drug should be stopped instead, and an alternative used. In Great Britain there are reports of deaths among asthmatics below twenty years of age which were thought to be related to the overuse of aerosols containing high doses of isoproterenol and similar drugs. It has been suggested that the use of these aerosols should not be repeated within the hour, and if relief is not obtained, an alternative drug should be used. *Dose* By mouth (suck under tongue), 10 to 15 mg. three or four times daily. By spray inhalation, 125 to 250 mcg. as a 0.25% solution when necessary. By subcutaneous or intramuscular injection, 200 mcg. By intravenous injection, 10 to 20 mcg.

*ISOPTO CARPINE   See pilocarpine.

*ISORDIL   See isosorbide dinitrate.

*isosorbide dinitrate (ISORDIL; SORBITRATE)   Effects and uses similar to those described under nitroglycerin.

*isoxsuprine (DUVADILAN, VASODILAN; isoxsuprine hydrochloride)
A vasodilator drug. Read Drugs Used to Treat Disorders of Circulation, p. 94. *Adverse effects* May cause transient dizziness, nausea, and
vomiting. *Precautions* Should be used with caution in patients with
rapid heartbeat or disorders of blood pressure. *Dose* By mouth, 10 to
20 mg. three to four times daily.

*ISUPREL  See isoproterenol.

*IZS  An insulin preparation. Read Drugs Used to Treat Diabetes, p.
182.

*JECTOFER  See iron sorbitex.

*KABIKINASE  See streptodornase.

*KAFOCIN  See cephaloglycin.

*kanamycin (KANTREX; kanamycin sulfate)  An antibiotic. It is used
to treat serious infections caused by organisms resistant to the more
commonly used antibiotics, certain infections of the urinary tract,
and tuberculosis. It is not absorbed when taken by mouth and may
therefore be used to treat infections of the gut. Read Antibiotics, p.
210. *Adverse effects* Occur with sufficient frequency to make kanamycin of use only in treating infections resistant to other antibiotics.
Skin rashes, nausea, and vomiting may occur. Reversible kidney
damage is relatively common. The most serious adverse reaction is
deafness. This can be irreversible and may follow intramuscular or
intravenous injections, particularly if the patient has impaired kidney function or if the drug is used for a prolonged period, as in the
treatment of tuberculosis. Some organisms develop resistance to
kanamycin. *Precautions* Should be given by intramuscular or intravenous injection only when there is no safer alternative. If the patient
develops noises in the ears (tinnitus) or dizziness, the drug should
be stopped immediately. It should be used with caution in patients
with impaired kidney function. Adverse reactions may be greatly
reduced by keeping the blood level at no more than 30 mg. per ml.
The total dose in acute infections should not exceed 15 G. over
fourteen days—provided the patient is not allowed to become dehydrated. *Dose* By mouth in the treatment of infection of the gut, 15
to 30 mg. per kg. of body weight in divided doses. By intramuscular
or intravenous injection, 0.5 to 1.5 G. every twelve hours.

*KANTREX  See kanamycin.

kaolin  Read Drugs Used to Treat Diarrhea, p. 80.

*KAON  See potassium.

KAOPECTATE  Suspension contains 5.83 G. of kaolin and 130 mg. of
pectin in each 30 ml. See pectin, and read Drugs Used to Treat
Diarrhea, p. 80.

karaya (sterculia, karaya gum)  Used as a bulk laxative, since by
taking up moisture it swells and increases the volume of the feces,

thus encouraging bowel movement. It is used in the food industry to make pastes and various foods. Read Drugs Used to Treat Constipation, p. 82.

**karaya gum** See karaya.

*\*KEFLEX** See cephalexin.

*\*KEFLIN** See cephalothin.

*\*KEFZOL** See cefazolin.

*\*KEMADRIN** See procyclidine.

*\*KENACORT** See triamcinolone.

*\*KENALOG** See triamcinolone.

*\*K-LOR** See potassium.

*\*K-LYTE** See potassium bicarbonate.

**KOLANTYL** Gel contains d ied aluminum hydroxide gel 150 mg., magnesium hydroxide 150 mg., dicyclomine hydrochloride 2.5 mg., and methylcellulose 50 mg. Tablets contain aluminum hydroxide 300 mg., magnesium oxide 185 mg., methylcellulose 100 mg., and dicyclomine hydrochloride 5 mg. Read Drugs Used to Treat Indigestion and Peptic Ulcers, p. 74. Also see dicyclomine. *Dose* By mouth, gel, 1 to 4 teaspoonfuls (5 to 20 ml.) 30 minutes to 1 hour after meals and at bedtime. 1 to 2 tablets 30 minutes to 1 hour after meals and at bedtime.

*\*KONAKION** See phytonadione.

*\*KWELL** See gamma benzene hexachloride.

*\*KYNEX** See sulfamethoxypyridazine.

**lactic acid** Used to prepare compound sodium lactate injections which are given for acidosis, a condition in which the blood acid/ base balance is disturbed. It may be used in vaginal douches for the treatment of vaginal discharge.

*\*LACTINEX** See lactobacillus.

*\*lactobacillus (LACTINEX)** *Lactobacillus bulgaricus* and *L. acidophilus* produce lactic acid and acidify the gut. This is said to be of use in cases of enteritis and colitis. They are used to make yogurt.

*\*lanatoside C (CEDILANID)** See general discussion on digitalis under Drugs Used to Treat Heart Failure and Heart Rhythm Disorders, p. 86.

*\*LANOXIN** See digoxin.

*\*LARGACTIL** See chlorpromazine.

*\*LAROCIN** See amoxicillin.

*\*LARODOPA** See levodopa.

*\*LASIX** See furosemide.

*\*l-asparaginase (CRASNITIN; colaspase)** An anticancer drug. Read Drugs Used to Treat Cancer, p. 225. *Adverse effects* These include fever, nausea, vomiting, liver damage, allergic reactions, alterations in the

levels of various chemicals in the blood, and a fall in white blood cells. *Precautions* It should not be used in pregnancy, and it should be given with caution to patients with impaired liver function. *Dose* Depends upon the treatment program being followed.

*LERITINE    See anileridine.

*LETTER    See levothyroxine.

*LEUKERAN    See chlorambucil.

*levallorphan (LORFAN; levallorphan tartrate)    An antagonist of morphine and similar drugs. Its effects are similar to nalorphine, but it is more potent. Both can produce respiratory depression on their own, and both have largely been replaced by the pure narcotic antagonist naloxone. Levallorphan has been used in childbirth in combination with meperidine with the object of reducing respiratory depression, but there is no convincing evidence that this object is achieved. Read Morphine and Narcotic Pain Relievers, p. 115.

*levamisole (levamisole hydrochloride)    Used to treat roundworm and hookworm infections. Read Drugs Used to Treat Worm Infections, p. 229. *Dose* By mouth, 2.5 mg. per kg. of body weight.

*levarterenol (LEVOPHED; levarterenol bitartrate; norepinephrine; noradrenaline tartrate)    The chemical released by adrenergic nerves. Read Drugs Which Act on the Autonomic Nervous System, p. 145. It is used to treat clinical shock in order to try to keep the blood pressure up and the circulation diverted to the heart and brain. *Adverse effects and precautions* See epinephrine. *Dose* 2 to 20 mcg. per minute by intravenous infusion according to the blood pressure of the patient.

*levodopa (BENDOPA; DOPAR; LARODOPA)    Used to treat Parkinsonism. Read Drugs Used to Treat Parkinsonism, p. 149. *Adverse effects* May produce loss of appetite, nausea, vomiting, dizziness, and faintness (due to a fall in blood pressure when the patient stands up), and irregularities of heart rate. Dosage requirements and side effects, particularly those related to the gut, have been substantially reduced by the addition of an inhibitor in the tablet which prevents the conversion of inactive levodopa to active dopamine until the drug reaches the brain (see Sinemet). Levodopa may also produce involuntary movements of the tongue, jaw, and neck. These are dose-related. It may produce mental disturbances and depression; psychosis and mania have been reported. *Precautions* Should not be used in patients with disorders of the heart or circulation. It should be used with caution in patients with mental disorders. Its effects may be reduced by phenothiazines, pyridoxine, methyldopa, and reserpine. Its effects may be increased by atropinelike drugs and by monoamine oxidase inhibitors. It should not be used while taking, or within two weeks of stopping, an MAO inhibitor drug. *Dose* By mouth, 500 mg. to 8 G. daily in divided doses.

**\*LEVO-DROMORAN** See levorphanol.

**\*LEVOPHED** See levarterenol.

**\*LEVOPROME** See methotrimeprazine.

**\*levopropoxyphene (NOVRAD)** Used as a cough suppressant. See Drugs Used to Treat Coughs, p. 135. *Adverse effects* Include headache, nausea, diarrhea, vomiting, and blurred vision. *Dose* By mouth, 50 to 100 mg. every four hours.

**\*levorphanol (LEVO-DROMORAN; levorphanol tartrate)** Effects and uses similar to those described under morphine, but it differs from morphine by being almost as effective by mouth as by injection. *Adverse effects, precautions, and drug dependence* See morphine. Read Morphine and Narcotic Pain Relievers, p. 115. *Dose* By mouth, 1.5 to 4.5 mg.; by intravenous injection, 1 to 1.5 mg.

**\*levothyroxine (SYNTHROID; LETTER)** A thyroid hormone used to treat underworking of the thyroid gland. Read Drugs Used to Treat Thyroid Disorders, p. 187. *Adverse effects* Too large a dose may produce sweating, rapid heartbeat, diarrhea, restlessness, excitability, irregularities of heart rhythm, and angina. It may also produce pain in the arms or legs and worsen the symptoms of osteoarthritis. *Precautions* It has a delayed and cumulative effect and may take up to two weeks to be effective; therefore the dose must be controlled carefully. It should be used with caution in patients with heart disorders. It may increase the effects of drugs used to prevent blood clotting, and its effects may be increased by phenytoin and aspirin. *Dose* By mouth, 50 to 300 mcg. daily.

**\*LEXAVITE** A vitamin B complex used to treat pernicious anemia. See Vitamins, p. 155.

**\*LIBRAX** Each tablet contains chlordiazepoxide 5 mg. and clidinium bromide 2.5 mg. See chlordiazepoxide, and read Minor Tranquilizers, p. 51. See clidinium, and read Drugs Used to Treat Indigestion and Peptic Ulcers, p. 74. *Dose* By mouth; varies with individual response. Usual dose is 1 or 2 capsules three or four times daily before meals and at bedtime.

**\*LIBRITABS** See chlordiazepoxide.

**\*LIBRIUM** See chlordiazepoxide.

**licorice root** See glycirrhiza.

**\*lidocaine (XYLOCAINE; lidocaine hydrochloride)** A local anesthetic. It is now used to treat disorders of heart rhythm. Read Local Anesthetics, p. 191.

**lime water** A calcium hydroxide solution, used in skin lotions and soaps. It has been used as an antacid and as an astringent.

*LINCOCIN See lincomycin.

*lincomycin (LINCOCIN; lincomycin hydrochloride) An antibiotic. It is sometimes used in patients sensitive to penicillin. It is active against a narrow range of bacteria. Since it penetrates bone, it is used for the treatment of bone infections (osteomyelitis). Bacterial resistance is induced easily, but cross-resistance is rare except with erythromycin. Read Antibiotics, p. 210. *Adverse effects* May produce diarrhea and colitis, nausea, and abdominal cramps, an itching anus (pruritis ani), and occasionally sore gums (stomatitis). Allergic reactions may produce skin rashes. Sensitivity of the skin to sunlight and supra-added infection with yeasts may occur. Rarely, blood disorders and liver damage may occur. *Precautions* Should not be given in pregnancy or to women who are breast-feeding. It should be given with caution to patients with impaired kidney function. *Dose* By mouth, 1.5 G. daily in divided doses, half an hour before food. By intramuscular injection, 0.6 to 1.2 G. daily in divided doses (12-hourly).

*liothyronine (CYTOMEL; liothyronine sodium; L-triiodothyronine sodium) A hormone produced by the thyroid gland, it has the effects and uses of thyroxine. It is effective in smaller doses, and works more quickly, but its effects do not last as long. Read Drugs Used to Treat Thyroid Disorders, p. 187. *Dose* By mouth, starting with 10 to 20 mcg. daily and gradually increasing by 10 mcg. daily every week up to a total of 80 to 100 mcg. daily.

*liotrix (EUTHYROID; THYROLAR) A 4-to-1 mixture of levothyroxine and triiodothyronine (liothyronine). See liothyronine and levothyroxine.

*LIQUAMAR See phenprocoumon.

*liquid nitrogen Used to destroy warts.

LIQUIPRIN Each tablet contains 325 mg. aspirin. See aspirin. Liquid contains acetaminophen 60 mg. per 1.75 ml. See acetaminophen.

LISTERINE—lozenges Contain hexylresorcinol 2.4 mg. and thymol, eucalyptol, methylsalicylate, and menthol. See each constituent drug.

LISTERINE—mouthwash Contains menthol, boric acid, thymol, eucalyptol, methylsalicylate, benzoic acid, alcohol. See each constituent drug, and read Antiseptics, p. 201.

*LITHANE See lithium.

*lithium (LITHANE; LITHONATE; lithium carbonate) Used to treat manic and depressive disorders. Read Antidepressants, p. 56. *Adverse effects* Develop slowly as the drug accumulates in the body; they are related to dosage. They include transient nausea, trembling, weakness, and drinking and passing a lot of water (polydipsia and polyuria). Higher dosage results in higher blood levels, which produce more serious adverse effects—confusion, slurred speech, diarrhea, drowsiness, trembling, and ataxia. It may also precipitate goiter. Changes on electrocardiograms have been reported. *Precautions* Should not be given to patients with impaired heart or kidney function and preferably not during pregnancy. Since lithium competes with sodium in the body, it alters the salt-water balance and patients therefore need added salt (sodium chloride) in their diet. *Dose* By mouth, 0.25 to 1.5 G. daily in divided doses.

*LITHONATE** See lithium.

*liver extracts** Formerly used widely in the treatment of pernicious anemia. They have now been largely replaced by Vitamin $B_{12}$ injections.

*lobeline (lobeline hydrochloride)** Produces effects in the body similar to those caused by nicotine. See Tobacco Dependence, p. 28. It may cause nausea, vomiting, coughing, headache, dizziness, trembling, and rapid heartbeat. Its effectiveness in helping patients to reduce the amount they smoke has not been proved.

*LOESTRIN** Contains norethindrone and ethinylestradiol. Read Oral Contraceptive Drugs, p. 173.

*LOMOTIL** Each tablet and each 5 ml. of liquid contain diphenoxylate hydrochloride 2.5 mg. and atropine sulfate 0.025 mg. See diphenoxylate, and read Drugs Used to Treat Diarrhea, p. 80. See atropine, and read Drugs Which Act on the Autonomic Nervous System, p. 145. *Dose* By mouth, 1 or 2 tablets or 5 to 10 ml. liquid up to four times daily.

*LOPRESS** See hydralazine.

*LORFAN** See levallorphan.

*LORIDINE** See cephaloridine.

*LOTRIMIN** See clotrimazole.

*LOTUSATE** See talbutal.

LSD A hallucinogenic drug. Read section on LSD in Dependence on Drugs, p. 23.

*L-triiodothyronine sodium** See liothyronine.

*LUMINAL** see phenobarbital.

*LURITINE** See anileridine.

*LYSODREN** See mitotane.

MAALOX Contains a colloidal suspension of aluminum and magnesium hydroxides. Read Drugs Used to Treat Indigestion and Peptic Ulcers, p. 74. *Dose* By mouth, as directed on container label or by physician.

*MACRODANTIN** See nitrofurantoin.

*MADRIBON** See sulfadimethoxine.

**magaldrate (RIOPAN)**   An antacid. Read Drugs Used to Treat Indigestion and Peptic Ulcers, p. 74.

**MAGCYL**   See poloxalkol.

**magenta**   Used as a skin antiseptic.

**magnesium carbonate (heavy magnesium carbonate, heavy mag. carb.; and light magnesium carbonate, light mag. carb.)**   Has antacid (see p. 76) and laxative (see p. 84) properties. Magnesium carbonate is less effective than magnesium hydroxide in neutralizing gastric acid, and it liberates carbon dioxide. Read Drugs Used to Treat Indigestion and Peptic Ulcers, p. 74, and Drugs Used to Treat Constipation, p. 82. *Adverse effects* Releases carbon dioxide in the stomach, which may produce belching. It acts as a laxative. It is absorbed into the bloodstream and is rapidly excreted by the kidneys, but if kidney function is impaired, the blood level of magnesium may rise, resulting in magnesium intoxication (fall in blood pressure and paralysis of respiration). *Precautions* Magnesium salts should be used with caution in patients with impaired kidney function. *Dose* By mouth: antacid, 250 to 500 mg.; laxative, 2 to 5 G.

**magnesium hydroxide**   Used as an antacid (see p. 76) and as a laxative (see Drugs Used to Treat Constipation, p. 82). *Dose* By mouth: as antacid, 500 to 750 mg.; as laxative, 2 to 4 G.

**magnesium oxide**   Used as an antacid (see p. 76) and as a laxative (see Drugs Used to Treat Constipation, p. 82). *Dose* By mouth: as antacid, 250 to 500 mg.; as laxative, 2 to 5 G.

**magnesium silicate**   See magnesium trisilicate.

**magnesium sulfate (EPSOM SALTS)**   Used as a laxative (see Drugs Used to Treat Constipation, p. 82). The usual dose is 5 to 15 G.

**magnesium trisilicate (magnesium silicate)**   Used as an antacid (see p. 76). It is absorbent and slow-acting. *Dose* By mouth, 0.5 to 2 G.

**malachite green**   A brilliant dye used as an antiseptic in skin applications.

***MANDELAMINE**   See methenamine mandelate.

***MANISTAT cream**   See miconazole.

***mannitol (OSMITROL)**   An osmotic diuretic. Read Diuretics, p. 103. It may produce diarrhea when given by mouth. Rapid injection into a vein may cause headache, chest pains, and depressed respiration. It should be used with caution in patients with heart failure or impaired kidney function.

***MARAX**   Tablets contain 10 mg., 25 mg., and 130 mg. respectively of hydroxyzine, ephedrine, and theophylline. See each constituent drug, and read Drugs Used to Treat Bronchial Asthma, p. 138. *Dose* By mouth, 1 tablet two to four times daily.

***MARCAINE**   See bupivacaine.

**MAREZINE** See cyclizine.

**marijuana (Cannabis sativa, cannabis)** Read section on marijuana in Dependence on Drugs, p. 23.

*MARPLAN See isocarboxazid.

*MASSE cream Contains allantoin and hydroxyquinoline sulfate and aminacrine. See hydroxyquinoline and allantoin. Aminacrine is a nonstaining acridine dye used as an antiseptic.

MASSENGILL—vaginal douche liquid Contains sodium lactate, lactic acid, octylphenoxypolyethoxyethanol, and alcohol. See each constituent drug.

MASSENGILL—vaginal douche powder Contains boric acid, ammonium alum, berberine sulfate, thymol, menthol, and eucalyptol. See each constituent drug.

*MASTERONE See dromostanolone.

*MATULANE See procarbazine.

*MAXIBOLIN See ethylestrenol.

*MAXIPEN See phenethicillin.

*mazindol (SANOREX) Used as a reducing drug. It has amphetamine-like effects. Read Reducing Drugs, p. 68, and Stimulants: Amphetamines, p. 64. *Adverse effects* Include rapid heartbeat, dry mouth, constipation, insomnia, weakness, sweating, overactivity, and skin rash. *Precautions* Should not be used in patients with diabetes, heart disorder, raised blood pressure, pregnancy, history of drug abuse, glaucoma, or anxiety states. It should not be used in children under twelve years of age. *Drug dependence* It may cause drug dependence. It may interfere with the ability to operate moving machinery and drive a motor vehicle. *Dose* By mouth, 2 mg. one hour before lunch or 1 mg. one hour before each meal.

*MEBARAL See mephobarbital.

*mebendazole Used to treat roundworm. Read Drugs Used to Treat Worm Infections, p. 229. *Adverse effects* May occasionally cause abdominal pain and diarrhea. *Precautions* Should not be used in pregnancy. *Dose* By mouth, from a single dose of 100 mg. to 100 mg. twice daily for three days according to the infection being treated.

*MEBROIN Each tablet contains mephobarbital 90 mg. and phenytoin (diphenylhydantoin) 60 mg. See mephobarbital and phenytoin. Read Drugs Used to Treat Epilepsy, p. 142. *Dose* By mouth, 1 or 2 tablets three times daily.

*mecamylamine (INVERSINE; mecamylamine hydrochloride) Used to treat raised blood pressure. Read Drugs Used to Treat Raised Blood Pressure, p. 108. *Adverse effects* These include blurred vision, constipation, dryness of the mouth, diarrhea, nausea, difficulty in urinating, drowsiness, and impotence. Paralysis of the small bowel is a serious hazard of long-term treatment. *Dose* By mouth, initially 2.5 mg. twice daily, increasing to a maximum of 60 mg. daily according to patient's needs.

*mechlorethamine (MUSTARGEN; mustine hydrochloride)** An anticancer drug. Read Drugs Used to Treat Cancer, p. 225. *Adverse effects* Include nausea, vomiting, diarrhea, peptic ulceration, drowsiness, psychosis, loss of hair, deafness and noises in the ears, several months without a menstrual period, reduced sperm count, and skin rashes. Damage to the bone marrow may occur, leading to severe blood disorders. Injections may produce pain, irritation, and thrombophlebitis at the site. *Precautions* Should not be used in pregnancy or in the presence of any infection or blood disorder. Evidence of impaired bone-marrow function should give rise to utmost caution in its use. *Dose* Varies according to the disorder being treated.

**meclizine (BONINE; meclizine hydrochloride)** An antihistamine drug. It is used mainly to treat motion sickness, nausea and vomiting, nausea and vertigo due to disorders of the organ of balance, and pregnancy sickness. Read Antihistamine Drugs, p. 127, and Drugs Used to Treat Nausea, Vomiting, and Motion Sickness, p. 71. *Adverse effects and precautions* Similar to those discussed under promethazine. It is suggested that meclizine not be used during the first three months of pregnancy (similar caution is recommended in the use of chlorcyclizine and cyclizine). *Dose* By mouth, 25 to 50 mg. daily in divided doses. The effect of a single dose lasts up to 24 hours. For motion sickness the dose is taken one hour before traveling.

*MEDIHALER-EPI** See epinephrine.

*MEDIHALER-ISO** See isoproterenol.

*MEDROL** See methylprednisolone.

*medroxyprogesterone (PROVERA; medroxyprogesterone acetate)** A progestogen. Read Female Sex Hormones, p. 166, and Oral Contraceptive Drugs, p. 173.

*mefenamic acid (PONSTEL)** Relieves pain and reduces a high temperature. It is as potent as aspirin and has a weak anti-inflammatory action. It is used to relieve symptoms of rheumatic disorders and as a mild pain reliever. Read Aspirin, Nonnarcotic Pain Relievers, and Drugs Used to Treat Rheumatism and Arthritis, p. 118. *Adverse effects* May cause indigestion, constipation, diarrhea, and irritation of the stomach with bleeding. It may also cause drowsiness, skin rashes, and blood disorders. *Precautions* Should be given with caution to patients with a history of peptic ulcer or impaired kidney function. It should not be taken during pregnancy or when breast-feeding. It may increase the effects of certain anticoagulant drugs. *Dose* By mouth, 0.5 to 1 G. daily in divided doses.

\*MEGACE  See megestrol.

\*megestrol (MEGACE)  A synthetic progestogen. Read Female Sex Hormones, p. 166. It is used mainly in combination with estrogens, as an oral contraceptive agent. Read Oral Contraceptive Drugs, p. 173. *Adverse effects* May cause headaches, tension, depression, nausea, vomiting, fullness of the breasts, fluid retention, weight gain, and breakthrough bleeding. It may increase premenstrual tension, and its prolonged use may lead to damage of liver function.

\*melarsonyl  Used to treat trypanosomiasis. *Adverse effects* Similar to those described under melarsoprol. It may produce nerve damage in the arms and legs. *Dose* By intramuscular injection, 4 mg. per kg. of body weight, but according to condition of patient.

\*melarsoprol  Used to treat trypanosomiasis. *Adverse effects* Include vomiting and colic; it commonly affects the brain, producing "strokelike" effects. *Precautions* Patient should be hospitalized and kept in bed and fasting for several hours after an injection. It should not be used in influenza epidemics. *Dose* Varies according to patient's needs.

\*MELLARIL  See thioridazine.

\*melphalan (ALKERAN)  An anticancer drug (see p. 226). Read Drugs Used to Treat Cancer, p. 225. *Adverse effects* Include nausea, vomiting, diarrhea, mouth ulcers, bleeding from the gut, and loss of hair. It damages the bone marrow, producing blood disorders. *Precautions* Should not be used in pregnancy or in the presence of an infection. It should be used with caution in patients with blood disorders and evidence of impaired bone-marrow function. *Dose* By mouth, 2 to 30 mg. daily in divided doses up to a total dose of about 200 mg.

\*MELTROL  See phenformin.

\*menadione  Vitamin $K_3$. Read Vitamins, p. 155.

\*MENRIUM  Tablets contain a combination of chlordiazepoxide and conjugated estrogens in various doses. See chlordiazepoxide, and read Minor Tranquilizers, p. 51, and Female Sex Hormones, p. 166. *Dose* By mouth, 1 tablet three times daily (all strengths)

menthol  Used in numerous preparations for treating cough and common cold symptoms. It also relieves itching and is used in skin applications.

\*meperidine (DEMEROL; meperidine hydrochloride)  A synthetic narcotic pain reliever. It has actions and uses similar to those described under morphine, but it is not as powerful and its effects are less prolonged. It has little effect on coughs. Read Morphine and Narcotic Pain Relievers, p. 115. *Adverse effects* May cause a lift in mood, dizziness, sweating, dry mouth, nausea, vomiting, constipation, and retention of urine. These are all much less frequent than with morphine. Injection into a vein may cause a fall in blood pressure. Its use during childbirth may depress the respiration of the baby at birth. *Precautions* Should not be given to patients with severe liver disease or with gall bladder pains. Its effects are increased by monoamine oxidase inhibitor antidepressant drugs and possibly by some major tranquilizers (e.g., phenothiazines). *Drug dependence* May cause drug dependence of the morphine type. Tolerance is not always complete, and addicts develop twitching, trembling, mental confusion, and hallucinations. Sometimes convulsions and death result from meperidine dependence. Withdrawal symptoms come on quicker than with morphine. *Dose* By mouth, 50 to 100 mg.; by subcutaneous or intramuscular injection, 25 to 100 mg.; by intravenous injection, 25 to 50 mg.

*mephenesin A muscle relaxant which works through the spinal cord. It has been used for the treatment of spastic muscle disorders and muscle spasms due to tetanus. *Adverse effects* By mouth it may cause nausea and drowsiness, and when injected into a vein it may damage the red blood cells and cause pain and thrombosis at the site of injection. *Dose* By mouth, 1 to 2 G up to six times daily. By intravenous injection, 1 G., repeated according to need; this requires a careful balance between desired and undesired effects.

*mephenoxalone Used as a minor tranquilizer. Effects are similar to those caused by meprobamate. Read Minor Tranquilizers, p. 51.

*mephentermine (WYAMINE) A sympathomimetic drug which has been used to maintain blood pressure in shock. Read Drugs Which Act on the Autonomic Nervous System, p. 145.

*mephenytoin (MESANTOIN) An anticonvulsant drug. It has effects and uses similar to those described under phenytoin, but it produces less drowsiness. Read Drugs Used to Treat Epilepsy, p. 142. *Adverse effects* May cause drowsiness, dizziness, clumsiness, and ataxia. It may also produce a skin rash and blood disorders. *Precautions* If you develop a sore throat or fever, stop taking the drug immediately and report to your doctor. Mephenytoin should be given with caution to patients with allergy to any drug. *Dose* By mouth, 50 to 600 mg. daily in divided doses, starting with 50 to 100 mg. daily and increasing by 50 mg. at weekly intervals to a maximum of 600 mg. daily.

*mephobarbital (MEBARAL) A barbiturate with effects and uses similar to those described under phenobarbital. *Dose* By mouth, 400 to 600 mg. daily in divided doses.

*MEPHYTON See phytonadione.

*mepivacaine (CARBOCAINE; mepivacaine hydrochloride) A local anesthetic. Read Local Anesthetics, p. 191.

*meprobamate (EQUANIL; MILTOWN) A minor tranquilizer. Read

Minor Tranquilizers, p. 51. *Adverse effects* May produce loss of appetite, nausea, vomiting, diarrhea, and headache. Large doses cause dizziness, drowsiness, a fall in blood pressure, and ataxia. Some patients are allergic to meprobamate and develop rashes, swelling of the face and throat, and wheezing (bronchospasm). The drug should be stopped immediately if these adverse effects occur. Blood disorders have been reported. Some patients become excited instead of calm. *Precautions* May trigger convulsions in someone with a history of epilepsy. It may also increase the effects of alcohol. *Drug dependence* May produce drug dependence of the barbiturate/alcohol type. *Dose* By mouth, 400 to 1200 mg. daily in divided doses.

**merbromin (MERCUROCHROME)** A weak antiseptic. Read Antiseptics, p. 201.

**\*mercaptopurine (PURINETHOL)** An anticancer drug. Read Drugs Used to Treat Cancer, p. 225. Also used as an immunosuppressant. *Adverse effects* Include nausea, vomiting, diarrhea, and occasionally ulceration of the lining of the gut and liver damage. It causes bone-marrow damage which leads to blood disorders. *Precautions* Should not be given in early pregnancy. *Dose* By mouth, 50 to 200 mg. daily in a single dose.

**MERCUROCHROME** See merbromin.

**\*mercury salts** Widely used in the past as antibacterial and antifungal agents to be applied to skin, eyes, ears, nose, and wounds, to clean the skin for surgery, to wash out the bladder, and to treat syphilis. They were also used as purgatives, in contraceptive creams, and as teething powders. *Adverse effects* Mercury and its salts can damage the lining of the mouth, stomach, and gut, damage the kidneys, and produce bleeding from the gut. In children it can produce pink disease (acrodynia), typified by hot red skin and nerve damage. The use of mercury or its salts is seldom, if ever, necessary.

**\*MERTHIOLATE** See thimerosal.

**\*MESANTOIN** See mephenytoin.

**\*mesoridazine (SERENTIL)** A phenothiazine major tranquilizer. Read Major Tranquilizers, p. 53. *Dose* By mouth, 50 to 400 mg. daily.

**\*mesterolone** A male sex hormone. Read Male Sex Hormones, p. 163. See testosterone. *Dose* By mouth, 25 mg. two to four times daily.

**\*MESTINON** See pyridostigmine.

**\*mestranol** An estrogen. Read Female Sex Hormones, p. 166, and Oral Contraceptive Drugs, p. 173.

**METAMUCIL** see psyllium.

**\*METANDREN** See methyltestosterone.

**\*metaproterenol (ALUPENT)** Used to treat asthma. Its effects are similar to those described under isoproterenol. Read Drugs Used to Treat

Bronchial Asthma, p. 138. *Adverse effects* Rapid beating of the heart, headache, dizziness, and nausea may occur, though less often than with isoproterenol. These are brought on by large doses and soon disappear. Difficulty in urinating may also occur. *Precautions* See warnings under isoproterenol. *Dose* By mouth or deep intramuscular injection, 20 mg. four times daily. Or by a spray solution for inhalation.

*metaraminol (ARAMINE; metaraminol bitartrate)** A sympathomimetic drug which has been used to maintain blood pressure in shock. Read Drugs Which Act on the Autonomic Nervous System, p. 145.

*methacholine (methacholine chloride)** A parasympathomimetic drug. Read Drugs Which Act on the Autonomic Nervous System, p. 145.

*methacycline (RONDOMYCIN; methacycline hydrochloride)** A tetracycline antibiotic. It has effects and uses similar to those described under tetracycline. Read Antibiotics, p. 210. *Dose* By mouth, 150 to 300 mg. every six hours.

*methallenestril (VALLESTRIL)** A synthetic estrogen. Read Female Sex Hormones, p. 166.

*methamphetamine (desoxyephedrine hydrochloride; methamphetamine hydrochloride)** A stimulant. It has effects and uses similar to those described under amphetamine, but it acts quicker and lasts longer. Read Stimulants: Amphetamines, p. 64. *Dose* By mouth, 2.5 to 10 mg.

*methandienone (methandrostenolone)** An anabolic steroid with effects and uses similar to those described under testosterone. Read Anabolic Steroids, p. 165. *Adverse effects* These are similar to those described under testosterone. Methandienone may cause jaundice when given for prolonged periods. Patients may develop water retention and a high blood calcium. It may increase the effects of certain anticoagulant drugs and cause other blood level imbalances. *Precautions* It should not be used in patients with impaired liver function or in those with cancer of the prostate gland. *Dose* By mouth, initially 5 to 20 mg. daily; maintenance, 5 to 10 mg. daily.

*methandriol** A male sex hormone. See testosterone, and read Male Sex Hormones, p. 163, and Anabolic Steroids, p. 165. *Dose* By mouth, 50 to 150 mg. daily.

*methandrostenolone (DIANABOL)** An anabolic steroid with effects and uses similar to those described under testosterone. Read Anabolic Steroids, p. 165. *Adverse effects* Similar to those described under testosterone. Methandrostenolone may cause jaundice when given for prolonged periods. Patients may develop water retention and a high blood calcium. It may increase the effects of certain anticoagulant drugs and increase the plasma level of oxyphenbutazone (a metabolite of phenylbutazone which is used to treat rheumatic disorders). *Precautions* Should not be used in patients with impaired liver function or cancer of the prostate gland. *Dose* By mouth, initially, 5 to 20 mg. daily; maintenance, 5 to 10 mg. daily for four to six weeks with breaks of two to four weeks.

*methantheline (BANTHINE; methantheline bromide) Closely related to propantheline. See propantheline. *Dose* By mouth, 50 to 100 mg. four times daily initially; maintenance dose, 25 to 50 mg. four times daily.

*methapyrilene (HISTADYL; methapyriline hydrochloride) An antihistamine drug. It is frequently sold as a sleeping drug. Read Antihistamine Drugs, p. 127, and Sleeping Drugs and Sedatives, p. 43. *Dose* By mouth, 50 to 100 mg. four times daily.

*methaqualone (QUAALUDE; PAREST; SOPOR) Used as a sleeping drug and sedative. Read Sleeping Drugs and Sedatives, p. 43. *Adverse effects* May produce headache, dizziness, drowsiness, nausea, and stomach discomfort. Dry mouth and rapid beating of the heart may occur. Some patients develop transient pins and needles before going to sleep, and there is a suspicion that methaqualone may produce nerve damage. *Precautions* Should be used with caution in patients with impaired liver function. It can interfere with ability to drive motor vehicles and operate machinery, and its effects are increased by alcohol, barbiturates, and other sedative drugs. It should be used with caution in pregnancy. *Drug dependence* May produce dependence of the barbiturate/alcohol type. *Dose* By mouth, sleeping dose, 150 to 300 mg.; sedative dose, 75 mg. three times daily.

*methdilazine (TACARYL; methdilazine hydrochloride) An antihistamine drug. Read Antihistamine Drugs, p. 127.

*methenamine hippurate (HIPREX) Uses and effects similar to methenamine mandelate. See methenamine mandelate. *Dose* By mouth, 1 G. twice daily.

*methenamine mandelate (MANDELAMINE; URITONE) Used to treat chronic and recurrent infections of the urinary system (see p. 224). It only works if the urine is first made acid by the taking of a preparation such as ammonium chloride, ascorbic acid (vitamin C), or sodium biphosphate. The urine should be regularly tested for acidity every morning. *Adverse effects* If taken in large doses, it may cause painful and frequent urination, cystitis, and blood in the urine due to its conversion into formaldehyde. Skin rashes may occasionally occur. *Precautions* It should not be given with sulfonamides, since crystals may develop in the urine. It should not be given to patients with impaired kidney function. *Dose* By mouth, 250 to 1000 mg. up to four times daily.

*METHERGINE See methylergonovine.

*METHIOCIL See methylthiouracil.

*methicillin (CELBENIN; STAPHCILLIN; methicillin sodium) A semi-synthetic penicillin. It is given by injection because it is not well absorbed by mouth. It is used to treat infections produced by bacteria which produce a substance which destroys penicillin (penicillinase). See Penicillins, p. 213. *Adverse effects and precautions* Similar to those described under penicillin G. *Dose* By intramuscular injection, 1 G. every four to six hours.

*methimazole (TAPAZOLE) Used to treat overworking of the thyroid glands. Read Drugs Used to Treat Thyroid Disorders, p. 187. *Dose* By mouth, 15 to 60 mg. daily in divided doses, initially; 5 to 15 mg. daily for maintenance therapy.

*methixine (TREMONIL; TREST; methixine hydrochloride) Has atropinelike effects and is used to treat Parkinsonism. Read Drugs Used to Treat Parkinsonism, p. 149. See atropine. *Dose* By mouth, 2.5 mg. three to six times daily, increasing according to patient's response.

*methocarbamol (ROBAXIN) Used as a muscle relaxant. It produces drowsiness. *Dose* By mouth, 1 to 2 G. daily in divided doses.

*methotrexate An anticancer drug. Read Drugs Used to Treat Cancer, p. 225. *Adverse effects* Include nausea, vomiting, diarrhea, abdominal pain, skin rashes, and loss of hair. Ulceration of the mouth and gut may occur with high doses. Severe allergic reactions, sometimes fatal, may occur. It may cause sensitivity of the skin to sunlight, and bone-marrow damage leading to serious blood disorders. *Precautions* Should not be given in early pregnancy, and should be used with caution in patients with impaired kidney, liver, or bone-marrow function. Its effects may be increased by aminobenzoic acid, aspirin, sulfonamides, and thiazide diuretics. *Dose* Varies with patient and disorder being treated.

*methotrimeprazine (LEVOPROME) A major tranquilizer. Read Major Tranquilizers, p. 53. It has effects, uses, and adverse effects similar to those described under chlorpromazine. *Precautions* May have a marked effect in dropping blood pressure, and patients on large doses should be kept lying down. It should therefore be used with caution in the elderly and not given to patients on drugs used for lowering blood pressure. *Dose* By mouth, 25 to 1000 mg. daily in divided doses.

*methoxyphenamine (ORTHOXINE) A sympathomimetic drug used to treat bronchial asthma. Read Drugs Used to Treat Bronchial Asthma, p. 138, and Drugs Which Act on the Autonomic Nervous System,

p. 145. *Adverse effects* May cause nausea, dizziness, and dry mouth. *Precautions* Should not be given to patients who are receiving, or who have received in the preceding two weeks, monoamine oxidase inhibitor drugs. *Dose* By mouth, 50 to 100 mg. every four hours.

*methscopolamine An atropinelike drug used to treat gut spasm. See atropine.

*methsuximide (CELONTIN) An anticonvulsant drug with effects and uses similar to those described under ethosuximide. Additional adverse effects include sweating and double vision. Read Drugs Used to Treat Epilepsy, p. 142.

*methyclothiazide (ENDURON) A diuretic with effects, uses, and adverse effects similar to those described under chlorothiazide. Read Diuretics, p. 103. *Dose* By mouth, 2.5 to 10 mg. once daily.

methylcellulose An emulsifying agent that swells in water and is used as a bulk laxative. Read Drugs Used to Treat Constipation, p. 82. It has also been used as a weight-reducing drug because its tendency to absorb water makes the stomach feel full. Read Reducing Drugs, p. 68.

*methyldopa (ALDOMET) Used to treat raised blood pressure. Read Drugs Used to Treat Raised Blood Pressure, p. 108. *Adverse effects* Drowsiness may occur in the first few days of treatment; this usually disappears on its own or on reduction of the dose. Other adverse effects include diarrhea, dryness of the mouth, nausea, depression, mental disturbances, nightmares, edema, stuffiness of the nose, fever, dizziness, and failure to ejaculate. Rarely, joint and muscle pains, impotence, skin rashes, and weakness may occur. Blood disorders have been reported, and liver function may be impaired in the first few weeks of treatment. Methyldopa may occasionally make the urine dark. *Precautions* Should be used with caution in patients with impaired kidney or liver function or with a history of liver disease or mental depression. It should preferably not be used in pregnancy. A severe fall in blood pressure may occur during anesthesia in patients on methyldopa. Amphetamines and antidepressant drugs decrease the effects of methyldopa. *Dose* By mouth, 500 to 3000 mg. daily in divided doses.

*methylergonovine (METHERGINE; methylergonovine maleate) Effects and uses similar to those described under ergonovine, but it is effective in smaller doses. It contracts the uterus and is used in childbirth, but usually not before the expulsion of the afterbirth (placenta). *Dose* By mouth, 250 to 500 mcg. By subcutaneous, intramuscular, or intravenous injection, 100 to 200 mcg.

methylmorphine See codeine.

methyl nicotinate Used in irritating skin applications (rheumatic rubs—see p. 202).

*methylphenidate (RITALIN; methylphenidate hydrochloride) A sympathomimetic drug which stimulates the central nervous system. Read Drugs Which Act on the Autonomic Nervous System, p. 145, and Stimulants: Amphetamines, p. 64. *Adverse effects* May cause loss of appetite, dry mouth, dizziness, headache, insomnia, nausea, nervousness, and palpitations. *Precautions* Should be used with caution in patients with epilepsy or high blood pressure. Its effects may be increased by monoamine oxidase inhibitor antidepressant drugs. *Dose* By mouth, 5 to 30 mg. daily in divided doses.

*methylprednisolone (MEDROL) A corticosteroid. Its effects and uses are similar to those of prednisone. Read Corticosteroids, p. 160. *Dose* By mouth, 8 to 80 mg. daily in divided doses.

methylsalicylate Has the action and uses of salicylates (see aspirin). It is used in rheumatic rubs and liniments. Read Drugs Used to Treat Skin Disorders, p. 193.

*methyltestosterone (ANDROID; METANDREN; ORETON) A male sex hormone. It has effects and uses similar to those described under testosterone. It has the advantage that it is absorbed when taken by mouth or sucked under the tongue. Read Male Sex Hormones, p. 163. *Adverse effects* Jaundice may occur after prolonged use. In women, excessive libido may develop, and with larger doses masculinization may occur—deep voice, facial hair, male-type baldness, and body hair. Acne may also occur. *Precautions* Should not be used in patients with impaired liver function or in pregnancy. For other precautions, see testosterone. *Dose* By mouth, 25 to 50 mg. daily.

*methylthiouracil (ANTIBASON; METHIOCIL) Used to treat overworking of the thyroid gland. It has effects and uses similar to those described under propylthiouracil. Read Drugs Used to Treat Thyroid Disorders, p. 187. *Adverse effects and precautions* Similar to those described under propylthiouracil. It may produce rashes, sore throat, fever, and blood disorders. *Dose* By mouth, initially, 100 to 200 mg. daily in divided doses; maintenance, 50 to 150 mg. daily in divided doses.

*methyprylon (NOLUDAR) Used as a sleeping drug. Read Sleeping Drugs and Sedatives, p. 43. *Adverse effects* Minor adverse effects which may occasionally occur include drowsiness, dizziness, headache, excitation, skin rashes, nausea, and vomiting. *Precautions* Methyprylon may interfere with the ability to drive motor vehicles and operate machinery. It increases the effects of alcohol. *Drug dependence* Methyprylon may produce drug dependence of the barbiturate/alcohol type. *Dose* By mouth, 200 to 400 mg. at night; for sedation, 50 to 100 mg. three times daily.

*methysergide (SANSERT; methysergide maleate) Used to treat migraine. Read Drugs Used to Treat Migraine, p. 125. *Adverse effects* May produce nausea, stomach pains, drowsiness, dizziness, restlessness, cramps in the legs, and mood changes. It may also cause vomiting, diarrhea or constipation, ataxia, weakness, weight gain, disorders of circulation in the arms and legs, confusion, insomnia, skin rashes, loss of hair, painful joints and muscles, fall in blood pressure when the patient stands up, rapid beating of the heart, and blood disorders. Prolonged use may produce fibrosis (scar tissue) of tissues at the back of the abdomen (retroperitoneal). *Precautions* Should not be taken during pregnancy or be used in patients with heart or circulatory disorders, high blood pressure, impaired kidney or liver function, edema, or peptic ulcers. *Dose* By mouth, 2 to 6 mg. daily in divided doses.

*metolazone (ZAROXOLYN)** A diuretic drug. Read Diuretics, p. 103. See chlorothiazide. *Dose* By mouth, 5 to 20 mg. once daily.

**METRECAL** Products contain protein, fat, carbohydrates, and vitamins. They are used in weight control. See Reducing Drugs, p. 68.

*metronidazole (FLAGYL)** Used to treat inflammation of the vagina and penis (trichomonas vaginitis and urethritis). It is also effective against amoebic infections, infections of the mouth (Vincent's angina), and giardiasis of the gut. It has no effect on thrush *(Candida albicans)*. Many relapses of vaginitis may be due to reinfection by the male, and therefore both sexual partners should be treated. Gonorrhea should be tested for and excluded. *Adverse effects* May cause loss of appetite, nausea, headache, malaise, coated tongue, dryness of the mouth, and skin rashes. Less often it may cause drowsiness, vertigo, depression, and insomnia. It may cause the urine to be stained brown. *Precautions* Recently it has been shown to cause cancer in mice and mutations in bacteria, although these effects have not been observed in humans. It should accordingly be reserved for serious amebiasis and trichomonas infections resistant to other treatments. It should not be taken by patients with blood disorders or during pregnancy. When taken with alcohol the patient may experience flushing of the face, headache, dizziness, and nausea. *Dose* By mouth, vaginal (trichomonas) infections, and Vincent's disease of the mouth, 250 mg. three times daily for ten days. For amebiasis, by mouth, 750 mg, three times daily for five to ten days. Vaginal inserts may be used to treat vaginal infections in a dose of one 500 mg. insert daily along with 250 mg. tablets twice daily by mouth for ten days.

*MICATIN** See miconazole.

*MICATIN creams** See miconazole.

**MI-CEBRIN T** A multiple vitamin and mineral preparation. Read Vitamins, p. 155, and Tonics, p. 65.

*miconazole (MICATIN; MANISTAT; MONISTAT) An antifungal antibacterial drug. Read Drugs Used to Treat Skin Disorders, p. 193.

*MICRONOR See norethindrone.

*MIDICEL See sulfamethoxypyridazine.

MIDOL Each tablet contains aspirin 450 mg., caffeine 32 mg., and cinnamedrine 15 mg. See aspirin, caffeine, and cinnamedrine. Used to treat menstrual pain.

*MIGRAL Each tablet contains ergotamine tartrate 1 mg., cyclizine hydrochloride 25 mg., and caffeine hydrate 50 mg. See ergotamine, and read Drugs Used to Treat Migraine, p. 125. See cyclizine, and read Drugs Used to Treat Nausea, Vomiting, and Motion Sickness, p. 71. See caffeine, and read Stimulants: Caffeine, p. 63. Dose By mouth, 1 tablet at the beginning of an attack of migraine. Take additional tablets at half-hour and one-hour intervals until successful relief of pain. No more than 6 tablets per attack or 10 tablets per week.

MILES' NERVINE See Nervine.

milk of magnesia See magnesium hydroxide.

*MILONTIN See phensuximide.

*MILTOWN See meprobamate.

mineral oil See petrolatum, liquid.

*MINOCIN See minocycline hydrochloride.

*minocycline hydrochloride (MINOCIN) A tetracycline antibiotic. Read Antibiotics, p. 210. Dose By mouth, 200 mg. initially, followed by 100 mg. every 12 hours.

*MIRADON See anisindione.

*MITHRACIN See mithramycin.

*mithramycin (MITHRACIN) An anticancer drug. Read Drugs Used to Treat Cancer, p. 225. Adverse effects Include nausea, vomiting, diarrhea, sore gums and mouth, headache, and skin rashes. Blood levels of potassium, calcium, and phosphorus may be reduced. It may cause damage to the bone marrow, leading to blood disorders and bleeding, and reversible damage to the kidneys and liver. Precautions Should not be used in pregnancy and should be given with caution to patients with impaired kidney, liver, or bone-marrow function. Dose Varies according to disorder being treated.

*mitobronitol An anticancer drug. Read Drugs Used to Treat Cancer, p. 225. Adverse effects It may produce nausea, vomiting, and diarrhea, loss of hair, skin rashes, irregular menstrual periods, and bone-marrow damage leading to severe blood disorders. Precautions It should be given with utmost caution to patients suspected of having impaired bone-marrow function. Dose Varies according to treatment program being followed.

*mitotane (LYSODREN) An anticancer drug. Read Drugs Used to Treat

Cancer, p. 225. *Adverse effects* Nausea, vomiting, diarrhea, drowsiness, ataxia, and vertigo have been reported. Mitotane inhibits the production of adrenal cortex hormones; in cases of trauma or shock, corticosteroids by injection should be given. *Precautions* It should not be used in pregnancy and it should be given with caution to patients with liver disease. Patients should not drive motor vehicles or operate moving machinery while taking mitotane. *Dose* By mouth, 3 to 10 G. daily in three or four divided doses.

\*MOBAN   See molindone.

\*MODERIL   See rescinnamine.

\*molindone (MOBAN)   Used as a major tranquilizer. Read Major Tranquilizers, p. 53. It is not a phenothiazine but produces similar effects and adverse effects (see chlorpromazine). *Dose* By mouth, 15 to 225 mg. daily in divided doses.

MOL-IRON   Preparations contain various mixtures of iron and vitamins. Read Iron, p. 152, and Vitamins, p. 155.

\*MONISTAT   See miconazole.

\*morphine (morphine hydrochloride; morphine sulfate)   A narcotic pain reliever. Read Morphine and Narcotic Pain Relievers, p. 115. It is the most valuable of all pain relievers; it reduces anxiety and sleeplessness due to pain, and in fact it reduces all disagreeable sensations except skin irritation. Unfortunately it is liable to give rise to nausea and constipation. It is more effective when injected than by mouth. Morphine is used in the treatment of shock and as a preoperative medication combined with hyoscine or atropine. *Adverse effects* Nausea, loss of appetite, constipation, vomiting, and confusion may occur. It may also produce difficulty in passing urine, vertigo, drowsiness, restlessness, and change in mood. These effects occur more often if the patient is up and about rather than in bed. Sneezing and skin rashes may occur. *Precautions* Babies and young children are very sensitive to the effects of morphine, and it is not usually given to children under one year of age. Alarming and unusual reactions may occur in the elderly and the debilitated. It should not be used by patients with severe respiratory disorders, or after operations on the gall bladder. It should not be used in acute alcoholism and convulsive disorders. Its effects may be increased by monoamine oxidase inhibitor antidepressant drugs and depressant drugs such as anesthetics, sleeping drugs, sedatives, and phenothiazine major tranquilizers. Tolerance quickly develops. *Drug dependence* Drug dependence of the morphine type is a state arising from repeated use of morphine or a morphinelike drug. It is characterized by an overwhelming desire to continue taking the drug, by a tendency to increase the dose, and by psychic and physical dependence.

Withdrawal symptoms include running eyes and nose, sneezing, trembling, headache, weakness, sweating, anxiety, insomnia, restlessness, nausea, loss of appetite, vomiting, diarrhea, muscle cramps, and a rise in temperature. *Dose* By intramuscular injection, 8 to 20 mg.

*MOTRIN See ibuprofen.

*MUCOMYST See acetylcysteine.

*muscarine Read about acetylcholine in Drugs Which Act on the Autonomic Nervous system, p. 145.

*MUSTARGEN See mechlorethamine.

*mustine (mustine hydrochloride; mechlorethamine) An anticancer drug. Read Drugs Used to Treat Cancer, p. 225. *Adverse effects* These include nausea, vomiting, diarrhea, peptic ulcers, drowsiness, psychosis, loss of hair, deafness and noises in the ears, suspension of menstruation, reduced sperm count, and skin rashes. Damage to the bone marrow may occur, leading to severe blood disorders. Injections may produce pain, irritation, and thrombophlebitis at the site. *Precautions* Mustine should not be used in pregnancy, or in the presence of any infection or blood disorder. Evidence of impaired bone-marrow function should give rise to utmost caution in its use. *Dose* Varies according to the treatment program being followed.

*MYAMBUTOL See ethambutol.

*MYCHEL See chloramphenicol.

*MYCIFRADIN See neomycin.

*MYCIGUENT (ophthalmic) See neomycin.

MYCIL See chlorphenesin.

*MYCOLOG Cream and ointment contain triamcinolone, neomycin, gramicidin, and nystatin. See triamcinolone, neomycin, gramicidin, and nystatin, and read Drugs Used to Treat Skin Disorders, p. 193.

*MYCOSTATIN See nystatin.

*MYDRIACYL See tropicamide.

MYLANTA Contains magnesium hydroxide 200 mg., aluminum hydroxide 200 mg., and simethicone 20 mg. in each chewable tablet or 5 ml. See magnesium hydroxide, aluminum hydroxide, and simethicone. Read Drugs Used to Treat Indigestion and Peptic Ulcers, p. 74.

*MYLERAN See busulfan.

MYLICON See simethicone.

*MYOCHRYSINE (gold sodium thiomalate; gold) Used to treat rheumatoid arthritis. See gold, and read Aspirin, Nonnarcotic Pain Relievers, and Drugs Used to Treat Rheumatism and Arthritis, p. 118. *Dose* By intramuscular injection, according to a complex schedule depending on response.

*MYSOLINE See primidone.

*MYSTECLIN-F Capsules contain tetracycline hydrochloride 250 mg. and amphotericin B 50 mg. See tetracycline and amphotericin, and read Antibiotics, p. 210. *Dose* By mouth, one capsule four times daily.

*NACTON See poldine.

*nafcillin (UNIPEN) Similar to oxacillin in its antibacterial actions. It is not as well absorbed orally. *Adverse effects* Similar to penicillin G. *Dose* By mouth, 250 mg. to 1 G. every four to six hours. By intravenous injection, 500 mg. to 1 G. every four to six hours.

*NALDECON Each tablet contains phenylephrine hydrochloride 10 mg., phenylpropanolamine hydrochloride 40 mg., phenyltoloxamine citrate 15 mg., and chlorpheniramine 5 mg. See each constituent drug, and read Drugs Used to Treat Common Colds, p. 132. *Dose* By mouth, 1 tablet three times daily.

*NALLINE See nalorphine.

*nalorphine (NALLINE; nalorphine hydrochloride) Reduces or abolishes most of the effects produced by morphine and related substances, although it has some depressant activity of its own. It is used to treat poisoning by these drugs. Read Morphine and Narcotic Pain Relievers, p. 115. *Adverse effects* May cause drowsiness, irritability, sweating, restlessness, nausea, slowing of the heart rate, and a fall in blood pressure. Given alone it may produce severe mental disturbance, and when given to narcotic addicts it may trigger withdrawal symptoms. *Dose* 5 to 10 mg. intravenously up to a maximum of 40 mg.

*naloxone (NARCAN; naloxone hydrochloride) A narcotic antagonist with no depressant activity. It is now the drug of choice in treating narcotic overdose. Read Morphine and Narcotic Pain Relievers, p. 115. *Dose* By intravenous injection, 0.4 mg.

*nandrolone (DECA-DURABOLIN; nandrolone decanoate) An anabolic (body-building) steroid. It has effects and uses similar to those described under methandrostenolone, but it is not active when given by mouth. Read Anabolic Steroids, p. 165. *Adverse effects and precautions* Similar to those discussed under testosterone. Jaundice has not been reported after its use. *Dose* By intramuscular injection, 50 to 100 mg. every three or four weeks. Durabolin (nandrolone phenylpropionate), by intramuscular injection, 25 to 50 mg. weekly.

naphazoline (PRIVINE; naphazoline hydrochloride) Constricts small blood vessels and is used in nose drops to reduce stuffiness and running noses. It is also used in eye drops to relieve eye inflammation. Read Drugs Which Act on the Autonomic Nervous System, p. 145, and Drugs Used to Treat Common Colds, p. 132. *Adverse effects* Overdose or accidental swallowing may produce drowsiness or coma. *Precautions* Frequent or prolonged use of naphazoline nose drops may produce congestion in the nose, and therefore the smallest dose, at not less than four- or six-hour intervals, should be used.

*NAQUA   See trichlormethiazide.

*NARCAN   See naloxone.

narcotine   See noscapine.

*NARDIL   See phenelzine.

NASOCON NASAL SPRAY   Nasal spray containing antazoline phosphate 0.5%, naphazoline hydrochloride 0.025%, sodium chloride (salt) 0.8%, phenylmercuric acetate 0.002%. See antazoline, naphazoline, and phenylmercuric acetate. Read Drugs Used to Treat Common Colds, p. 132.

*NATULAN   See procarbazine.

*NATURETIN   See bendroflumethiazide.

*NAVANE   See thiothixene.

*NAVIDRIX   See cyclopenthiazide.

NECTADON   See noscapine.

*NEFROLAN   See clorexolone.

*NEMBUTAL   See pentobarbital.

*NEOBIOTIC   See neomycin

*NEODECADRON   Preparations contain dexamethasone and neomycin. See dexamethasone and neomycin. Read Drugs Used to Treat Skin Disorders, p. 193, Antibiotics, p. 210, and Corticosteroids, p. 160.

*NEO-MERCAZOLE   See carbimazole.

*neomycin (MYCIFRADIN; NEOBIOTIC)   An antibiotic. Its use is restricted to treating infections of the skin, ears, and eyes, and also bowel infections. Read Antibiotics, p. 210. *Adverse effects* Should not be given by injection because it causes kidney damage, deafness, and disorders of balance after a few days of treatment. The deafness may be permanent. Allergy may occur, producing skin rashes and itching after local application to the eye, ears, or skin. Neomycin increases the effects of drugs used to treat blood pressure, thiazide diuretics, and certain neuromuscular blocking agents used in surgical anesthetics. *Precautions* Should not be given by injection, applied to raw areas or wounds, or given by mouth for prolonged periods. Prolonged use in creams, ointments, and drops should be avoided because it leads to allergy, which may be obscured but not prevented by the use of preparations of neomycin containing corticosteroids. *Dose* As an intestinal antiseptic, by mouth 2 to 8 G. daily in divided doses.

*NEO-POLYCIN   Ointment contains neomycin sulfate, zinc bacitracin, and polymixin B sulfate in a special base. See neomycin, bacitracin, and polymixin B, and read Antibiotics, p. 210, and Drugs Used to Treat Skin Disorders, p. 193.

*NEOSPORIN Topical applications contain polymixin B, neomycin, and gramicidin. See polymixin B, neomycin, and gramicidin, and read Antibiotics, p. 210, and Drugs Used to Treat Skin Disorders, p. 193.

*neostigmine (PROSTIGMIN; neostigmine methylsulfate) Acts on the parasympathetic division of the autonomic nervous system. Read Drugs Which Act on the Autonomic Nervous System, p. 145. Its effects and uses are similar to those described under physostigmine. It is used to treat patients with myasthenia gravis, and also in the treatment of urinary retention and paralysis of the bowel after surgical operations. *Dose* 0.5 to 1 mg. by intramuscular injection.

NEO-SYNEPHRINE Elixir, 5 ml., contains phenylephrine hydrochloride 5 mg. and alcohol 8%. See phenylephrine.

NERVINE (MILES' NERVINE) Each tablet or capsule contains 615.4 mg. sodium, potassium, and ammonium bromide, plus B vitamins, niacinamide 7 mg., and thiamine 1 mg. For sodium, potassium, and ammonium bromide, see potassium bromide, and read Vitamins, p. 155.

*neutral insulin Read Drugs Used to Treat Diabetes, p. 182.

niacin (nicotinic acid) A member of the vitamin B group. Read Vitamins, p. 155. It is also used to treat disorders of the circulation, since it causes vasodilation (see p. 96). *Adverse effects* In doses used to treat disorders of the circulation it may cause flushing, dry skin, itching, skin rashes, nausea, vomiting, diarrhea, headache, abdominal cramps, debility, loss of appetite, flare-up of peptic ulcers, jaundice, and may increase blood sugar and uric acid levels. It may increase the effects of drugs used to treat raised blood pressure. *Dose* By mouth, to treat disorders of circulation, 50 to 250 mg. daily in divided doses. Higher doses have been used to treat high blood fat levels (see p. 99).

niacinamide See nicotinamide.

*nialamide (NIAMID) A monoamine oxidase inhibitor antidepressant drug. It has effects and uses similar to those described under phenelzine. Read Antidepressants, p. 56. *Adverse effects and precautions* See phenelzine. The most frequent of these are headaches, nausea, vertigo, dryness of the mouth, and sweating. *Dose* By mouth, 75 to 150 mg. daily in divided doses.

*NIAMID See nialamide.

*niclosamide Used to treat tapeworm. Read Drugs Used to Treat Worm Infections, p. 229. *Adverse effects* May occasionally cause stomach upset. *Precautions* A purgative must be given within one to two hours of treatment to clear the bowel of dead segments of tapeworms before the parasites can be digested and release their eggs. *Dose* By mouth, 2 G.; tablets should be chewed or swallowed with a large drink of water.

**nicotinamide (niacinamide)** Has the effects of niacin. It is a member of the vitamin B group. Read Vitamins, p. 155.

**nicotine** See section on tobacco in Dependence on Drugs, p. 23.

**nicotinic acid** See niacin.

**nicotinic acid amide** See nicotinamide.

*****nicotinyl (RONIACOL, nicotinyl tartrate)** A vasodilator drug. Read Drugs Used to Treat Disorders of Circulation, p. 93. *Adverse effects* May produce flushing and faintness, slight swelling of the face, nausea, vomiting, and a fall in blood pressure. *Precautions* It should be given with caution to patients with disorders of the arteries supplying the brain. *Dose* By mouth, 25 to 50 mg. four times daily.

*****nikethamide** Stimulates the respiratory center in the brain and also improves the circulation. It was previously used to treat clinical shock.

*****NILSTAT** See nystatin.

*****NIPRIDE** See nitroprusside.

*****niridazole** Used to treat schistosomiasis. *Adverse effects* Include nausea, vomiting, colic, loss of appetite, diarrhea, headache, insomnia, skin rash, and pins and needles. It may affect the heart and produce changes on the electrocardiograph. *Precautions* Should be used with utmost caution in patients with impaired liver function, psychological disorders, epilepsy, malnutrition, and certain anemias. Patients should be treated in a hospital. *Dose* By mouth, 25 mg. per kg. of body weight daily for five to seven days.

*****NISENTIL** See alphaprodine.

*****nitrofurantoin (FURADANTIN; MACRODANTIN)** An antibacterial drug. Its mode of action is unknown. It is excreted in high concentration in the urine, and its principal use is in the treatment of infections of the urine which are prolonged and cannot be treated by other drugs. Read Drugs Used to Treat Infections of the Urinary System, p. 223. *Adverse effects* Nausea, abdominal discomfort, and drowsiness may occur on full dosage; these disappear on reduction of the dose. Skin rashes, nerve damage (peripheral neuritis), and an acute respiratory disorder (asthma) have been reported. These are more common in patients with impaired kidney function and patients on prolonged treatment with large doses. Blood disorders and liver damage may occur. *Precautions* Should not be taken by patients with impaired kidney function or a genetic disease which causes a fault in glucose metabolism (deficiency of glucose-6-phosphate-dehydrogenase), since they may develop hemolytic anemia. It should never be used in patients who have previously developed allergy or asthma while on nitrofurantoin. *Dose* By mouth, 50 to 150 mg. four times daily or 5 to 8 mg. per kg. of body weight for seven to fourteen days.

*nitrofurazone (FURACIN)  An antibacterial drug used in skin applications. Read Drugs Used to Treat Skin Disorders, p. 193. It has been used with other drugs to treat trypanosomiasis. *Adverse effects* Continuous application for five days or more may produce allergic skin reactions. By mouth, it may produce polyneuritis, nausea, vomiting, joint pains, and headaches.

*nitroglycerin (trinitrin; glyceryl trinitrate)  Principally used to treat angina. Read Drugs Used to Treat Angina, p. 100. It may also be used to relieve pain from kidney stones or gallstones. *Adverse effects* Large doses cause flushing of the face, severe throbbing headache, and faintness. In severe cases restlessness, blueness, vomiting, and fainting may occur, but these last only for a short time. *Precautions* Should be used with caution in patients with marked anemia, head injury, or acute coronary thrombosis. *Dose* Tablets dissolved in the mouth, 0.15 to 0.6 mg. as required.

*nitroprusside (NIPRIDE; sodium nitroprusside, sodium nitroferricyanide)  Lowers the blood pressure. See Drugs Used to Treat Raised Blood Pressure, p. 108. Very powerful and short-acting dilator of blood vessels. Used only as initial short-term treatment of emergency cases of high blood pressure and certain heart diseases. *Adverse effects* Primarily due to low blood pressure: nausea, vomiting, sweating, restlessness, headache, palpitation, angina, fainting. The elderly and those taking other drugs for high blood pressure or heart disease are more sensitive. *Dose* Varies according to disease, and requires constant supervision and monitoring.

*NOCTEC  See chloral hydrate.

NO DOZ  Tablets contain caffeine 100 mg. Read Stimulants: Caffeine, p. 63.

*NOLUDAR  See methyprylon.

*noradrenaline  See levarterenol.

norephedrine  See phenylpropanolamine.

*norepinephrine  See levarterenol.

*norethindrone (MICRONOR, NORLUTIN; NOR-Q.D.; norethindrone acetate; NORLUTATE)  A synthetic female hormone. It is used to treat menstrual irregularities, to delay menstruation, to treat painful periods, and for birth control. Read Female Sex Hormones, p. 166. *Adverse effects* May cause headache, tension, depression, nausea, vomiting, breast fullness, fluid retention, weight gain, bleeding between periods, deep voice, acne, hairiness, and masculinization of the unborn baby when doses of more than 15 mg. a day are taken. Prolonged use may cause liver damage. It prevents conception when taken with estrogens (see Oral Contraceptive Drugs, p. 173). *Precautions* Should be taken with caution by patients with impaired liver function or a history of serious thrombosis. *Dose* By mouth, 10 to 20 mg. daily in divided doses.

*norethynodrel (ENOVID; ENOVID E) Has effects, uses, and adverse effects similar to those described under norethindrone. *Dose* By mouth, 5 to 30 mg. daily in divided doses.

*NORFLEX See orphenadrine.

*NORGESIC Each tablet contains orphenadrine citrate 25 mg., aspirin 225 mg., phenacetin 160 mg., and caffeine 30 mg. See orphenadrine, and read Drugs Used to Treat Parkinsonism, p. 149. See aspirin and phenacetin, and read Aspirin, Nonnarcotic Pain Relievers, and Drugs Used to Treat Rheumatism and Arthritis, p. 118. Also read Stimulants: Caffeine, p. 63. *Dose* By mouth, 1 to 2 tablets three to four times daily.

*norgestrel A progestogen. Read Female Sex Hormones, p. 166, and Oral Contraceptive Drugs, p. 173.

*NORINYL Tablets contain norethindrone and mestranol. Read Female Sex Hormones, p. 166, and Oral Contraceptive Drugs, p. 173.

*NORLESTRIN Tablets contain norethindrone and ethinylestradiol in various strengths. Read Female Sex Hormones, p. 166, and Oral Contraceptive Drugs, p. 173.

*NORLUTATE See norethindrone.

*NORLUTIN See norethindrone.

*NORMENON See chlormadinone.

*NORPRAMIN See desipramine.

*NOR-Q.D. See norethindrone.

*NORQUEN Tablets contain norethindrone and mestranol. Read Female Sex Hormones, p. 166, and Oral Contraceptive Drugs, p. 173.

*nortriptyline (AVENTYL; nortriptyline hydrochloride) A tricyclic antidepressant drug. It has effects and uses similar to those described under amitriptyline, but it produces less drowsiness. Read Antidepressants, p. 56. *Adverse effects and precautions* Similar to those listed under amitriptyline. Nortriptyline should not be given to patients with glaucoma, patients who may develop retention of urine, patients with coronary artery disease, or patients with disordered heart rhythm. *Dose* By mouth, 20 to 100 mg. daily in divided doses.

noscapine (NECTADON; narcotine) A cough suppressant. It is obtained from opium, but it does not relieve pain or alter mood, and it is unlikely to cause drug dependence. Read Drugs Used to Treat Coughs, p. 135. *Adverse effects* Drowsiness, dizziness, headache, nausea, and skin rash may occasionally occur. *Dose* By mouth, 15 to 30 mg.

*NOVAHISTINE-DH 5 ml. contains phenylephrine hydrochloride 10 mg., chlorpheniramine maleate 2 mg., codeine phosphate 10 mg., chloroform 13.5 mg., and alcohol 5%. See each constituent drug, and read Drugs Used to Treat Common Colds, p. 132, Drugs Used to Treat Coughs, p. 135, and Antihistamine Drugs, p. 127. *Dose* By mouth, 2 teaspoonfuls (10 ml.) four times daily.

\*NOVAHISTINE EXPECTORANT 5 ml. contains phenylephrine hydrochloride 10 mg., chlorpheniramine maleate 2 mg., codeine phosphate 10 mg., glyceryl guaiacolate 100 mg., chloroform 13.5 mg., and alcohol 5%. See each constituent drug and read Drugs Used to Treat Coughs, p. 135, and Antihistamine Drugs, p. 127. *Dose* By mouth, 2 teaspoonfuls (10 ml.) four times daily.

\*novobiocin (ALBAMYCIN; novobiocin calcium, novobiocin sodium) An antibiotic. Bacterial resistance and adverse effects are common; its use should be restricted to certain infections by organisms resistant to other antibiotics and to infections of the gall bladder by organisms sensitive to novobiocin. Read Antibiotics, p. 210. *Adverse effects* Nausea, vomiting, diarrhea, abdominal colic, skin rashes, and fever are fairly common. Novobiocin may produce blood disorders and impair liver function. *Precautions* Novobiocin should not be given to children under six months of age, and it should be given with caution during pregnancy. *Dose* By mouth, 1 to 2 G. daily in divided doses.

\*NOVOCAIN See procaine.

\*NOVRAD See levopropoxyphene.

NOXZEMA Medicated cream is used to treat burns and contains phenol, menthol, camphor, oil of cloves, eucalyptus oil, and lime water in a water-dispersible base. See each constituent drug, and read Drugs Used to Treat Skin Disorders, p. 193.

\*NUPERCAINAL Suppositories, cream, ointment, and aerosol contain dibucaine as the active ingredient. See dibucaine, and read Drugs Used to Treat Skin Disorders, p. 193.

\*NUPERCAINE See dibucaine.

nux vomica Has the effects, uses, and adverse effects of strychnine. (See strychnine.) It is present in numerous tonics.

\*nylidrin (ARLIDIN, nylidrin hydrochloride) A vasodilator drug. Read Drugs Used to Treat Disorders of Circulation, p. 94. It may cause palpitations, and it should be given with caution to patients with coronary artery disease, overworking of the thyroid gland, or peptic ulcers. *Dose* By mouth, 6 mg. three or four times daily.

NYQUIL Contains dextromethorphan hydrobromide 15 mg., ephedrine sulfate 8 mg., doxylamine succinate 7.5 mg., acetaminophen 600 mg., and alcohol 25% in each ounce. See each constituent drug, and read Drugs Used to Treat Common Colds, p. 132, Drugs Used to Treat Coughs, p. 135, and Antihistamine Drugs, p. 127.

*nystatin (MYCOSTATIN; NILSTAT) An antibiotic which is active against a wide range of fungi and yeasts. When given by mouth, little is absorbed. It is mainly used to treat candida infections (e.g., thrush) of the skin, mouth, genitals, and intestine. Read Antibiotics, p. 210. *Adverse effects* May rarely cause nausea, vomiting, and diarrhea. *Dose* For intestinal infection, by mouth, 1 to 2 million units per day in divided doses. For vaginal moniliasis, suppositories containing 100,000 units, one or two at night for two weeks.

NYTOL Contains methapyrilene 25 mg. and salicylamide 200 mg. See each constituent drug, and read Sleeping Drugs and Sedatives, p. 43.

octylphenoxypolyethoxyethanol An ether used in making water and oil emulsions, and other drug preparations.

*OGEN See estrone.

oil of cloves Obtained from dried buds of *Caryophyllus aromaticus*. It is used in mixtures to treat gas and indigestion.

*oleandomycin An antibiotic. Read Antibiotics, p. 210. *Dose* 250 to 500 mg. four times daily.

*OMNIPEN See ampicillin.

*ONCOVIN See vincristine.

*OPHTHOCHLOR See chloramphenicol.

*opium Read Morphine and Narcotic Pain Relievers, p. 115. It has effects and uses similar to those described under morphine, which it contains. It is more constipating than morphine.

*ORACON Tablets contain dimethisterone and ethinyl estradiol. See Oral Contraceptive Drugs, p. 173.

*ORA-TESTRYL See fluoxymesterone.

*ORATROL See dichlorphenamide.

*ordinary insulin Read Drugs Used to Treat Diabetes, p. 182.

*ORETIC See hydrochlorothiazide.

*ORETON-M See methyltestosterone.

*ORINASE See tolbutamide.

*ORISUL See sulfaphenazole.

*ORNADE Each spansule contains isopropamide iodide 2.5 mg., phenylpropanolamine hydrochloride 50 mg., and chlorpheniramine maleate 9 mg. See isopropamide, chlorpheniramine, and phenylpropanolamine, and read Drugs Used to Treat Common Colds, p. 132. *Dose* By mouth, 1 capsule every twelve hours.

ORNEX Each capsule contains acetaminophen 325 mg. and phenylpropanolamine hydrochloride 18 mg. See acetaminophen and phenylpropanolamine. Read Drugs Used to Treat Common Colds, p. 132.

*orphenadrine (NORFLEX; orphenadrine citrate, and DISIPAL; orphenadrine hydrochloride) Closely related to the antihistamine drug diphenhydramine, but it has only weak antihistamine properties; it lifts the mood and relaxes spasm of skeletal muscles. It is used to treat Parkinsonism and muscle spasms due to injury (often combined with a pain reliever). Read Drugs Used to Treat Parkinsonism, p. 149. *Adverse effects* Insomnia, mental excitement, increased trembling (tremor), and nausea may occur. These are usually dose-related. Anxiety, confusion, and tremors have followed its combined use with dextropropoxyphene (propoxyphene). *Precautions* Should be used with caution in patients with glaucoma or urinary retention. *Dose* By mouth, orphenadrine citrate, 200 to 400 mg. daily in divided doses. By injection (intramuscular or intravenous), 60 mg. once or twice a day. Orphenadrine hydrochloride, by mouth, 200 to 400 mg. daily in divided doses.

*ORTHO-NOVUM Tablets contain norethindrone and mestranol in various strengths. Read Female Sex Hormones, p. 166, and Oral Contraceptive Drugs, p. 173.

*ORTHOXINE See methoxyphenamine.

*OSMITROL See mannitol.

*OTRIVIN See xylometazoline.

*ouabain (strophanthin-G) Read Drugs Used to Treat Heart Failure and Heart Rhythm Disorders, p. 86.

*OVRAL Tablets contain norgestrel and ethinyl estradiol in various strengths. Read Female Sex Hormones, p. 166, and Oral Contraceptive Drugs, p. 173.

*OVULEN Tablets contain ethynodiol diacetate and mestranol in various strengths. Read Female Sex Hormones, p. 166, and Oral Contraceptive Drugs, p. 173.

*oxacillin (BACTOCILL; PROSTAPHILIN) Has uses and effects similar to those of cloxacillin. See cloxacillin. *Dose* By mouth, 2 to 4 G. daily in four divided doses. By intramuscular injection, 2 to 12 G. daily.

*OXALID See oxyphenbutazone.

*oxanamide A minor tranquilizer with effects and uses similar to those described under meprobamate. Read Minor Tranquilizers, p. 51.

*oxandrolone (ANAVAR) A male sex hormone. Read Male Sex Hormones, p. 163, and Anabolic Steroids, p. 165. *Adverse effects* These are similar to those described under testosterone. If given for prolonged periods, it may cause jaundice, and it should not be used in patients with impaired liver function. *Dose* By mouth, 2.5 to 10 mg. daily.

*oxazepam (SERAX) A minor tranquilizer. Its effects and uses are similar to those described under chlordiazepoxide. Read Minor Tranquilizers, p. 51. *Adverse effects* Similar to those described under chlordiazepoxide. Edema, nightmares, lethargy, slurred speech, and blood disorders have also been reported. *Precautions and drug dependence* See chlordiazepoxide. *Dose* By mouth, 10 to 30 mg. daily in divided doses.

*oxethazaine A local anesthetic. Read Local Anesthetics, p. 191.

*oxtriphylline (CHOLEDYL; choline theophyllinate) Used to relax bronchial muscles in patients suffering from asthma and other respiratory disorders. Read Drugs Used to Treat Bronchial Asthma, p. 138. *Adverse effects* Produces irritation of the stomach and may cause nausea and vomiting, but less frequently than aminophylline. *Precautions* Should be given with caution to young children. *Dose* By mouth, 400 to 1600 mg. daily in divided doses.

*oxycodone (oxycodone hydrochloride) Produces effects similar to those of morphine. See morphine, and read Morphine and Narcotic Pain Relievers, p. 115. *Adverse effects* Similar to those described under morphine. *Drug dependence* Prolonged use may produce drug dependence of the morphine type. *Dose* By mouth, 5 to 20 mg. By subcutaneous injection, 5 mg. Maximum in 24 hours, 100 mg.

*oxymetazoline (in AFRIN nasal spray) Used as a nasal decongestant. Read Drugs Used to Treat Common Colds, p. 132. It may cause local stinging, sneezing, and dry throat and mouth. It should not be used in children under six years of age.

*oxymetholone (ADROYD; ANADROL) An anabolic (body-building) steroid with effects, uses and adverse effects similar to those described under methandrostenolone. Read Anabolic Steroids, p. 165. It may impair liver function. *Dose* By mouth, 5 to 30 mg. daily.

*oxyphenbutazone (OXALID; TANDEARIL) An antirheumatic drug. Its effects, uses, and adverse effects are similar to those described under phenylbutazone, of which it is a breakdown product within the body. Read Aspirin, Nonnarcotic Pain Relievers, and Drugs Used to Treat Rheumatism and Arthritis, p. 118. *Dose* By mouth, after meals, initially 400 to 600 mg. daily in divided doses; maintenance, 200 to 300 mg. daily.

*oxyphencyclimine (DARICON; oxyphencyclimine hydrochloride) An atropinelike drug. Its effects and uses are similar to those described under propantheline. It reduces gastric acidity and spasm and is used to treat patients with peptic ulcers. It has a long duration of action. Read Drugs Which Act on the Autonomic Nervous System, p. 145, and Drugs Used to Treat Indigestion and Peptic Ulcers, p. 74. *Adverse effects* May cause a fall in blood pressure, retention of urine, and constipation. It lacks the effects of atropine on the brain and is less likely to produce dry mouth, rapid heart rate, and blurred vision. *Precautions* Should be used with caution in patients with glaucoma or enlarged prostate glands. *Dose* By mouth, 20 to 40 mg. daily in divided doses.

**oxyphenisatin** Used to treat constipation. Read Drugs Used to Treat Constipation, p. 82. It may possibly cause jaundice.

*__oxytetracycline (TERRAMYCIN; oxytetracycline dihydrate) and oxytetracycline hydrochloride (DALIMYCIN; TERRAMYCIN HYDROCHLORIDE)__ A tetracycline antibiotic. Read Antibiotics, p. 210. Its effects, uses, and adverse effects are similar to those described under tetracycline. *Dose* Oxytetracycline dihydrate, by mouth, 1 to 3 G. daily in divided doses. Oxytetracycline hydrochloride, by mouth, 1 to 3 G. daily in divided doses.

*__oxytocin (PITOCIN; SYNTOCINON)__ Injection contains the active principle from the posterior lobe of the pituitary gland. It may either be prepared from animal glands or synthesized. It is used to stimulate the uterus to contract during labor. Oxytocin may also be given by tablet to suck in the mouth, or by nose spray.

PABAFILM See Suntan and Sunburn Applications, p. 196.

PABANOL Contains 5% para-aminobenzoic acid. See Suntan and Sunburn Applications, p. 196.

*PABESTROL See diethylstilbestrol.

*PAGITANE HYDROCHLORIDE See cycrimine.

*PALUDRINE See chloroguanide.

*__pamabrom__ Related to theophylline. See theophylline.

*PAMINE See scopolamine.

PAMPRIN Each tablet contains phenacetin 125 mg., pamabrom 25 mg., pyrilamine maleate 12.5 mg., and salicylamide 250 mg. See phenacetin, pamabrom, pyrilamine, and salicylamide. Used to treat menstrual pain.

*__pancreatic dornase__ An enzyme extracted from beef pancreas. It is used as a liquefier, e.g., to liquefy sticky sputum. Read Drugs Used to Treat Coughs, p. 135. It may produce allergic reactions. *Dose* Inhalation by aerosol, 50,000 to 400,000 units daily.

*__pancreatin__ A preparation extracted from the pancreas of certain animals and used to treat patients suffering from a disease of the pancreas characterized by a deficient production of pancreatic digestive enzymes. *Dose* By mouth with meals, 0.5 to 3 G.

*__pancrelipase (COTAZYM)__ Used in pancreatic digestive enzyme deficiency. It contains lipase, protease, amylase, trypsin, and other pancreatic enzymes.

*__pancuronium (PAVULON; pancuronium bromide)__ A muscle-relaxant drug used along with general anesthetics in surgical operations. Read Drugs Which Act on the Autonomic Nervous System, p. 145.

*PANMYCIN See tetracycline.

*PANWARFIN  See warfarin.

*papaverine  Obtained from opium, and because it relaxes involuntary muscles it was used to treat colic of the gut or gall bladder, bronchial asthma, and to dilate blood vessels in the limbs and brain. It has never been proven to be of therapeutic value in any condition, although it is currently being studied in relation to certain brain syndromes in the elderly which are due to decreased blood flow. *Adverse effects* It may cause disorders of heart rhythm.

**para-aminobenzoic acid**  Used in suntan creams.

*para-aminosalicylic acid  See aminosalicylic acid.

PARACODIN  See dihydrocodeine.

*PARADIONE  See paramethadione.

*PARAFLEX  See chlorzoxazone.

*PARAFON FORTE  Each tablet contains chlorzoxazone 250 mg. and acetaminophen 300 mg. See chlorzoxazone and acetominophen, and read Aspirin, Nonnarcotic Pain Relievers, and Drugs Used to Treat Rheumatism and Arthritis, p. 118. *Dose* By mouth, 2 tablets four times daily.

*paraldehyde  A quick-acting sleeping drug and anticonvulsant. Because of its nasty smell, taste, and partial excretion in the breath, it is seldom used except in hospitals. Read Sleeping Drugs and Sedatives, p. 43. *Adverse effects* Because it irritates the stomach it is usually given by injection, which may be painful. Adverse effects are not common. Skin rashes may occur, and rarely it may cause liver and kidney disorders. Nerve damage may occur if it is injected close to a main nerve. *Precautions* If given by mouth or by rectum it should be well diluted. Intramuscular injections should not exceed more than 5 ml. into any one site. It should not be given in plastic syringes and should be given with caution to patients with impaired liver function. It decomposes in light and heat to form acetic acid. Deaths have occurred from the use of old paraldehyde; it should always be tested for acidity and discarded if acid. *Drug dependence* May produce dependence of the barbiturate/alcohol type. *Dose* By intramuscular injection or by mouth, 5 to 10 ml.

*paramethadione (PARADIONE)  An anticonvulsant drug used to treat petit mal epilepsy. Read Drugs Used to Treat Epilepsy, p. 142. *Adverse effects* Similar to but less severe than those described under trimethadione. It may produce kidney and blood disorders. *Precautions* Should not be given to patients with severely impaired kidney or liver function, disorders of the retina or optic nerve, or anemia or other blood disorders. *Dose* By mouth, 900 to 2100 mg. daily in divided doses.

*paregoric  Camphorated tincture of opium which contains 0.04%

morphine. Read Morphine and Narcotic Pain Relievers, p. 115. It is used to treat diarrhea. Read Drugs Used to Treat Diarrhea, p. 80. *Dose* 5 to 50 ml. daily in divided doses.

*PAREST See methaqualone.

*PARNATE See tranylcypromine.

*paromomycin (HUMATIN; paromomycin sulfate) An antibacterial and antiamoebic drug used to treat infections of the gut. It is taken by mouth and should never be given by injection because of its adverse effects, which are similar to those produced by neomycin. Read Antibiotics, p. 210. *Dose* By mouth, 25 to 66 mg. per kg. of body weight daily in divided doses for at least five days.

*PARSIDOL See ethopropazine.

*PAS See aminosalicylic acid.

*PATHILON See tridihexethyl.

*PATHOCIL See dicloxacillin.

*PAVABID See papaverine.

*PAVULON See pancuronium.

pectin Read Drugs Used to Treat Diarrhea, p. 80.

*PEDIAMYCIN See erythromycin.

*PEGANONE See ethotoin.

*PENBRITIN See ampicillin.

*penicillamine (CUPRIMINE; penicillamine hydrochloride) Used to treat toxic metal poisoning (e.g., lead) and also to treat a disorder of copper metabolism found in Wilson's disease. It has been used to treat rheumatoid arthritis and other disorders. Read Aspirin, Non-narcotic Pain Relievers, and Drugs Used to Treat Rheumatism and Arthritis, p. 118. *Adverse effects* May produce headache, nausea, sore throat, fever, muscle and joint pains, skin rash, swollen glands, and blood and kidney disorders. Severe allergic reactions may occur rarely, and also in some patients allergic to penicillin. *Precautions* Frequent blood and urine tests should be carried out during treatment. *Dose* 1 to 5 G. daily in four divided doses.

*penicillin See penicillin G.

*penicillin G (benzyl penicillin, penicillin) A very effective antibiotic from which a group of semisynthetic penicillins have been developed. It is usually given by injection. Read Penicillins, p. 213. *Adverse effects* All penicillins carry the risk of hypersensitivity (what most doctors and patients call allergy). This allergy is more likely to develop if the penicillin is applied to the skin. Allergic reactions include nettle rash (urticaria), dermatitis, swelling of the throat (angioneurotic edema), fever, and occasionally swollen joints. Very rarely death may occur in an allergic person. These allergic reactions are more likely to occur after injections but may occur if the penicillin is taken by mouth in a patient who has been made sensitive to penicillin. Patients allergic to one type of penicillin are allergic to *all* penicillins, and frequently also to cephalosporins. Penicillin skin rashes may occur in allergic patients after drinking milk from cows treated with penicillin for mastitis. Onset of allergic symptoms may occur immediately, within a few hours, after a few days, or not until the next course of penicillin treatment. Penicillin taken by mouth may cause nausea, diarrhea, and an itching anus (pruritis ani). If sucked, penicillin tablets can cause a sore tongue (glossitis), and sore gums and lips with small ulcers (angular and aphthous stomatitis). There is no suitable test for sensitivity to penicillin. *Precautions* Penicillin should not be used for trivial infections. If you have ever had an allergic reaction to penicillin or any drug, *you* should tell the doctor. Penicillin ointment or lozenges should *never* be used. Caution is necessary when giving a large dose of potassium or sodium salts of penicillin to patients with impaired kidney function or congestive heart failure. *Dose* By mouth, 125 to 500 mg. every *four* hours, on an empty stomach. By intramuscular injection, 150 to 600 mg. every four hours or every twelve hours. (Penicillin G dosage is often expressed in units: 125 mg. = 200,000 units; 250 mg. = 400,000 units; 500 mg. = 800,000 units.)

*penicillin V See phenoxymethylpenicillin.

*penicillin VK See phenoxymethylpenicillin.

*pentaerythritol (PERITRATE; pentaerythritol tetranitrate) Used to treat angina. Its effects and uses are similar to those described under nitroglycerin. It is taken by mouth, takes about one hour to work, and lasts for about five hours. Read Drugs Used to Treat Angina, p. 100. *Adverse effects and precautions* Similar to those described under nitroglycerin. *Dose* By mouth, 10 to 40 mg.

*pentamidine Used to treat leishmaniasis and trypanosomiasis. *Adverse effects* Intravenous injections can cause sudden fall of blood pressure, producing breathlessness, fainting, headache, dizziness, vomiting, and rapid heartbeat. It may affect blood sugar levels and kidney function. *Dose* By intramuscular injection, 4 mg. per kg. of body weight daily on alternate days up to 12 to 15 doses, and repeated in two weeks according to the disorder being treated.

*pentazocine (TALWIN) Related to the narcotic analgesics. Read Morphine and Narcotic Pain Relievers, p. 115. *Adverse effects* May produce nausea, vomiting, dizziness, changes in mood, and sweating. Headache, confusion, and hallucinations may occur if the drug is taken by mouth or by injection. Injection may also cause constipation, pins and needles, breathlessness, a fall in blood pressure, retention of urine, allergic skin rashes, and, rarely, depression of breathing.

These adverse effects are more likely to occur if the patient is up and about rather than in bed. The precautions which apply to morphine also apply to pentazocine. Its prolonged use may lead to drug dependence. *Dose* By mouth, 25 to 100 mg. every three to four hours up to a maximum of 600 mg. in 24 hours. By subcutaneous or intramuscular injection, 20 to 60 mg. every three to four hours.

\*PENTIDS   See penicillin G.

\*pentobarbital (NEMBUTAL; pentobarbital sodium)   A barbiturate sleeping drug. Read Sleeping Drugs and Sedatives, p. 43. *Dose* By mouth, 100 to 200 mg. at night.

pentobarbital sodium   See pentobarbital.

\*pentolinium (ANSOLYSEN, pentolinium tartrate)   Used to lower blood pressure. Read Drugs Used to Treat Raised Blood Pressure, p. 108. *Adverse effects* These include dry mouth, constipation, blurred vision, fall in blood pressure on standing, impotence, difficulty in urinating, diarrhea, nausea, and drowsiness. It may cause a severe fall in blood pressure in patients receiving a general anesthetic, and it may produce sensitivity to epinephrinelike drugs. *Dose* By subcutaneous injection, initially 1 mg. every twelve hours, increasing the dose according to need.

\*pentothal   See thiopental.

\*PEN-VEE   See phenoxymethylpenicillin.

\*PEN-VEE K   See phenoxymethylpenicillin.

peppermint   Used in preparations to prevent intestinal colic and gas. It is a common flavoring agent in mixtures.

PEPTO-BISMOL—liquid   Contains bismuth subsalicylate, sabol, and zinc phenolsulfonate. See each constituent drug, and read Drugs Used to Treat Indigestion and Peptic Ulcers, p. 74.

PEPTO-BISMOL—tablets   Each tablet contains calcium carbonate 350 mg., bismuth subsalicylate (strength not available), and glycocoll. See calcium carbonate, bismuth salts, and glycocoll, and read Drugs Used to Treat Indigestion and Peptic Ulcers, p. 74.

\*PERAZIL   See chlorcyclizine.

\*PERCODAN   Each tablet contains oxycodone hydrochloride 4.5 mg., oxycodone terephthalate 0.38 mg., aspirin 224 mg., phenacetin 160 mg., and caffeine 32 mg. See oxycodone, phenacetin, and aspirin. Read Aspirin, Nonnarcotic Pain Relievers, and Drugs Used to Treat Rheumatism and Arthritis, p. 118.

PERCOGESIC   Each tablet contains phenyltoloxamine citrate 30 mg. and acetaminophen 325 mg. See phenyltoloxamine and acetaminophen.

\*PERIACTIN   See cyproheptadine.

PERI-COLACE   Contains dioctyl sodium sulfosuccinate 100 mg. and casanthranol 30 mg. See the constituent drugs, and read Drugs Used to Treat Constipation, p. 82.

**PERISTIM** See casanthranol.

*PERITRATE See pentaerythritol.

*PERITRATE SA (sustained action) See pentaerythritol.

*PERMAPEN See benzathine penicillin G.

*PERMITIL See fluphenazine.

*perphenazine (TRILAFON) A major tranquilizer. It may also be used in treating nausea and vomiting. Read Major Tranquilizers, p. 53, and Drugs Used to Treat Nausea, Vomiting, and Motion Sickness, p. 71. *Adverse effects* Similar to those described under chlorpromazine, but perphenazine produces less sedation. It may produce dryness of the mouth, blurred vision, restlessness, fatigue, headache, and symptoms like those seen in Parkinsonism; at high doses these symptoms become more marked. *Precautions* Similar to those discussed under chlorpromazine. *Dose* By mouth, for mental disorders, 8 to 32 mg. daily in divided doses. For nausea and vomiting, 4 to 8 mg.

*PERSANTINE See dipyridamole

*PERTOFRANE See desipramine.

**PERTUSSIN EIGHT-HOUR COUGH FORMULA** 5 ml. contain 7.5 mg. dextromethorphan, 25 mg. ammonium chloride, chloroform 0.3%, sodium citrate 75 mg., and alcohol 9.5%. See dextromethorphan, ammonium chloride, chloroform, and sodium citrate, and read Drugs Used to Treat Coughs, p. 135.

**petrolatum, white (VASELINE)** Used in many skin applications. Read Drugs Used to Treat Skin Disorders, p. 193.

**petrolatum gauze** Sterilized absorbent cotton gauze saturated with sterilized white soft petroleum jelly.

**petrolatum liquid (mineral oil)** Used to treat constipation. Read Drugs Used to Treat Constipation, p. 82.

*PHELANTIN Each capsule contains phenytoin 100 mg., phenobarbital 30 mg., and methamphetamine 2.5 mg. It is used to treat epilepsy. See each constituent drug, and read Drugs Used to Treat Epilepsy, p. 142. *Dose* By mouth; must be determined in each individual patient. Usually three to four capsules daily.

*phenacemide (PHENURONE) An anticonvulsant drug used to treat grand mal and psychomotor epilepsy. Read Drugs Used to Treat Epilepsy, p. 142. *Adverse effects* Include skin rashes and ataxia; occasionally it may produce albumin and sugar in the urine. *Dose* By mouth, 2 to 3 G. daily in divided doses.

**phenacetin (acetophenetidin)** A mild pain reliever, and it reduces fever. It has no anti-inflammatory effects. It is broken down in the body to acetaminophen, which is widely used as a mild pain reliever. Read Aspirin, Nonnarcotic Pain Relievers, and Drugs Used to Treat Rheumatism and Arthritis, p. 118. *Adverse effects* May cause sweating and rarely skin rashes and jaundice. Blood disorders may occur, and patients may turn blue due to an alteration in the pigment which carries oxygen in red blood cells (methemoglobinemia and sulfemoglobinemia). Prolonged use may cause kidney damage, and large doses may damage the liver. *Precautions* Should be given with caution to patients with impaired kidney or liver function. *Dose* By mouth, 300 to 600 mg. as a single dose. Often combined with other pain relievers. *Warning* Because of the link between kidney damage and pain relievers containing phenacetin, it is suggested that phenacetin alone or in combination should be used with caution.

\*PHENAPHEN **with codeine** Each tablet contains phenacetin 194 mg., aspirin 162 mg., phenobarbital 15 mg., hyoscyamine sulfate 0.031 mg., and codeine phosphate: 15 mg. in Phenaphen No. 2, 30 mg. in Phenaphen No. 3, and 60 mg. in Phenaphen No. 4. See each constituent drug, and read Aspirin, Nonnarcotic Pain Relievers, and Drugs Used to Treat Rheumatism and Arthritis, p. 118. *Dose* By mouth, Phenaphen No. 2 and No. 3, one or two capsules every three to four hours as needed; Phenaphen No. 4, one capsule every three to four hours.

\*phenazopyridine (PYRIDIUM) Used to treat painful disorders of the bladder and urinary tract. It often colors the urine orange to red. *Adverse effects* May cause headache, vertigo, and abdominal colic. It may damage the red blood cells if given in high doses to patients with impaired kidney function. *Precautions* Should not be given to patients with severe impairment of liver or kidney function. *Dose* By mouth, 50 to 200 mg. three or four times daily.

\*phenelzine (NARDIL; phenelzine sulfate) A monoamine oxidase inhibitor antidepressant drug. Read Antidepressants, p. 56. *Adverse effects* Causes a fall in blood pressure and giddiness. It may cause headache, trembling, restlessness, constipation, difficult urination, dry mouth, blurred vision, skin rash, edema, and impotence. Severe reactions may occur with certain foods and drugs, and liver damage may occur. *Precautions* Should not be given to patients with impaired liver or heart function, disorders of the arteries supplying the brain (e.g., patients who have had a stroke), or epilepsy. A severe rise in blood pressure may occur, resulting in brain hemorrhage or heart failure, if patients on phenelzine or other monoamine oxidase inhibitor drugs take certain drugs. The following drugs should not be used: amphetamine, atropine, carbamazepine, chloroquine, dexamphetamine, ephedrine, ethamivan, fenfluramine, guanethidine, mephentermine, methoxamine, methoxyphenamine, methamphetamine, morphine, orciprenaline, meperidine, phenmetrazine, phenylephrine, phenylpropanolamine, pseudoephedrine, and reserpine. These drugs should not be given within two weeks of stopping monoamine oxidase inhibitor drugs. Certain foods contain tyramine, which can produce dangerous reactions in patients who are taking monoamine oxidase inhibitors; these include cheese, pickled herring, broad bean pods, ripe bananas, wines, beer, chicken liver, and protein extracts prepared from meal or yeast. Certain tricyclic antidepressant drugs should not be given at the same time or within two weeks of stopping MAO inhibitor drugs, and the effects of other drugs may be increased: antihistamines, barbiturates, some oral antidiabetic drugs, and nonbarbiturate hypnotics. Sensitivity to insulin may be increased, and meperidine and other narcotic pain relievers have produced severe reactions. In general, no drugs should be taken with phenelzine or other monoamine oxidase inhibitors without first consulting a physician or pharmacist. *Dose* By mouth, 15 to 45 mg. daily in divided doses.

*PHENERGAN See promethazine.

*PHENERGAN EXPECTORANT 5 ml. contains promethazine hydrochloride 5 mg., ipecac 2.3 mg., potassium guaiacolsulfonate 44 mg., chloroform, citric acid, sodium citrate, and alcohol. See each constituent drug, and read Drugs Used to Treat Coughs, p. 135, and Antihistamine Drugs, p. 127. *Dose* By mouth, 1 teaspoonful (5 ml.) every four to six hours.

*PHENERGAN EXPECTORANT with codeine Phenergan Expectorant with added codeine phosphate 8 mg. in each 5 ml. See codeine, and read Drugs Used to Treat Coughs, p. 135. *Dose* By mouth, 1 teaspoonful (5 ml.) every four to six hours.

*PHENERGAN VC EXPECTORANT 5 ml. contains promethazine hydrochloride 5 mg., phenylephrine hydrochloride 5 mg., potassium guaiacolsulfonate 44 mg., sodium citrate 197 mg., and ipecac, chloroform, and alcohol. See each constituent drug, and read Drugs Used to Treat Coughs, p. 135, and Antihistamine Drugs, p. 127. *Dose* By mouth, 1 teaspoonful (5 ml.) every four to six hours.

*PHENERGAN VC EXPECTORANT with codeine Phenergan VC Expectorant with added codeine phosphate 10 mg. per 5 ml. See Phenergan VC Expectorant and codeine, and read Drugs Used to Treat Coughs, p. 135. *Dose* By mouth, 1 teaspoonful (5 ml.) every four to six hours.

*phenethicillin (DARCIL; MAXIPEN; SYNCILLIN) A penicillin drug. It has effects, uses, and adverse effects similar to those described under phenoxymethylpenicillin. Although it gives rise to higher blood levels than phenoxymethylpenicillin, it is less potent, and therefore the effects of the two penicillins are similar. Read Penicillins, p. 213. *Dose* By mouth, 500 to 1500 mg. daily in divided doses.

*phenformin (DBI; MELTROL; phenformin hydrochloride)** An oral antidiabetic drug. Read Drugs Used to Treat Diabetes, p. 182. *Adverse effects* A bitter taste, loss of appetite, nausea, vomiting, and diarrhea are common and related to the dose. Loss of weight and lack of energy may occur. *Precautions* In light of possible heart damage, it should be considered only for rare cases of maturity onset diabetes where dietary or insulin control has proven either unacceptable or ineffective. It should not be used in patients with impaired liver or kidney function or congestive heart failure. It should not be used in pregnancy, before or after surgery, or in acute infections when insulin will be required. Alcohol should be taken only in moderation by patients on phenformin. *Dose* By mouth, 25 to 300 mg. daily in divided doses.

*phenindamine (THEPHORIN; phenindamine tartrate)** An antihistamine drug. Unlike other antihistamine drugs, it does not produce drowsiness but may cause stimulation. Read Antihistamine Drugs, p. 127. *Adverse effects* May cause nausea, dryness of the mouth, dizziness, and stomach upsets. Insomnia and convulsions may occur. *Precautions* As for antihistamine drugs. *Dose* By mouth, 75 to 150 mg. daily in divided doses.

*phenindione (DANILONE; HEDULIN)** Used to stop the blood from clotting. Read Drugs Used to Prevent Blood from Clotting, p. 90. *Adverse effects* Early signs of overdose are bleeding from the gums or nose or elsewhere and red blood cells in the urine. It may cause vomiting, diarrhea, skin rashes, and fever. Sore throat may be an early sign of allergy, which may lead to blood disorders, liver damage, kidney damage, and death. Phenindione may cause a brownish pigmentation of the fingernails, fingers, and palms of the hands of persons handling it. It sometimes colors the urine red. *Precautions* Blood-clotting tests should be carried out at frequent intervals. It should be given with great caution to patients with impaired liver or kidney function. It should not be used in the later months of pregnancy or within three days of surgery. Mothers who are taking phenindione should not breast-feed their babies. Its effects may be increased by other drugs: methandrostenolone, clofibrate, phenylbutazone, and similar antirheumatic drugs. Its effects may be reduced by barbiturates, chloral hydrate, glutethimide, and meprobamate. Aspirin and other salicylates may increase the danger of hemorrhage. *Dose* By mouth, initially 200 to 300 mg. daily, reducing to 25 to 100 mg. daily according to response.

**pheniramine (INHISTON; pheniramine maleate)** An antihistamine drug. Read Antihistamine Drugs, p. 127. *Dose* By mouth, 25 to 50 mg. daily.

*****phenmetrazine (PRELUDIN; phenmetrazine hydrochloride)** A reducing drug which suppresses the appetite for a few weeks. In large doses it has stimulating effects like amphetamine. Read Reducing Drugs, p. 68. *Adverse effects* Similar to those produced by amphetamine. Large doses or prolonged use may produce severe mental depression. *Precautions* Read Reducing Drugs, p. 68, and Stimulants: Amphetamines, p. 64. *Drug dependence* Produces drug dependence of the amphetamine type. *Dose* By mouth, 25 to 75 mg. daily in divided doses.

*****phenobarbital (LUMINAL; and phenobarbital sodium)** A barbiturate drug. It is used as a sedative and anticonvulsant. Read Sleeping Drugs and Sedatives, p. 43. *Adverse effects* Drowsiness may occur, and elderly patients may become confused. Allergic reactions are rare and include skin rashes. *Precautions* Should be given with caution to the elderly and those with impaired liver or kidney function. It should not be given to patients with acute intermittent porphyria. It may cause confusion in the presence of severe pain. Phenobarbital may interfere with ability to drive motor vehicles and operate machinery. It increases the effects of alcohol and may make patients depressed. It affects enzymes in the liver, increasing the breakdown of certain drugs, for example, folic acid, griseofulvin, phenylbutazone, phenytoin, and some anticoagulants. The effects of phenobarbital and other barbiturates may be increased by other sedatives, diphenoxylate, mephenesin, and possibly tricyclic antidepressant drugs. The blood level of the latter may be reduced by barbiturates. *Drug dependence* May produce drug dependence of the barbiturate/alcohol type, which is characterized by a strong psychological dependence, intoxication resulting in sedation, sleep, coma, stupor, impaired judgment, and ataxia, the development of tolerance, and a dangerous physical dependence manifested by anxiety, insomnia, weakness, trembling, convulsions, and delirium upon its withdrawal. Cross-tolerance with hypnosedative drugs may occur. *Dose* By mouth, 30 to 125 mg. daily in divided doses.

**phenol** Used as a disinfectant (see p. 201).

**phenolphthalein** An irritant laxative. Read Drugs Used to Treat Constipation, p. 82. *Adverse effects and precautions* Adverse effects produced by laxatives are discussed in Drugs Used to Treat Constipation, p. 82. Phenolphthalein may cause abdominal cramps, rarely produce a skin rash, and color the urine and feces red. It has occasionally caused protein to appear in the urine (albuminuria) and also free hemoglobin (the pigment in red blood cells); this is called hemoglobinuria. *Dose* By mouth, 50 to 300 mg.

*PHENOXENE See chlorphenoxamine.

*phenoxybenzamine (DIBENZYLINE; phenoxybenzamine hydrochloride) A vasodilator drug. Read Drugs Used to Treat Disorders of Circulation, p. 94. *Adverse effects* May cause a fall in blood pressure when the patient stands up, and large doses may produce rapid beating of the heart. It may also produce a stuffy nose, dry mouth, and drowsiness. *Precautions* Should be given with care to patients with raised blood pressure, impaired kidney function, or coronary artery disorders. *Dose* By mouth, 20 to 240 mg. daily in divided doses.

*phenoxymethylpenicillin (COMPOCILLIN-V; V-CILLIN; PEN-VEE; penicillin V) One of a group of penicillins that are not destroyed by the acid in the stomach and can be taken by mouth. It should not be given by injection because it is relatively insoluble, and it should not be applied to the skin. Read Penicillins, p. 213. *Adverse effects and precautions* Similar to those discussed under penicillin G. *Dose* By mouth, 0.5 to 1.5 G. daily in divided doses. The calcium and potassium salts of phenoxymethylpenicillin are absorbed more readily and are used in capsules, tablets, mixtures, and elixirs.

*phenprocoumon (LIQUAMAR) An anticoagulant drug related to warfarin but much longer-acting. Read Drugs Used to Prevent Blood from Clotting, p. 90. *Dose* By mouth, 1 to 4 mg. daily.

*phensuximide (MILONTIN) An anticonvulsant drug used to treat petit mal epilepsy. Read Drugs Used to Treat Epilepsy, p. 142. *Adverse effects* Similar to those described under ethosuximide. They include loss of appetite, nausea, dizziness, and drowsiness. Rarely, blood disorders and kidney damage may occur. *Precautions* See ethosuximide. Blood and urine tests should be carried out periodically. *Dose* By mouth, 1 to 3 G. daily in divided doses.

*phentermine (WILPO) A sympathomimetic drug used as a reducing drug. Read Reducing Drugs, p. 68. Also see amphetamine, and read Stimulants: Amphetamines, p. 64. *Adverse effects* Similar to those described under amphetamine. *Precautions* Should be given with caution to patients with heart disease, overworking of the thyroid glands, and psychological disturbances. *Dose* By mouth, 15 to 30 mg. daily in one dose in the morning.

*phentolamine (REGITINE MESYLATE; phentolamine hydrochloride; phentolamine mesylate) A vasodilator drug. Read Drugs Used to Treat Disorders of Circulation, p. 94. Phentolamine (5 mg. intravenously) is used to diagnose a rare tumor of the adrenal glands, pheochromocytoma, in which the blood pressure increases. It may also be given by mouth. *Adverse effects* May cause rapid beating of the heart, anginal pain, flushing, and occasionally vertigo. *Precautions* Should be used with caution in patients with coronary artery disease.

\*PHENURONE See phenacemide.

\*phenylbutazone (AZOLID; BUTAZOLIDIN) An anti-inflammatory drug used to treat rheumatic disorders and acute thrombophlebitis. It has pain-relieving properties and reduces a high temperature. It is metabolized and excreted slowly, and therefore its effects are prolonged. Read Aspirin, Nonnarcotic Pain Relievers, and Drugs Used to Treat Rheumatism and Arthritis, p. 118. *Adverse effects* Causes salt retention, blocks iodine uptake by the thyroid gland, and interferes with several enzyme processes in the body. Adverse effects are common and occur even when the dose does not exceed 400 mg. daily. They include rashes, nausea, stomach upset, fluid retention (edema), blurred vision, insomnia, and diarrhea. Ulceration of the mouth, esophagus, stomach, or duodenum may occur, leading to hemorrhage from these sites. Phenylbutazone may also cause damage to the liver, and blood disorders are not uncommon, occasionally resulting in death. Enlarged glands (including salivary glands) may occur, and a generalized allergic reaction and kidney failure have been reported. Adverse effects may occur within a few days of starting phenylbutazone, and some patients may become sensitized, so that a subsequent course of the drug may trigger adverse effects. *Precautions* Should not be given to patients with a history of peptic ulcers. It should be used with caution in patients with impaired heart, liver, or kidney function and by those with high blood pressure. The appearance of abdominal pains, fever, sore throat, or ankle swelling should be reported to a doctor. Phenylbutazone increases the effects of acetohexamide, tolbutamide, and certain anticoagulant drugs, and it may also increase the effects of phenytoin and some sulfonamides. *Dose* By mouth, 200 to 400 mg. daily.

phenylephrine (NEO-SYNEPHRINE; phenylephrine hydrochloride) A sympathomimetic drug included in numerous cold remedies and nasal drops and sprays. It constricts blood vessels and is used in anesthesia, shock, and other states to combat a fall in blood pressure. It is also used with local anesthetics to prolong their effects, and in eye drops. Read Drugs Which Act on the Autonomic Nervous System, p. 145, and Drugs Used to Treat Common Colds, p. 132. *Adverse effects* May cause pain and irritation at the site of injection. Overdose may cause headache, palpitation, and vomiting. Nose drops may cause local irritation, and eye drops may trigger glaucoma. *Precautions* Injections should not be given to patients with severe heart disease or raised blood pressure. It should be used with caution in patients with overworking thyroid glands, and it should not be given during or within two weeks of stopping treatment with monoamine oxidase inhibitor antidepressant drugs. *Dose* By intravenous injection, 50 mcg. By subcutaneous or intramuscular injection, 5 mg.

**phenylmercuric acetate** Used in some nose drops and in spermicides. It may irritate the skin, producing blisters and redness. See mercury salts.

**phenylmercuric nitrate** Used as a preservative for injection solutions and eye drops and to sterilize instruments. It is also used as a spermicide in contraceptive creams and foams. *Adverse effects* See mercury salts. It is irritating to the skin and causes redness and blistering 6 to 12 hours after application. Eye drops containing phenylmercuric nitrate should not be used for prolonged periods.

**phenylpropanolamine** (PROPADRINE; norephedrine; phenylpropanolamine hydrochloride) Effects similar to those described under ephedrine, but it is more active in constricting blood vessels and less active in dilating bronchi and as a stimulant. It is given by mouth in the treatment of snuffy noses, hay fever, and other allergic disorders. Read Drugs Used to Treat Common Colds, p. 132. *Dose* By mouth, 25 to 50 mg. in single doses only when required.

*phenyltoloxamine An antihistamine. Read Antihistamine Drugs, p. 127.

*PHENYTOIN (diphenylhydantoin) An anticonvulsant drug used to treat grand mal epilepsy. Read Drugs Used to Treat Epilepsy, p. 142. *Adverse effects* May irritate the lining of the stomach and should be taken with plenty of water, preferably after meals (although it is more effective if given before meals). Adverse effects, fairly frequent and occasionally severe, include dizziness, nausea, and skin rashes; these may be overcome by reducing the dose for a few days and then slowly increasing it. Tenderness and thickening of the gums may occur, as well as hairiness (hirsutism). Other adverse effects include fever, ataxia, double vision, trembling, hallucinations, and mental confusion. Severe blood disorders and skin rashes may occur. It may cause anemia (megaloblastic anemia) by interfering with folic acid metabolism (see p. 157). *Precautions* Should be given with caution to patients on thyroid drugs and in pregnancy. Increases in dosage must be made carefully, as disproportionately high blood levels of phenytoin may occur in some patients. *Dose* By mouth, 50 to 200 mg. three times daily.

PHILLIPS' MILK OF MAGNESIA See magnesium hydroxide.

*PHISOHEX An antiseptic detergent containing hexachlorophene. See hexachlorophene.

PHOSPHALJEL See aluminum phosphate gel.

*phospholine (echothiophate iodide, phospholine iodide)  An ingredient in eye drops used to treat certain types of glaucoma. It inhibits cholinesterase. Read Drugs Which Act on the Autonomic Nervous System, p. 145. *Adverse effects* Pain, headaches, and blurred vision may occur during the first four days of treatment. It may occasionally cause acute inflammation of the iris and set off an attack of glaucoma. It may cause cysts to develop on the iris, particularly in children. *Precautions* It should be used with caution in patients who are sensitive to iodine or in patients with a history of detached retina. It should be stopped immediately if the patient develops diarrhea, sweating, and weakness, signs that it is affecting the autonomic nervous system.

*phthalylsulfathiazole (SULFATHALIDINE)  Has the antibacterial actions of the sulfonamides. It is slowly broken down in the gut, the bulk being excreted in the feces. It is still sometimes used to treat bowel infections. Read Sulfonamides, p. 220. *Adverse effects* Allergic reactions may occur in patients sensitized to sulfonamides, and skin disorders (erythema multiforme and Stevens-Johnson syndrome) may occur. *Precautions* Prolonged use may lead to a thrush *(Candida albicans)* infection of the gut and interference with vitamin B and vitamin K production in the intestine. *Dose* By mouth, 5 to 10 G. daily in divided doses.

*physostigmine (physostigmine salicylate; eserine salicylate)  Acts on the sympathomimetic division of the autonomic nervous system. Read Drugs Which Act on the Autonomic Nervous system, p. 145. It is used principally in eye drops to constrict the pupil and reduce the pressure inside the eyeball in the treatment of glaucoma. *Adverse effects* By mouth, it may cause nausea, vomiting, diarrhea, and abdominal pain. With large doses, muscle twitching, weakness, and paralysis of breathing may occur.

*phytonadione (MEPHYTON; vitamin K)  Occurs naturally and is involved in blood clotting. It is an antidote to overdosage with anticoagulant drugs and is used in bleeding disorders. Overdose may cause jaundice in newborn babies. If injected into a vein it should be given very slowly because it may produce sweating, flushing, a sense of suffocation, and collapse. Read Vitamins, p. 155. *Dose* 5 to 20 mg. as a suspension for intravenous injection. By mouth, 5-mg. tablet once daily.

*pilocarpine (ISOPTO CARPINE; pilocarpine hydrochloride; pilocarpine nitrate)  Effects and uses similar to those described under physostigmine. It is used in eye drops to constrict the pupil and decrease the pressure inside the eyeball in patients with glaucoma. Its effect on the eye is less complete and of shorter duration than that produced by physostigmine, and a slight increase in pressure in the eye may occur at first. Read Drugs Which Act on the Autonomic Nervous System, p. 145.

*PIPANOL see trihexyphenidyl.

*piperacetazine (QUIDE) A major tranquilizer. Read Major Tranquilizers, p. 53. *Dose* By mouth 10 mg. two to four times daily initially, then increasing up to 160 mg. if needed.

*piperazine (ANTEPAR; piperazine citrate, hydrate, and phosphate) Used to treat threadworm and roundworm infection. Read Drugs Used to Treat Worm Infections, p. 229. *Adverse effects* Very rare unless high and prolonged dosage is used, when the patient may develop dizziness, clumsiness, vomiting, pins and needles, and blurred vision. *Dose* By mouth, over twelve years of age, 2 G. daily in divided doses for one week.

*piperidolate (DACTIL) An atropinelike drug used to relieve intestinal colic and other disorders of the stomach and gut. Read Drugs Used to Treat Indigestion and Peptic Ulcers, p. 74, and Drugs Used to Treat Diarrhea, p. 80. *Dose* By mouth, 50 mg. four times daily.

*PITOCIN See oxytocin.

*PITRESSIN See vasopressin.

*PLACIDYL See ethchlorvynol.

plantago seed See psyllium.

*PLAQUENIL See hydroxychloroquine.

podophyllum A purgative. Read Drugs Used to Treat Constipation, p. 82. It is an irritant and is also used as a keratolytic to treat warts. See Drugs Used to Treat Skin Disorders, p. 193.

*POLARAMINE See dexchlorpheniramine.

*poldine (NACTON; poldine methylsulfate) An atropinelike drug. It reduces gastric secretion, is long-acting, and is used to treat peptic ulcers and conditions associated with an increased production of acid in the stomach. Read Drugs Used to Treat Indigestion and Peptic Ulcers, p. 74. *Adverse effects* Similar to those described under atropine. Blurred vision, constipation, difficulty in beginning urination, and rapid heartbeat may occur. *Precautions* Similar to those described under atropine. *Dose* By mouth, 2 to 6 mg. every six hours.

poloxalkol (MAGCYL; POLYKOL) Reduces surface tension and is used to treat constipation. Read Drugs Used to Treat Constipation, p. 82.

*POLYCILLIN See ampicillin.

POLYKOL See poloxalkol.

*polymyxin B (AEROSPORIN; polymyxin B sulfate) An antibiotic. It is used in ointments, sprays, drops, and powders and is taken by mouth to treat infections of the gut. It may also be given by injection. Read Antibiotics, p. 210. *Adverse effects* When given by injection it may cause dizziness and sensory sensations, particularly over the face, hands, and feet (this suggests that it is toxic to nerves), and rarely it may damage the kidneys and produce nerve damage leading to paralysis of respiration. These adverse effects do not occur when the drug is taken by mouth; but adverse effects may occur when it is applied to large raw areas, especially burns. Fever and pain at the site of injection may occur. *Precautions* Should be given with caution to patients with impaired kidney function. *Dose* By mouth, 750,000 to 1,000,000 units daily in divided doses. By intramuscular injection, 500,000 units every eight hours.

*POLYSPORIN Contains polymyxin B sulfate and bacitracin in ointment base or ophthalmic (eye) solution. See each constituent drug, and read Drugs Used to Treat Skin Disorders, p. 193.

*polythiazide (RENESE) A diuretic. Read Diuretics, p. 103. Its effects, uses, and adverse effects are similar to those described under chlorothiazide. *Dose* By mouth, 1 to 4 mg. daily.

*PONDIMIN See fenfluramine.

*PONSTEL See mefenamic acid.

*PONTOCAINE See tetracaine

*potassium Diuretic drugs used to treat fluid retention (edema) caused by heart, liver, or kidney disorders may result in a loss of potassium salts. This loss is usually corrected by giving potassium salts by mouth. Sufficient potassium can also usually be given in special diets. Read Diuretics, p. 103. Potassium citrate makes the urine less acid and is used to treat inflammation of the bladder. *Adverse effects* Potassium salts are irritant when taken by mouth; they may cause ulceration of the stomach or intestine with bleeding and obstruction. When included in a thiazide diuretic preparation they may cause similar effects. *Precautions* Enteric-coated tablets should be avoided where possible. Liquid formulations should be used if dietary sources are ineffective. The salts should be taken well diluted and given with caution to patients with impaired kidney function or adrenal insufficiency. *Dose* Depends upon the salt used and the patient's requirements.

potassium acid tartrate See cream of tartar.

*potassium bicarbonate (K-LYTE) Used as a potassium supplement. See potassium.

potassium bitartrate (cream of tartar) Used as a saline laxative.

potassium bromide Once widely used as a sedative. Read Sleeping Drugs and Sedatives, p. 43. *Adverse effects* During prolonged use, accumulation of bromide occurs in the body, which may give rise to symptoms of bromide intoxication (bromism), including skin rashes, nausea, vomiting, mental dullness, poor memory, apathy, loss of appetite, constipation, and drowsiness. These symptoms disappear if the drug is stopped, but if it is continued, insomnia, restlessness, disorientation, hallucinations, delirium, stupor, and coma may result.

*potassium chloride  Potassium salt. It is used to treat deficiency of potassium which may occur with patient's taking certain diuretic drugs. Read Diuretics, p. 103.

potassium guaiacolsulfonate  Formerly used in cough medicines and as an intestinal antiseptic. It is of doubtful value.

potassium iodide  Used in cough expectorants. Read Drugs Used to Treat Coughs, p. 135. It is also used to treat overworking of the thyroid gland in preparation for surgery. Read Drugs Used to Treat Thyroid Disorders, p. 187.

*POVAN  See pyrvinium.

povidone-iodine  Used in skin and mouth applications as an antiseptic. See iodine.

*pramoxine (TRONOTHANE; pramoxine hydrochloride)  A local anesthetic. Read Local Anesthetics, p. 191.

*prednisolone  Prednisone (see below) is converted in the liver to prednisolone; there is no significant difference between the effects of the two substances.

*prednisone  A corticosteroid. It has effects and uses similar to those described under cortisone, but it is effective in a much smaller dose and has weaker salt-retention effects. Because of this it is preferred to cortisone as an anti-inflammatory drug in the treatment of such disorders as rheumatoid arthritis, rheumatic fever, and asthma. Read Corticosteroids, p. 160. *Adverse effects and precautions* Similar to those described under cortisone. It may produce indigestion and peptic ulcers. *Dose* By mouth, 10 to 100 mg. daily in divided doses.

*PRELUDIN  See phenmetrazine.

*PREMARIN  Contains estrogens from the urine of pregnant mares. Read Female Sex Hormones, p. 166.

PREPARATION H  Ointment and suppositories for hemorrhoids, containing phenylmercuric nitrate 1 part in 10,000, shark liver oil 3%, and live yeast cells. See phenylmercuric nitrate and yeast, and read about applications used to treat hemorrhoids on p. 209.

*PRESAMINE  See imipramine.

*PRE-SATE  See chlorphentermine.

PRE-SUN  Contains 5% para-aminobenzoic acid. See Suntan and Sunburn Applications, p. 196.

*prilocaine (CITANEST; prilocaine hydrochloride)  A local anesthetic with effects and uses similar to those of lidocaine. *Adverse effects and* *precautions* Overdose may cause chemical change inside the red blood cells (methemoglobinemia), and it should therefore not be used in patients with anemia; similarly, it should not be used in pregnancy because of this risk. Read Local Anesthetics, p. 191.

\*primaquine (primaquine phosphate)  An antimalarial drug. Read Drugs Used to Treat Malaria, p. 227. *Adverse effects* Common adverse effects of high dosage are nausea, abdominal pain, and blood disorders. Adverse effects on the blood occur more frequently in patients with a genetic fault which leads to an abnormality of glucose metabolism. *Dose* By mouth, prevention, 30 to 60 mg. once a week along with 300 mg. of chloroquine; treatment, 15 mg. daily for fourteen days.

\*PRIMATENE MIST  See epinephrine.

\*primidone (MYSOLINE)  An anticonvulsant used to treat grand mal epilepsy. Read Drugs Used to Treat Epilepsy, p. 142. *Adverse effects* May cause drowsiness, ataxia, nausea, vomiting, vertigo, irritability, headache, visual disturbances, fatigue and general debility, and occasionally skin rashes. These are usually mild and disappear with reduction of dosage. Other adverse effects include thirst, frequent urination, edema, and impaired sexual function. Anemia may occur; it responds to folic acid treatment (see p. 157). *Dose* By mouth, 500 to 2000 mg. daily in divided doses.

\*PRINCIPEN  See ampicillin.

\*PRISCOLINE  See tolazoline.

PRISTEEN  A vaginal deodorant (see p. 206).

\*PRIVINE  See naphazoline.

\*PRO-BANTHINE  See propantheline.

\*probenecid (BENEMID)  Used to treat gout. It increases the excretion of urates by the kidneys, which results in a reduction of the raised blood uric acid level (which occurs in gout) and slowly causes removal of urate deposits (tophi) from the tissues. It is of no value in treating an acute attack of gout and is used only to prevent, or reduce the frequency of, acute attacks. Treatment must usually be continued for life. Probenecid reduces the excretion of penicillins and the antibiotics cephalexin and cephalothin. It therefore increases the plasma level of these drugs, which is directly related to their effectiveness. Read Drugs Used to Treat Gout, p. 124. *Adverse effects* Rare with doses up to 1 G. daily. Above this dose nausea, vomiting, skin rashes, and fever may occur, particularly in patients with impaired kidney function. *Precautions* Acute attacks of gout may be precipitated in the first few weeks or months of treatment with probenecid, particularly with high doses. Daily dosage should not be interrupted, because this allows the blood uric acid level to rise. Aspirin, citrates, and salicylates should not be given with probenecid, since they antagonize its effects. *Dose* By mouth, 1 to 2 G. daily.

*procainamide (PRONESTYL; procainamide hydrochloride) Has effects on the heart rate and rhythm. Read Drugs Used to Treat Heart Failure and Heart Rhythm Disorders, p. 86. *Adverse effects* After high dosage it may cause loss of appetite, nausea, vomiting, and diarrhea. Rapid injections into a vein may cause a sudden fall in blood pressure and disorders of heart rhythm. Prolonged administration may produce joint pains, skin rashes, chest pains, and a blood disorder (these signs and symptoms are known as lupus erythematosus). It may also cause abdominal pain, enlargement of the liver, confusion, itching, and allergic reactions—fever and skin rashes. *Precautions* Should not be given to patients with bronchial asthma, allergy to the drug, impaired kidney function, or heart disorders affecting the conduction of nervous impulses, or during treatment with sulfonamide drugs. It should be used with caution in patients with digitalis intoxication. *Dose* By mouth, 0.5 to 1 G. every four to six hours. By slow intravenous injection, up to 1 G. in a 2.5% solution.

*procaine (ANUCAINE; NOVOCAIN; UNICAINE; procaine hydrochloride) A short-acting local anesthetic. Read Local Anesthetics, p. 191.

*procaine penicillin (procaine benzylpenicillin; procaine penicillin G) A salt of penicillin G. Read Penicillins, p. 213. Given by intramuscular injection, it creates a depot from which the penicillin G. is slowly released into the bloodstream. It should therefore be given only once daily. Large doses given more than once daily may cause adverse effects due to release of procaine and leave painful lumps at the site of injection. *Dose* 600,000 to 4,800,000 units as a single dose daily by deep intramuscular injection.

*procaine penicillin G See procaine penicillin

*procarbazine (MATULANE; NATULAN) An anticancer drug. Read Drugs Used to Treat Cancer, p. 225. *Adverse effects* Include loss of appetite, nausea, vomiting, sore mouth and gums, diarrhea, pain, fever, and infections. Skin rashes, bleeding, disorders of the heart and circulation, loss of hair, impaired liver function, and general itching have been recorded. Mood changes and nerve damage may occasionally occur, and trembling, convulsions, and unconsciousness have been reported in children. *Precautions* Should not be used in pregnancy. It should be used with caution in patients with impaired kidney and liver function, and it should not be used if there is evidence of impaired bone marrow function. It is a monoamine oxidase inhibitor drug, and therefore special precautions about food and other drugs should be taken (see phenelzine). It may increase the brain-depressant effects of antihistamines, narcotic pain relievers, and phenothiazine major tranquilizers. It can produce a disulfiram-like effect with alcohol. See disulfiram. *Dose* Varies according to disorder being treated.

*prochlorperazine (COMPAZINE; prochlorperazine maleate)* A major tranquilizer. It has effects and uses similar to those described under chlorpromazine, but it is less sedating and is more effective in treating nausea and vomiting. It is also effective in treating vertigo and Ménière's disease. Read Major Tranquilizers, p. 53, and Drugs Used to Treat Nausea, Vomiting, and Motion Sickness, p. 71. *Adverse effects* Similar to those described under chlorpromazine. Adverse effects occur less frequently than with chlorpromazine, but Parkinsonism is more common. Dryness of the mouth, dizziness, fall in blood pressure, and rapid heartbeat may occur occasionally. Drowsiness is frequent, and jaundice and blood disorders have been reported. Severe Parkinsonism may occur in ill children and can be very alarming. *Precautions* Should not be given to ill children; other precautions are similar to those described under chlorpromazine. *Dose* By mouth, for nausea, vomiting, or vertigo, 10 to 30 mg. daily in divided doses, or by suppository or intramuscular injection, 5 to 10 mg. For psychological disorders, by mouth, 15 to 150 mg. daily in divided doses.

*procyclidine (KEMADRIN; procyclidine hydrochloride)* Used to treat Parkinsonism. It decreases rigidity and tremor and improves muscle coordination and mobility. It has little effect on salivation. It is an atropinelike drug. Read Drugs Used to Treat Parkinsonism, p. 149, and Drugs Which Act on the Autonomic Nervous System, p. 145. *Adverse effects and precautions* Similar to those described under atropine. Drowsiness, ataxia, giddiness, blurred vision, confusion, nausea, and vomiting may occur. These usually disappear when the dose is reduced. *Dose* By mouth, 7.5 to 30 mg. daily in divided doses.

**proflavine** An antiseptic and disinfectant.

*progesterone* A female sex hormone produced by the ovaries which works on the lining of the uterus. Read Female Sex Hormones, p. 166. It was previously used to treat habitual miscarriages and disorders of menstruation but has now been mainly replaced by preparations effective by mouth which have fewer adverse effects (acne, greasy hair, tenderness of the breasts, premenstrual depression, and disorders of liver function). *Adverse effects* Progesterone drugs used in oral contraceptives may cause changes of appetite, cramps in the legs and abdomen, changes in libido, fluid retention, a white vaginal discharge, dry vagina, or reduced menstrual loss. Large doses in pregnancy may cause masculinization of the unborn baby.

*proguanil* See chloroguanide.

\*PROLIXIN   See fluphenazine.

\*PROLOID   See thyroid.

\*promazine (SPARINE: promazine hydrochloride)   A major tranquil-
izer with effects and uses similar to those described under chlorpromazine. Read Major Tranquilizers, p. 53. *Adverse effects and precautions* Similar to those described under chlorpromazine. Dizziness and
drowsiness occur frequently, but a fall in blood pressure and Parkinsonism are not as frequent. *Dose* By mouth or intramuscular or intravenous injection, 50 to 800 mg. daily.

\*promethazine (PHENERGAN; promethazine hydrochloride)   A pow-
erful and long-acting antihistamine drug. Read Antihistamine
Drugs, p. 127, and Drugs Used to Treat Nausea, Vomiting, and
Motion Sickness, p. 71. *Adverse effects* Include dryness of the mouth,
throat, and nose, abdominal pain with vomiting, and diarrhea. The
most common adverse effect is drowsiness, which can interfere with
the ability to drive a motor vehicle or operate machinery. Other
adverse effects include inability to concentrate, lassitude, dizziness,
muscle weakness, incoordination, headache, blurred vision, irritability, loss of appetite, and noises in the ears (tinnitus). Stimulation
may occur particularly in children and infants, causing excitability
and nightmares even after one dose. Blood disorders and jaundice
have been reported, and skin sensitivity to sunlight may occur.
*Precautions* May increase the sedation effects of alcohol, barbiturates,
sleeping drugs, sedatives, and tranquilizers. The effects of antidepressant drugs and atropinelike drugs may also be increased. It
should be used with caution in patients with impaired liver function.
Patients should be warned about the dangers of driving motor vehicles and operating machinery and of the dangers of taking alcohol
while on promethazine. *Dose* By mouth, 25 to 50 mg. daily (usually
at night). By deep intramuscular injection, up to 50 mg.

\*PRONESTYL   See procainamide.

PROPADRINE   See phenylpropanolamine.

\*propantheline (PRO-BANTHINE; ROPANTH; propantheline bromide)
An atropinelike drug. It does not produce the effects of atropine on
the brain and is used to treat peptic ulcers because it reduces gastric
secretions and spasm. It may also be used to treat intestinal colic,
spasms of the gall bladder ducts, spasm of the ureters, and excessive
salivation. Read Drugs Which Act on the Autonomic Nervous System, p. 145, and Drugs Used to Treat Indigestion and Peptic Ulcers,
p. 74. *Adverse effects* Similar to those described under atropine. Propantheline may cause a fall in blood pressure, retention of urine, and
constipation. It is less likely than atropine to produce dryness of the
mouth, rapid heartbeat, and blurred vision. *Precautions* Similar to

those described under atropine. It should be used with caution in patients with glaucoma or an enlarged prostate. *Dose* By mouth, 15 mg. three times daily.

**propionic acid** An antifungal drug used as a preservative.

\***propoxyphene (DARVON: dextropropoxyphene hydrochloride; propoxyphene hydrochloride and also DARVON-N: propoxyphene napsylate)** A mild pain reliever. Read Morphine and Narcotic Pain Relievers, p. 115, and Aspirin, Nonnarcotic Pain Relievers, and Drugs Used to Treat Rheumatism and Arthritis, p. 118. *Adverse effects* May cause dizziness, headache, drowsiness, excitation, raised mood (euphoria), insomnia, skin rashes, nausea, vomiting, abdominal pains, and constipation. Symptoms of overdose are similar to those produced by morphine, except convulsion may occur. *Precautions* Should be given with caution to patients with severe respiratory disorders. It may increase the effects of other respiratory depressant drugs (e.g., sedatives and hypnotics). *Dose* Propoxyphene hydrochloride, by mouth, up to 260 mg. daily in divided doses. Propoxyphene napsylate, by mouth, up to 400 mg. daily in divided doses.

\***PROPOXYPHENE COMPOUND 65** Each pulvule contains propoxyphene hydrochloride 65 mg., acetylsalicylic acid (aspirin) 227 mg., phenacetin 162 mg., and caffeine 32.4 mg. See propoxyphene, aspirin, phenacetin, and caffeine, and read Aspirin, Nonnarcotic Pain Relievers, and Drugs Used to Treat Rheumatism and Arthritis, p. 118. *Dose* By mouth, 2 capsules every four hours as needed for pain.

\***propranolol (propranolol hydrochloride)** A beta-receptor blocking drug. Used to treat disorders of heart rhythm and angina. Read Drugs Used to Treat Angina, p. 100, and Drugs Used to Treat Heart Failure and Heart Rhythm Disorders, p. 86. *Adverse effects* Nausea, vomiting, diarrhea, insomnia, lassitude, and ataxia may occur. Various sensations in the hands, blood disorders, skin rashes, and visual hallucinations also may occur, though less frequently. Heart failure and wheezing (bronchospasm) may also occur. *Precautions* Should not be given to patients with bronchial asthma, bronchospasm, or partial heart block. It should be given to patients with congestive heart failure only when they have been treated with digoxin. It should not be used during pregnancy and it should be given only with caution to patients on antidiabetic drugs. It should not be withdrawn abruptly. *Dose* By mouth: for disordered heart rhythm, 10 to 30 mg. three or four times daily; for angina, 60 to 240 mg. daily in divided doses.

**propylene glycol** Used as a vehicle for drugs and for flavoring agents in food.

**propylhexedrine (BENZEDREX)** A vasoconstrictor drug used in inhalers to relieve stuffy or runny noses. Read Drugs Used to Treat Common Colds, p. 132.

*propylthiouracil  Used to treat overworking of the thyroid gland. It has effects, uses, and adverse effects similar to those described under methimazole. Read Drugs Used to Treat Thyroid Disorders, p. 187. *Dose* By mouth, initially 200 to 600 mg. daily in divided doses, reducing to a maintenance dose of 50 to 200 mg. daily.

*PROSTAPHILIN  See oxacillin.

*PROSTIGMINE  See neostigmine.

*protamine  Neutralizes the anti-blood-clotting effects of heparin. Read Drugs Used to Prevent Blood from Clotting, p. 90.

*protriptyline  (VIVACTIL; protriptyline hydrochloride)  A tricyclic antidepressant drug. Its effects and uses are similar to those described under imipramine, although it has a more rapid onset of action, varying from four to eight days. Read Antidepressants, p. 56. *Adverse effects* Similar to those discussed under imipramine. Rashes may develop due to sunlight sensitivity of the skin. *Precautions* Similar to those described under imipramine. Exposure to strong sunlight should be avoided. *Dose* By mouth, 15 to 60 mg. daily in divided doses.

*PROVERA  See medroxyprogesterone.

pseudoephedrine  (SUDAPHED; pseudoephedrine hydrochloride)  Has effects and uses similar to those described under ephedrine. It is used to relieve nasal and bronchial congestion, particularly in bronchial asthma. *Adverse effects and precautions* The same adverse effects as ephedrine. It should not be given to patients with high blood pressure or enlarged prostate glands because it may cause retention of urine. Read Drugs Used to Treat Bronchial Asthma, p. 138, and Drugs Used to Treat Common Colds, p. 132. *Dose* By mouth, 60 to 180 mg. daily in divided doses.

psyllium  (METAMUCIL; plantago seed; EFFERSYLLIUM)  Absorbs and retains water and is therefore used as a bulk laxative. Read Drugs Used to Treat Constipation, p. 82. *Dose* By mouth, 5 to 15 G.

*pteroylglutamic acid  See folic acid.

*PURINETHOL  See mercaptopurine.

*PURODIGIN  See digitoxin.

*PYOPEN  See carbenicillin.

*pyrantel (pyrantel pamoate)  Used to treat roundworm infection. Read Drugs Used to Treat Worm Infections, p. 229. *Adverse effects* May produce nausea, diarrhea, headache, and dizziness. *Precautions* Should not be used in pregnancy or in children under one year of age. *Dose* By mouth, 11 mg. per kg. of body weight in one dose (maximum 1 G.).

\***pyrazinamide** Used to treat tuberculosis. Read Drugs Used to Treat Tuberculosis, p. 224. It has uses similar to those described under sodium aminosalicylate. It should be used along with other antituberculous drugs in order to prevent the development of resistant strains of bacteria. *Adverse effects* Loss of appetite, malaise, nausea, vomiting, fever, painful joints, difficult urination, rashes, and sunlight sensitivity of the skin may occur. Liver damage and jaundice may occasionally occur in patients receiving 3 G. or more each day. The blood level of uric acid may increase, leading to attacks of gout. *Precautions* Should not be given to patients with impaired liver function, and frequent liver function tests should be carried out during treatment. It should be given with caution to patients with a history of gout or with impaired kidney function. If given to patients with diabetes it may cause difficulty in controlling the diabetes. *Dose* By mouth, up to 35 mg. per kg. of body weight per day up to a maximum of 3 G. daily, given in divided doses three to four times daily at equally spaced intervals.

\***PYRIBENZAMINE** See tripelennamine.

\***PYRIDIUM** See phenazopyridine.

\***pyridostigmine** (**MESTINON; pyridostigmine bromide**) Primarily used to treat myasthenia gravis. Read Drugs Which Act on the Autonomic Nervous System, p. 145. *Dose* By mouth, 120 to 300 mg. every four hours up to 6 G. per day.

**pyridoxine** (**HEXA-BETALIN; pyridoxine hydrochloride**) Vitamin $B_6$. Read Vitamins, p. 155.

\***pyrilamine (pyrilamine maleate)** An antihistamine drug. Read Antihistamine Drugs, p. 127. *Dose* By mouth, 300 to 600 mg. daily in divided doses, 25 to 50 mg. by intramuscular or intravenous injection.

\***pyrimethamine** (**DARAPRIM**) An antimalarial drug. Read Drugs Used to Treat Malaria, p. 227. *Adverse effects* High doses may cause rashes and affect blood formation. Very large doses may cause vomiting, convulsions, and respiratory failure. *Dose* By mouth as a suppressive, 25 to 50 mg. daily.

\***pyrrobutamine** An antihistamine drug. Read Antihistamine Drugs, p. 127. *Dose* By mouth, 15 to 30 mg. two to three times daily.

\***pyrvinium** (**POVAN; pyrvinium pamoate**) Used to treat pinworm infection. Read Drugs Used to Treat Worm Infections, p. 229. *Adverse effects* Are rare, but include nausea and vomiting. *Dose* By mouth, 5 mg. per kg. up to 350 mg. as a single dose. A second dose should be administered two weeks later. The drug will color the stools red.

\***QUAALUDE** See methaqualone.

\***QUANTRIL** See benzquinamide.

*QUESTRAN See cholestyramine.

*QUIDE See piperacetazine.

*quinacrine (quinacrine hydrochloride) Has effects and uses similar to those described under chloroquine, which has largely replaced quinacrine in the suppression and treatment of malaria. Read Drugs Used to Treat Malaria, p. 227, and Drugs Used to Treat Worm Infections, p. 229. *Adverse effects* May cause pains in the stomach, dizziness, and headache. Large doses may cause nausea, vomiting, and diarrhea. It may also produce yellow pigmentation of the skin and, rarely, skin rashes, transient mental disturbances, and blood disorders. *Precautions* Increases the toxicity of certain drugs, such as pamaquin and primaquine. *Dose* By mouth, malaria, suppressive, 100 mg. daily in divided doses. Treatment, 200 to 500 mg. daily in divided doses. Giardiasis, 300 mg. daily in divided doses for one week. Tapeworm, 1 G. in divided doses (100 mg. every five minutes).

*QUINAGLUTE (quinidine gluconate) Sustained-release form of quinidine. See quinidine.

*quinethazone (HYDROMOX) A diuretic drug. Read Diuretics, p. 103. It produces effects similar to those described under chlorothiazide. *Dose* By mouth, 50 to 200 mg. daily.

*QUINIDEX See quinidine.

*quinidine (QUINIDEX; QUINORA; quinidine sulfate) Prolongs the resting period of the heart and reduces its rate. It is used to treat disorders of heart rhythm. Read Drugs Used to Treat Heart Failure and Heart Rhythm Disorders, p. 86. *Adverse effects* Patients allergic to quinidine may develop noises in the ears, vertigo, visual disturbances, headache, confusion, skin rash, loss of appetite, nausea, vomiting, diarrhea, pain in the chest, abdominal cramps, and fever. Fall in blood pressure, difficulty in breathing, blueness (cyanosis), and collapse may also occur. Quinidine accumulates in the body and may affect the heart rate and sometimes cause death. *Precautions* Should not be given to allergic patients; allergy should be tested for by giving a small dose initially. Quinidine should not be used in severe heart disorders or to treat irregular heart rhythms due to overworking of the thyroid gland. It may increase the effects of some anticoagulants and some muscle-relaxant drugs. *Dose* By mouth, to prevent disorders of rhythm, 200 mg. three or four times daily. To treat atrial fibrillation, 200 to 400 mg. every two to four hours up to a total daily dose of 3 G. If there is no improvement after ten days, the drug should be stopped.

*quinine (quinine bisulfate; quinine acid sulfate; quinine hydrochloride) Previously used to treat malaria, but has largely been replaced by less toxic and more effective drugs. Read Drugs Used to

Treat Malaria, p. 227. *Adverse effects* Deafness, noises in the ears, visual disturbances, giddiness, and trembling may occur. Excessively high doses may cause headache, vomiting, fever, excitement, confusion, permanent blindness and deafness, coma, and abortion in pregnant women. Repeated average doses may cause cinchonism, which is characterized by noises in the ears, headache, nausea, abdominal pain, skin rashes, disturbed vision, and blindness. The use of quinine by patients who have chronic and inadequately treated malaria may cause the development of black water fever (red blood cells are destroyed and the urine turns black).

*QUINORA See quinidine.

*racephedrine See ephedrine.

*RAUDIXIN See reserpine.

*rauwolfia See reserpine.

*rauwolfia alkaloids See reserpine.

*RAUZIDE Each tablet contains rauwolfia 50 mg. and bendroflumethiazide 4 mg. See reserpine, and read Drugs Used to Treat Raised Blood Pressure, p. 108. See bendroflumethiazide, and read Diuretics, p. 103. *Dose* By mouth, 1 to 4 tablets daily.

*REGITINE MESYLATE See phentolamine.

*REGROTON Contains chlorthalidone 50 mg. and reserpine 0.25 mg. per tablet. See reserpine, and read Drugs Used to Treat Raised Blood Pressure, p. 108. See chlorthalidone, and read Diuretics, p. 103. *Dose* By mouth, 1 or 2 tablets daily.

*regular insulin Read Drugs Used to Treat Diabetes, p. 182.

*RELA See carisoprodol.

*RENESE See polythiazide.

*rescinnamine (MODERIL) Has effects and uses similar to those described under reserpine. Read Drugs Used to Treat Raised Blood Pressure, p. 108. *Dose* By mouth, 0.5 mg. two or three times daily, increasing slowly according to need.

*reserpine (obtained from the roots of rauwolfia) Depresses the brain, produces sedation, lowers the blood pressure, and slows the heart rate. It is used to treat patients with high blood pressure. It takes about three to six days to work, then accumulates in the body, and its effects continue for some time after it is stopped. It should not be used as a tranquilizer to treat patients with anxiety or psychoses (see p. 55). Read Drugs Used to Treat Raised Blood Pressure, p. 108. *Adverse effects* Commonly include lethargy, stuffiness of the nose, drowsiness, increased dreaming, stomach upsets, diarrhea, and vertigo. Breathlessness, increase in weight, and skin rashes may occur. High doses may cause flushing, insomnia, redness of the eyes, slowing of the pulse, and occasionally Parkinsonism and severe depression which may lead to suicide. Salt retention with swelling (edema), blurred vision, disturbances of ejaculation, peptic ulcers, and nose-bleeds have been reported. There is controversy over whether it causes a small increase in the incidence of breast cancer. On the whole, adverse effects are mild and pass off on reduction of dosage or if the drug is stopped. *Precautions* Should be used with caution in patients with psychological symptoms, particularly if they are depressed. It should also be used with caution in patients with peptic ulcers, ulcerative colitis, heart disorders, and asthma or bronchitis. It may cause a fall in blood pressure in patients under anesthetic. *Dose* By mouth, for raised blood pressure, 100 to 500 mcg. daily.

**resorcinol**  Stops itching and is used in skin ointments because it causes peeling. Prolonged use on the skin can cause underworking of the thyroid gland because it may be absorbed and interfere with the production of thyroid hormones. Read Drugs Used to Treat Skin Disorders, p. 193.

**\*RETIN-A**  See tretinoin.

**\*retinoic acid**  See tretinoin.

**rhubarb**  Obtained from *Rheum palmatum* grown in China and Tibet. Read Drugs Used to Treat Constipation, p. 82.

**riboflavin**  A member of the vitamin B group. Read Vitamins, p. 155.

**\*RIFADIN**  See rifampin.

**\*rifampin (RIFADIN)**  An antibiotic principally used to treat tuberculosis. Read Drugs Used to Treat Tuberculosis, p. 224. It is related to streptomycin. Read Antibiotics, p. 210. *Adverse effects* May cause nausea, jaundice, blood disorders, and allergy. It may color the urine red-orange. It should not be used in patients with obstructive disease of gall bladder ducts, and it should preferably not be used in the first three months of pregnancy.

**\*RIMACTANE**  See rifampin.

**\*RIOPAN**  See magaldrate.

**\*RITALIN**  See methylphenidate.

**\*ROBAXIN**  See methocarbamol.

**\*ROBINUL**  See glycopyrrolate.

**ROBITUSSIN**  See guaifenesin.

**ROCHELLE SALTS (sodium potassium tartrate)**  Used as a laxative. Read Drugs Used to Treat Constipation, p. 82.

**ROLAIDS**  See dihydroxyaluminum sodium carbonate.

**ROMILAR**  Children's cough syrup contains 7.5 mg. dextromethorphan, 25 mg. glyceryl guaiacolate, sodium citrate, and citric acid per 5 ml. See dextromethorphan, guaifenesin, and sodium citrate Adult syrup contains 15 mg. of dextromethorphan. Read Drugs Used to Treat Coughs, p. 135.

*RONDOMYCIN   See methacycline.

*RONIACOL   See nicotinyl.

*ROPANTH   See propantheline.

rosewater ointment   See cold cream.

saccharin (sodium saccharin)   An artificial noncaloric sweetener.

ST. JOSEPH ASPIRIN for children   See aspirin.

ST. JOSEPH COUGH SYRUP for children   5 ml. contains dextromethorphan hydrobromide 7.5 mg., sodium citrate 100 mg., and menthol. See dextromethorphan, sodium citrate, and menthol, and read Drugs Used to Treat Coughs, p. 135.

*salbutamol (VENTOLIN; salbutamol sulfate)   Has effects and uses similar to those described under isoproterenol. Its main effects, however, are on the bronchi rather than the heart. It is therefore used to treat asthma and bronchospasm. It does not cause the rapid heartbeat produced by isoproterenol and similar drugs. Read Drugs Used to Treat Bronchial Asthma, p. 138, and Drugs Which Act on the Autonomic Nervous System, p. 145. *Adverse effects* These are similar to, but less marked than, those produced by isoproterenol. Muscle trembling may occur after using salbutamol by mouth. *Precautions* It should not be given to patients with high blood pressure, heart disorders, or overworking of the thyroid gland. *Dose* By aerosol spray, 0.2 mg. (in one discharge); 1 to 2 inhalations at intervals of not less than four hours. Salbutamol sulfate is taken by mouth as tablets or elixir, 6 to 16 mg. daily in divided doses.

SAL HEPATICA   Granules contain 51% sodium phosphate, 44% sodium bicarbonate, and 5% anhydrous citric acid. See sodium phosphate, sodium bicarbonate, and citric acid. Read Drugs Used to Treat Constipation, p. 82.

salicylamide   Has effects and uses similar to those described under aspirin, but is less effective.

salicylic acid   Used in skin applications because it kills bacteria and fungi and causes peeling. Read Drugs Used to Treat Skin Disorders, p. 193. It is also used in rheumatic liniments. *Adverse effects* It can cause dermatitis, and prolonged extensive use may cause poisoning. See aspirin.

salol   Used in suntan creams. Read Drugs Used to Treat Skin Disorders, p. 193.

*SALURON   See hydroflumethiazide.

*SALUTENSIN   Each tablet contains hydroflumethiazide 50 mg. and reserpine 0.125 mg. See hydroflumethiazide, and read Diuretics, p. 103. See reserpine, and read Drugs Used to Treat Raised Blood Pressure, p. 108. *Dose* By mouth, 1 to 4 tablets daily.

*SANDOPTAL   See butalbital.

*SANOREX   See mazindol.

\*SANSERT    See methysergide.

\*scilla    See squill.

scoline (suxamethonium chloride; methscopolamine bromide)    See suxamethonium.

scopolamine (hyoscine hydrobromide; hyoscine; scopolamine hydrobromide)    Effects and uses similar to those described under atropine. It depresses the brain and produces drowsiness and is therefore used to treat patients who are excited. It is used along with morphine as a medication before surgical operations, and to produce "twilight sleep" in women in labor. It is also used to prevent motion sickness and in the treatment of Parkinsonism. Read Drugs Which Act on the Autonomic Nervous System; p. 145, Drugs Used to Treat Nausea, Vomiting, and Motion Sickness, p. 71, and Drugs Used to Treat Parkinsonism, p. 149. *Adverse effects and precautions* Similar to those listed under atropine. *Dose* Preoperative medication, 600 mcg. scopolamine with 10 to 15 mg. morphine by subcutaneous or intramuscular injection. Motion sickness, by mouth, 600 mcg. Parkinsonism, by mouth, 300 to 600 mcg. three times daily.

\*secobarbital sodium (SECONAL SODIUM)    A barbiturate sleeping drug. Read Sleeping Drugs and Sedatives, p. 43. *Dose* By mouth, 100 to 200 mg. at night.

\*SECONAL    See secobarbital sodium.

\*SECONAL SODIUM    See secobarbital sodium.

\*selenium (SELSUN; selenium sulfide)    Used as a shampoo. Read Drugs Used to Treat Skin Disorders, p. 193. When taken by mouth it is very dangerous. It should not be used on inflamed or broken skin, and it should not enter the eyes.

\*SELSUN    See selenium.

\*SEMIRITARD MC    An insulin preparation. Read Drugs Used to Treat Diabetes, p. 182.

senna    An irritant laxative. Read Drugs Used to Treat Constipation, p. 82. *Dose* By mouth, 0.5 to 2 G.

SENOKOT    Read Drugs Used to Treat Constipation, p. 82.

\*SEPTRA    Each tablet contains sulfamethoxazole 400 mg. and trimethoprim 80 mg. See each constituent drug, and read Sulfonamides, p. 220. It is used to treat infections. *Dose* By mouth, 2 tablets every 12 hours for 10 to 14 days.

\*SER-AP-ES    Each tablet contains reserpine 0.1 mg., hydralazine hydrochloride 25 mg. and hydrochlorothiazide 15 mg. See reserpine and hydralazine, and read Drugs Used to Treat Raised Blood Pressure, p. 108. See hydrochlorothiazide, and read Diuretics, p. 103. *Dose* By mouth, 1 to 2 tablets three times daily.

\*SERAX    See oxazepam.

*SERENTIL See mesoridazine.

*SEROMYCIN See cycloserine.

*SERPASIL See reserpine.

SILENCE IS GOLDEN Each lozenge and each 5 ml. of syrup contains dextromethorphan 15 mg. per 5 ml. See dextromethorphan, and read Drugs Used to Treat Coughs, p. 135.

silicone Used as a water-repellent in skin applications. Read Drugs Used to Treat Skin Disorders. p. 193.

SILICOTE Is 30% silicone oils. See silicone.

silver nitrate Used in solution as an astringent (see p. 205) and antiseptic (see p. 201). It causes tissue to stain black due to silver deposits. It is used in the eyes of newborn babies to prevent infection.

simethicone (MYLICON) An antifoaming agent promoted for the reduction of gas in the gastrointestinal tract. *Dose* By mouth, usually 150 to 400 mg. daily in divided doses.

SINAREST Each tablet contains phenylephrine hydrochloride 5 mg., chlorpheniramine maleate 1 mg., acetaminophen 300 mg., and caffeine 30 mg. See phenylephrine, chlorpheniramine, acetaminophen, and caffeine. Read Drugs Used to Treat Common Colds, p. 132.

*SINEMET Tablets come in two sizes. The smaller contain 10 mg. carbidopa and 100 mg. levodopa; the larger, 25 mg. carbidopa and 250 mg. levodopa. See carbidopa and levodopa. Read Drugs Used to Treat Parkinsonism, p. 149. *Dose* By mouth, initially according to patient's needs and previous drug treatment. Maintenance dose is 3 to 6 tablets daily.

SINE-OFF Each tablet contains phenylpropanolamine hydrochloride 12.5 mg., chlorpheniramine maleate 1 mg., and aspirin 325 mg. See phenylpropanolamine, chlorpheniramine, and aspirin. Read Drugs Used to Treat Common Colds, p. 132.

*SINEQUAN See doxepin.

*SINTROM See acenocoumarol.

*SK-ERYTHROMYCIN See erythromycin stearate.

slaked lime See calcium hydroxide.

SLENDER Condensed skim milk with added vegetable oil, saccharin, vitamins, and minerals. Read Reducing Drugs, p. 68.

SLENDER X Tablets contain phenylpropanolamine, methylcellulose, caffeine, and vitamins (strengths not available). See each constituent drug, and read Reducing Drugs, p. 68.

SLIM MINT chewing gum Contains benzocaine, methylcellulose, and dextrose. See each constituent drug, and read Reducing Drugs, p. 68.

*sodium aminosalicylate Used in the treatment of tuberculosis. Read Drugs Used to Treat Tuberculosis, p. 224. It is used only in conjunction with streptomycin or isoniazid or both to delay the development of resistance by the tuberculosis bacteria. It is rapidly absorbed and excreted, and therefore frequent doses are necessary to maintain an adequate blood level. *Adverse effects* May cause adverse effects such as fever, nausea, vomiting, diarrhea, and skin rashes. Jaundice, low blood potassium, liver and kidney damage, swollen glands, and blood disorders may also occur. Absorption of certain essential elements in food may be interfered with, and the urine of patients on this drug may give a positive test for sugar. *Precautions* Patients allergic to aminosalicylic acid may also be allergic to other compounds, including sulfonamide drugs and certain hair dyes. It should be used with caution in patients with impaired kidney function. Salicylates may partially inhibit its effects. The adverse effects of salicylates and aminosalicylate are additive. *Dose* By mouth, 10 to 15 G. daily in divided doses.

*sodium amobarbital  See amobarbital sodium.

*sodium aurothiomalate  See gold.

*sodium aurothiosuccinate  See gold.

sodium benzoate  Used as an antibacterial and antifungal drug in mouthwashes and in surgical instrument sterilization fluids and preservatives.

sodium bicarbonate  Used as an antacid. Read Drugs Used to Treat Indigestion and Peptic Ulcers, p. 74. *Dose* By mouth, 300 mg. to 2 G. one to four times daily.

sodium biphosphate  May be used to make the urine more acid, as during treatment with methenamine mandelate.

sodium borate  See borax.

sodium carbonate  Used in some skin lotions as a water softener and to relieve skin irritation.

sodium carboxymethylcellulose  Used in various drug preparations to encourage emulsification, and as a bulk laxative because it swells in water. It is widely used in the food industry. Read Drugs Used to Treat Constipation, p. 82.

sodium citrate  Used to make the urine less acid; as a very mild diuretic; as a constituent in some laxatives and enemas; to prevent milk from forming large curds when feeding infants; to stop blood from clotting in laboratory instruments; and to wash out the bladder after an operation.

*sodium cromoglycate  See cromolyn sodium.

*sodium cromolyn  See cromolyn sodium.

sodium hypochlorite solutions  These release chlorine and are used as disinfectants and antiseptics (see p. 201). They should be protected from the light, and not stored for more than three to four months.

*sodium lactate   Used to make the urine less acid. It is usually given by intravenous injection in a dose of 60 ml. of a sodium lactate solution per kg. of body weight for the treatment of acidosis and of 30 ml. per kg. for making the urine alkaline. It is also used intravenously to treat diabetic coma.

sodium phosphate   A saline laxative. Read Drugs Used to Treat Constipation, p. 82. *Dose* By mouth, 2 to 15 G.

sodium potassium tartrate (ROCHELLE SALTS)   A saline laxative. Read Drugs Used to Treat Constipation, p. 82. *Dose* By mouth, 8 to 16 G.

sodium propionate   An antifungal drug used in skin applications. Read Drugs Used to Treat Skin Disorders, p. 193.

sodium salicylate   A mild pain reliever, and it reduces fever. It is rapidly excreted, and frequent doses are required. It irritates the stomach, and therefore sodium bicarbonate is often given with it. However, this increases its rate of excretion and reduces its effectiveness. It is seldom used now except in acute rheumatic fever. *Adverse effects and precautions* Similar to those described under aspirin. After large doses most patients develop headache, noises in the ears, confusion, blurring of vision, sweating, rashes, and breathlessness. It should be given with caution to patients with severely impaired kidney function, or to patients on a low-sodium diet. *Dose* By mouth, for pain, 0.6 to 2 G. In acute rheumatism, 5 to 10 G. daily in divided doses.

sodium sulfate (GLAUBER'S SALTS)   Used as a saline laxative. Read Drugs Used to Treat Constipation, p. 82. *Dose* By mouth, 5 to 15 G.

sodium tetraborate   See borax.

*SOLGANAL   See gold.

*soluble insulin   Read Drugs Used to Treat Diabetes, p. 182.

*SOMA   See carisoprodol.

*SOMBULEX   See hexobarbital.

SOMINEX   Each tablet contains methapyrilene 25 mg., scopolamine 0.25 mg., and salicylamide 200 mg. See each constituent drug, and read Sleeping Drugs and Sedatives, p. 43, and Antihistamine Drugs, p. 127.

*SOMNAFAC   See methaqualone.

*SOMNOS   See chloral hydrate.

*SOPOR   See methaqualone.

sorbitol   Used as a sweetening agent.

*SORBITRATE   See isosorbide dinitrate.

*SPARINE   See promazine.

*spectinomycin   An antibiotic recommended for use only in the treatment of acute gonorrhea. *Adverse effects* Include skin rash, chills, fever, dizziness, and insomnia. *Dose* By intramuscular injection, 2 to 4 G. as a single dose.

**SPECTRABAN** See Suntan and Sunburn Applications, p. 196.

**spermaceti** A solid wax obtained from mixed oils of the sperm whale. It is a common ingredient of cold creams.

*\*spiramycin** Has antibiotic effects similar to erythromycin but is less potent. Read Antibiotics, p. 210.

*\*spironolactone (ALDACTONE)** Inhibits the effects of aldosterone, a naturally occurring corticosteroid in the body. Since aldosterone produces retention of sodium and loss of potassium from the urine, spironolactone does the reverse and thus increases sodium loss and potassium retention. It is therefore used as a diuretic to treat patients with fluid retention caused by certain heart and other disorders associated with an increased production of aldosterone by the adrenal glands. Read Diuretics, p. 103. *Adverse effects* May cause headache and, when taken in large doses, drowsiness. Skin rashes may also occur; these clear when the drug is stopped. Ataxia, mental confusion, hairiness (hirsutism), irregular menstrual periods, and swelling of the breasts have been reported. *Precautions* Should be given with caution to patients with impaired kidney function. *Dose* By mouth, 50 to 200 mg. daily in divided doses.

*\*SPOROSTACIN** See chlordantoin.

*\*squill (scilla)** Has an effect upon the heart like that of digitalis, but it is poorly absorbed and irritates the stomach, producing nausea and vomiting. In a small dose it is a constituent of some cough mixtures. Read Drugs Used to Treat Coughs, p. 135.

*\*stanozolol (WINSTROL)** An anabolic steroid with effects, uses, and adverse effects similar to those described under methandionone. Prolonged use may cause jaundice. Read Male Sex Hormones, p. 163, and Anabolic Steroids, p. 165. *Dose* By mouth, up to 6 mg. daily.

*\*STAPHCILLIN** See methicillin.

**starch** Polysaccharide granules from corn, rice, wheat, or potatoes, used as a dusting powder either alone or mixed with zinc oxide. It is also used in protective skin applications. Read Drugs Used to Treat Skin Disorders, p. 193.

*\*STELAZINE** See trifluoperazine.

*\*STERAZOLIDIN** Each capsule contains phenylbutazone 50 mg., prednisone 1.25 mg., dried aluminum hydroxide gel 100 mg., and magnesium trisilicate 150 mg. See phenylbutazone, and read Aspirin, Nonnarcotic Pain Relievers, and Drugs Used to Treat Rheumatism and Arthritis, p. 118. See prednisone, and read Corticosteroids, p. 160. See aluminum hydroxide and magnesium trisilicate, and read Drugs Used to Treat Indigestion and Peptic Ulcers, p. 74. *Dose* By mouth,

up to 12 capsules the first day and 6 to 8 capsules on succeeding days. The drug should not be used in children 14 years of age or less or in elderly debilitated patients. When the drug is used longer than one week, no more than 6 capsules per day should be taken.

**sterculia** See karaya.

*****stilbestrol** See diethylstilbestrol.

*****STOXIL** See idoxuridine.

*****streptodornase (KABIKINASE)** An enzyme produced by the bacteria hemolytic streptococci. It dissolves pus and is used in combination with streptokinase, a similar enzyme, to dissolve blood clots and pus. It is also used in inhalations to dissolve sputum.

*****streptokinase** See streptodornase.

*****streptomycin (streptomycin sulfate)** An antibiotic. It is effective against a wide range of bacteria, but is used particularly to treat pneumonia, tuberculosis, intestinal infections, and infections of the gall bladder and urinary tract. Read Antibiotics, p. 210. *Adverse effects* Are unlikely to occur when the drug is taken by mouth because it is not well absorbed. After intramuscular injections the patient may develop pain at the site of injection, peculiar sensory sensations around the mouth, vertigo, headache, and lassitude. Allergic reactions are common, and patients may develop skin rashes, swollen glands, and fever. This usually comes on after two weeks, but in patients who have previously received the drug it may develop immediately. Streptomycin may cause severe dermatitis in persons allergic to it and in pharmacists, nurses, and others who handle the drug frequently. They should wear masks and rubber gloves. More severe adverse effects may result from streptomycin's effects upon the nerves supplying the ear and organs of balance. Doses slightly above the minimum effective dose may cause vertigo, nausea, noises in the ears, and deafness. These may come on suddenly and disappear when the drug is withdrawn, but permanent deafness and damage to the organ of balance may develop slowly, and even after the drug has been stopped. In high doses, kidney damage, blood disorders, and liver damage may develop. *Precautions* Great caution is needed when giving streptomycin to patients with impaired kidney or liver function, to the elderly, and to premature infants. It should not be used in pregnancy because the baby could be born deaf. It should not be used in patients with ear disorders or disorders of their organ of balance or in patients who are allergic to it. (Desensitization is possible, but it is better to use an alternative drug.) To prevent the development of resistance bacteria, streptomycin should be used with other antituberculous drugs in the treatment of tuberculosis. It should not be used for more than five days in treatment of urine

infections. *Dose* By mouth for intestinal infections, 500 mg. of streptomycin every eight hours. By intramuscular injection, 0.5 to 1 G.
daily.

**STRESSTABS 600** A multivitamin preparation. See Vitamins, p. 155.

*__strophanthin-G__ See ouabain.

__strychnine__ A substance that stimulates all parts of the nervous system and was formerly used in tonics, bitters, and laxatives. *Adverse
effects* May cause convulsions, and it should not be used.

*__succinylcholine (ANECTINE; scoline; succinylcholine chloride; sux-
amethonium; suxamethonium chloride)__ A depolarizing voluntary-muscle relaxant used in surgery. Read Drugs Which Act on the
Autonomic Nervous System, p. 145, in which voluntary-muscle
relaxants are discussed. *Adverse effects* May cause slowing of the heart
rate, irregularities of heart rhythm, and heart arrest. Fever and allergic reactions may occur, and patients up and about soon after surgery may develop pains in their chest, abdomen, trunk, shoulders,
and neck. Prolonged absence of breathing (apnea) may occur in some
patients due to a low level of the enzyme cholinesterase, which
breaks down the chemical transmitter called acetylcholine. This low
level may occur in patients with impaired liver function and severe
anemia. The drug should not be used in such patients, and it should
not be used for eye surgery. Patients exposed to weed-killers and
insecticides may also have a low blood level of cholinesterase and
should not be given succinylcholine.

*__succinylsulfathiazole__ Has effects, uses, and adverse effects similar
to those described under phthalylsulfathiazole. It is an antibacterial
drug used to treat infections of the gut. Read Sulfonamides, p. 220.
*Dose* By mouth, 10 to 20 G. daily in divided doses.

**SUCRETS** Lozenges sold over the counter as oral antibacterial preparations. Contains hexylresorcinol 2.4 mg. See hexylresorcinol.

__sucrose__ Refined sugar.

**SUDAPHED** See pseudoephedrine.

*__sulfacetamide__ A sulfonamide drug. It is used chiefly to treat infec-
tions of the eye (conjunctivitis). Read Sulfonamides, p. 220.

*__sulfadiazine__ A sulfonamide. Read Sulfonamides, p. 220.

*__sulfadimethoxine (MADRIBON)__ A long-acting sulfonamide. Read
Sulfonamides, p. 220. *Dose* By mouth, 2 G. daily initially and then
1 G. daily.

*__sulfadoxide__ A sulfonamide drug. Read Sulfonamides, p. 220, and
Drugs Used to Treat Malaria, p. 227.

*__sulfadoxine (FANSIL)__ A long-acting sulfonamide. It may produce
itching, skin rashes, vomiting, and blood disorders. It has been used
to treat leprosy and also malaria (combined with pyrimethamine).

*sulfamethazine A sulfonamide. Read Sulfonamides, p. 220. *Adverse effects and precautions* Usually mild but may be severe. They are similar for the whole group of sulfonamides and are discussed in the section Sulfonamides, p. 220.

*sulfamethizole A sulfonamide drug. Read Sulfonamides, p. 220. *Dose* By mouth, 0.5 to 1 G. four times daily.

*sulfamethoxazole (GANTANOL) A sulfonamide. Read Sulfonamides, p. 220. It is now frequently used combined with trimethoprim, as in Bactrim or Septra. Patients on prolonged treatment with this combination should have repeated blood tests because there is a risk of blood disorders, and it should not be given during pregnancy. *Dose* By mouth, 2 G. initially and then 1 G. every twelve hours.

*sulfamethoxydiazine (SULLA) A long-acting sulfonamide. Read Sulfonamides, p. 220. *Dose* By mouth, 1 to 2 G. initially and then 500 mg. daily.

*sulfamethoxypyridazine (KYNEX, MIDICEL) A sulfonamide. Read Sulfonamides, p. 220. *Dose* By mouth, 1 G. initially and then 500 mg. daily.

*sulfanilamide A sulfonamide drug. Read Sulfonamides, p. 220. *Adverse effects* Stevens-Johnson syndrome has been reported. *Dose* By mouth, 3 G. initially and then 1 to 1.5 G. every four hours.

*sulfaphenazole (ORISUL) A sulfonamide. Read Sulfonamides, p. 220. *Dose* By mouth, 1 G. every twelve hours for two days, and 500 mg. every twelve hours for three days.

*sulfapyridine A sulfonamide now rarely used except in a serious skin disorder called dermatitis herpetiformis. Read Sulfonamides, p. 220.

*sulfasalazine A sulfonamide antibiotic used to treat ulcerative colitis. Read Sulfonamides, p. 220. *Dose* By mouth, 2 to 8 G. per day in four to eight divided doses.

*SULFATHALIDINE See phthalylsulfathiazole.

*sulfathiazole A sulfonamide. Read Sulfonamides, p. 220. *Adverse effects* These are frequent, and include fever and skin rashes. Blood disorders occur occasionally. *Dose* By mouth, 3 G. initially and then 1 G. every four hours.

*sulfinpyrazone (ANTURANE) Reduces the blood uric acid level and is used as a long-term treatment for gout. It increases uric acid excretion by the kidneys. It has little pain-relieving effect, and is no use for treating acute attacks of gout. Read Drugs Used to Treat Gout, p. 124. *Adverse effects* May cause nausea, vomiting, and abdominal pain and may aggravate peptic ulcers. At the beginning of treatment it may actually cause acute attacks of gout. Blood disorders may occasionally occur with prolonged treatment. *Precautions*

It should be given with caution to patients with impaired kidney function, or to those who have had peptic ulcers in the past. It should not be given to patients with active peptic ulcers. It may increase the effects of certain anti-blood-clotting drugs, and of insulin and other antidiabetic drugs; and its effects are diminished by aspirin and other salicylates. *Dose* By mouth, 200 to 500 mg. daily in divided doses.

**sulisobenzone** A sunscreen agent used in suntan and sunburn preparations. Read Drugs Used to Treat Skin Disorders, p. 193.

*****sulfisoxazole** A sulfonamide. Read Sulfonamides, p. 220.

**sulfur** Used in skin applications as a peeling agent and as an antifungal and antiseptic. Read Drugs Used to Treat Skin Disorders, p. 193.

*****SULLA** See sulfamethoxydiazine.

*****SUMYCIN** See tetracycline.

**SUPER ANAHIST** Each tablet contains phenylpropanolamine hydrochloride 12.5 mg., phenyltoloxamine citrate 6.25 mg., thonzylamine hydrochloride 6.25 mg., phenacetin 97.2 mg., aspirin 227 mg., caffeine, and ascorbic acid. See each drug and Drugs Used to Treat Common Colds, p. 132.

*****suramin** Used to treat trypanosomiasis. *Adverse effects* Depend upon the degree of nutrition of the patient. If the patient has malnutrition, adverse effects are worse. They include vomiting, edema, itching, skin rash, nerve damage and visional disturbances, kidney damage, and blood disorders. *Precautions* Should not be used in patients with kidney disorders or adrenal disorders. *Dose* By intravenous injection, 200 mg. initially, then 1 G. at intervals of one to two times weekly for five weeks.

**SURBEX PREPARATIONS** Contain B vitamins. See Vitamins, p. 155.

*****SURFACAINE** See cyclomethycaine.

**SURFADIL** Contains 2% methapyrilene and 0.5% cyclomethycaine. See each constituent drug, and read Antihistamine Drugs, p. 127, and Drugs Used to Treat Skin Disorders, p. 193.

**SURFAK** See dioctyl calcium sulfosuccinate.

*****SURMONTIL** See trimipramine.

*****suxamethonium** See succinylcholine.

*****SYMMETREL** See amantadine.

*****SYNALAR** See fluocinolone.

*****SYNCILLIN** See phenethicillin.

*****SYNKAYVITE (synthetic vitamin K)** Read Vitamins, p. 155.

*****SYNTHROID** See levothyroxine.

*****SYNTOCINON** See oxytocin.

*****TACARYL** See methdilazine.

*****TACE** See chlorotrianisene.

*talbutal (LOTUSATE) An intermediate-acting barbiturate. Read Sleeping Drugs and Sedatives, p. 43. *Dose* By mouth: for sleep, 120 mg. at night; for sedation, 30 to 60 mg. two or three times daily.

talc Purified magnesium silicate. It is used in dusting powders. Read Drugs Used to Treat Skin Disorders, p. 193. Prolonged and intense use may cause pneumonoconiosis.

*TALWIN See pentazocine.

*TANDEARIL See oxyphenbutazone.

tannic acid (tannin) Formerly used as an astringent in throat lozenges, gargles, and skin preparations, and to treat diarrhea and cases of poisoning by mouth. Deaths from liver damage have been reported following its use on burns and when it has been mixed with enemas for X-ray examinations.

tannin See tannic acid.

*TAPAZOLE See methimazole.

tar Used as an anti-itching drug in skin applications. Read Drugs Used to Treat Skin Disorders, p. 193. It is used to treat eczema and psoriasis.

*TARACTAN See chlorprothixene.

*TEDRAL Each tablet contains theophylline 130 mg., ephedrine hydrochloride 24 mg., and phenobarbital 8 mg. See theophylline and ephedrine, and read Drugs Used to Treat Bronchial Asthma, p. 138. See phenobarbital, and read Sleeping Drugs and Sedatives, p. 43. *Dose* One or 2 tablets four times daily. No more than 2 tablets in any four-hour period.

*TEGOPEN See cloxacillin sodium.

*TEGRETOL See carbamazepine.

TELDRIN See chlorpheniramine.

*TELEPAQUE See iopanoic acid.

*TEMARIL See trimeprazine.

TEMPRA See acetaminophen.

*TENSILON See edrophonium.

*TENUATE See diethylpropion.

*TEPANIL See diethylpropion.

*terbutaline (BRETHINE; BRICANYL) A bronchodilator drug. Similar to isoproterenol, but with less side effects on the heart. Read Drugs Used to Treat Bronchial Asthma, p. 138. It should not be used in patients with heart failure, high blood pressure, or overworking of the thyroid glands. *Dose* By subcutaneous injection, 0.25 mg.; repeat 0.25 mg. in half-hour if necessary. Maximum dose in one four-hour period is 0.5 mg. By mouth, 2.5 to 5 mg. (tablets) three times daily.

terpin hydrate Used as an expectorant. It is usually combined in an elixir along with codeine or dextromethorphan as a cough preparation. Read Drugs Used to Treat Coughs, p. 135.

*TERRAMYCIN   See oxytetracycline.

*testosterone   A male sex hormone. Read Male Sex Hormones, p. 163. *Adverse effects* May cause increase in skeletal weight, salt and water retention, edema, increased number of small blood vessels in the skin, raised blood calcium, and increased bone growth. Prolonged use of high doses (300 mg. monthly) in women produces masculinization: hairiness (hirsutism), deep voice, decrease in breast size, enlargement of the clitoris, and increased libido. It also produces acne. *Precautions* Should be used with extreme caution in pregnancy and in patients with cancer of the prostate, disorders of the circulation or kidneys, or any other condition in which increased retention of fluids would cause trouble. Phenobarbital may reduce its effects by increasing its breakdown in the liver. *Dose* By implant under the skin, 100 to 600 mg. Other preparations of testosterone may be taken by mouth or injection.

*tetracaine (PONTOCAINE; amethocaine, dimethylaminobenzoate)   A local anesthetic. Read Local Anesthetics, p. 191. It is more toxic than procaine by injection and cocaine by local application, but it is relatively safer because its local anesthetic action is greater and it can, therefore, be used in smaller concentrations. It does not produce the idiosyncratic reactions that may be caused by cocaine.

*tetrachloroethylene   Used to treat hookworm infection. Read Drugs Used to Treat Worm Infections, p. 229. *Adverse effects* Include nausea, vomiting, cramps in the abdomen, burning pain in the stomach, headache, vertigo, a feeling of drunkenness, and, rarely, unconsciousness. *Precautions* Patient must be kept at rest for four hours after treatment. Very anemic patients may collapse during treatment. Alcohol should not be taken one day before and one day after treatment. *Dose* By mouth, 0.12 ml. per kg. of body weight (maximum of 5 ml.).

*tetracycline (ACHROMYCIN; tetracycline hydrochloride)   An antibiotic. Read Antibiotics, p. 210. *Adverse effects* These, common to all tetracyclines, include nausea, gas, vomiting, and diarrhea. Overgrowth of resistant bacteria and fungi may cause thrush, sore tongue, sore lips, and irritation around the anus and the vagina. In undernourished adults, tetracyclines may delay blood coagulation and cause body wasting and weight loss. Alteration of the bacterial content of the bowel may cause diarrhea and vitamin B deficiency. The most serious adverse effect is enteritis, which is rare but has resulted in death when this drug has been used after abdominal surgery. Serious adverse effects may be produced in patients with impaired kidney function. These include loss of appetite, nausea, vomiting, and weakness. Large doses given intravenously have produced death due to liver damage in pregnant women. Tetracycline is deposited in the bone, teeth, and nails of children, causing discoloration. When given in late pregnancy or to young infants it may interfere with the growth of the child's bones and teeth. In young infants, also, it (and other tetracyclines) may cause increased brain pressure and tense bulging of the membranes between the skull bones. Allergic reactions may occur, producing fever and skin rashes. *Precautions* Should not be given to pregnant women or infants and preferably not to children under 12 years of age because of its effects on bone and teeth. It decomposes to toxic metabolites on storage and may cause nausea and alterations in the chemistry of the blood and urine. *Dose* By mouth, 1 to 2 G. daily in divided doses. Absorption from the gut is not complete, and it should be taken on an empty stomach. Do not take with milk or milk products, antacids, or iron preparations.

**tetrahydrozoline (TYZINE; VISINE; tetrahydrozoline hydrochloride)** Used in nasal drops and sprays. Read Drugs Used to Treat Common Colds, p. 132. *Adverse effects* May produce irritation at the site of use, and overdose may produce unconsciousness and a drop in body temperature, particularly in infants. *Precautions* Should be used with caution in patients with raised blood pressure, overworking of the thyroid glands, and glaucoma. It should not be used in children under two years of age.

**\*TETREX** See tetracycline.

**\*thebaine** In opium. Read Morphine and Narcotic Pain Relievers, p. 115.

**\*thenylpyramine** See methapyriline.

**\*theobromine** Has a weak diuretic effect on the kidneys; read Stimulants: Caffeine, p. 63. It has practically no stimulating effect upon the brain. It dilates coronary and other arteries, and was once widely used to treat angina. It was also used to treat high blood pressure, usually combined with phenobarbital. *Adverse effects* It may produce nausea and loss of appetite in high doses. *Dose* By mouth, 300 to 600 mg.

**\*theophylline** Has a diuretic effect on the kidneys. It relaxes involuntary muscles (e.g., bronchial muscles). It produces slight stimulation of the brain (see Stimulants: Caffeine, p. 63). It is widely used to treat asthma and bronchitis. Read Drugs Used to Treat Bronchial Asthma, p. 138. *Adverse effects* May cause irritation of the stomach, nausea, and vomiting. Toxic effects include rapid heart rates and convulsions. *Dose* By mouth, 100 to 200 mg. three or four times daily. There are substantial variations in dose requirements, particularly in infants, the elderly, and patients with reduced liver function.

*THEPHORIN See phenindamine.

THERAGRAN A multiple-vitamin preparation. See Vitamins, p. 155.

THERAGRAN-M A multiple-vitamin and mineral preparation. See Vitamins, p. 155.

*thiabendazole Used to treat certain roundworm infections. Read Drugs Used to Treat Worm Infections, p. 229. *Adverse effects* Include nausea, loss of appetite, vomiting, diarrhea, itching, drowsiness, headache, giddiness, and, rarely, noises in the ears (tinnitus), disturbed vision, numbness, raised blood sugar, and decrease in pulse rate and blood pressure. Fever, chills and conjunctivitis, swelling of the throat (angioneurotic edema), skin rashes, and swollen glands may occur. *Precautions* About half the patients treated experience incapacitating symptoms for several hours. It should be used with caution in patients with impaired liver function and because of its effects on the brain and mental function, patients should rest for half a day at least. *Dose* By mouth, usually 25 mg. per kg. of body weight daily for two days, but varies according to disorder being treated.

thiamine (thiamine hydrochloride) Vitamin $B_1$. Read Vitamins, p. 155.

*thiethylperazine (TORECAN; thiethylperazine maleate) Has effects similar to chlorpromazine and is used to treat nausea and vomiting. Read Drugs Used to Treat Nausea, Vomiting, and Motion Sickness, p. 71, and Major Tranquilizers, p. 53. *Adverse effects and precautions* May produce Parkinsonism and should not be used in children or in women under thirty years of age, who appear to be more prone to adverse effects than men or those over thirty years of age. *Dose* By mouth, 10 to 30 mg. daily.

thimerosal (MERTHIOLATE) A weak mercury-containing antiseptic. See Antiseptics, p. 201.

*thioguanine An anticancer drug. Read Drugs Used to Treat Cancer, p. 225. Also used as an immunosuppressant. *Adverse effects and precautions* Similar to those described under mercaptopurine. *Dose* By mouth, initially 2 mg. per kg. of body weight daily; maintenance dose according to patient's needs.

*thiopental (pentothal) A fast-acting barbiturate. See Sleeping Drugs and Sedatives, p. 43. Used by intravenous injection as a general anesthetic.

thiopental sodium See thiopental.

*thioridazine (MELLARIL; thioridazine hydrochloride) A major tranquilizer. Read Major Tranquilizers, p. 53. It has effects and uses similar to those described under chlorpromazine, but it has little effect in stopping nausea and vomiting or in reducing body temperature. It produces fewer Parkinsonism symptoms than chlorpromazine. *Adverse effects* May cause drowsiness, dizziness, dryness of the mouth, skin rashes, production of milk (galactorrhea), fall in blood pressure, disorders of heart rhythm, fluid retention, weight gain, blood disorders, irritation of the stomach, and nasal stuffiness. Large doses may damage vision by causing pigmentation of the retina (this may be produced within four to eight weeks of treatment with a dose of 1 G. or more daily). It may cause changes in the electric tracings of the heart, and it may produce sunlight sensitivity of the skin. *Precautions* See chlorpromazine. *Dose* By mouth, 50 to 800 mg. daily.

*thiotepa (THIO-TEPA) An anticancer drug. Read Drugs Used to Treat Cancer, p. 225. *Adverse effects* Include nausea, vomiting, headache, fever, allergic reactions, loss of hair, loss of menstrual periods, and reduced sperm production. It is very damaging to the bone marrow, producing severe blood disorders. *Precautions* Should not be used in pregnancy, in the presence of infection, or in patients with severe blood disorders. It should be used with utmost caution if impaired bone-marrow function is suspected. *Dose* Varies according to the disorder and patient being treated.

*thiothixene (NAVANE) Produces effects similar to chlorprothixene. Read Major Tranquilizers, p. 53. *Dose* By mouth, 6 to 60 mg. daily in three divided doses.

thonzylamine An antihistamine drug. Read Antihistamine Drugs, p. 127. It is used in skin applications. Read Drugs Used to Treat Skin Disorders, p. 193.

*THORAZINE See chlorpromazine.

thymol An antiseptic (see p. 201) used in mouthwashes, gargles, and skin applications. It is irritant.

*thyroid Read Drugs Used to Treat Thyroid Disorders, p. 187.

thyroid extracts Read Drugs Used to Treat Thyroid Disorders, p. 187.

*THYROLAR See liotrix.

*thyroxine (thyroxine sodium; levothyroxine sodium) A thyroid hormone used to treat underworking of the thyroid gland. Read Drugs Used to Treat Thyroid Disorders, p. 187. *Adverse effects* Too large a dose may produce sweating, rapid heartbeat, diarrhea, restlessness, excitability, irregularities of heart rhythm, and angina. It may also produce pain in the arms or legs and worsen the symptoms of osteoarthritis. *Precautions* Thyroxine has a delayed and cumulative effect and may take up to two weeks to be effective; the dose must therefore be controlled carefully. It should be used with caution in patients with heart disorders. It may increase the effects of drugs used to prevent blood-clotting, and its effects may be increased by phenytoin and aspirin. *Dose* By mouth, 0.05 to 0.3 mg. daily.

*thyroxine sodium See thyroxine.

*TIGAN See trimethobenzamide.

TINACTIN See tolnaftate.

titanium dioxide Used as a skin protective and also in suntan and antisunburn creams and in some face powders and cosmetics. Read Drugs Used to Treat Skin Disorders, p. 193.

TITRALAC Each tablet contains calcium carbonate 420 mg. and glycine 180 mg. It is used as an antacid. See calcium carbonate, and read Drugs Used to Treat Indigestion and Peptic Ulcers, p. 74.

*tobramycin An antibiotic. Read Antibiotics, p. 210. It has effects similar to those of gentamicin.

tocopherol Vitamin E. Read Vitamins, p. 155.

*TOFRANIL See imipramine.

*tolazamide (TOLINASE) An oral antidiabetic drug. Read Drugs Used to Treat Diabetes, p. 182. *Adverse effects* May cause nausea, vomiting, diarrhea, loss of appetite, dizziness, weakness, nervousness, and skin rashes. *Dose* By mouth, initially 100 to 250 mg.; dose is then adjusted every four to six days until response is satisfactory or toxicity requires discontinuation. Doses larger than 1 G. per day usually will not increase the response. If the daily dose exceeds 500 mg. it should be given in two divided doses.

*tolazoline (PRISCOLINE) Used to treat disorders of the circulation. It dilates small arteries and capillaries and increases the circulation and skin temperature. It also increases stomach secretions. Read Drugs Used to Treat Disorders of Circulation, p. 94. *Adverse effects* May produce nausea, vomiting, diarrhea, and a fall in blood pressure when the patient stands up. It may also cause flushing, rapid heartbeat, tingling, shivering, and pain in the stomach. *Precautions* Should not be given to patients with coronary artery disease, other severe heart disorders, or peptic ulcers. *Dose* By mouth, 25 to 50 mg. four times daily.

*tolbutamide (ORINASE) A drug used to treat diabetes. It is taken by mouth and has effects and uses similar to those described under chlorpropamide, but it works for a shorter time. Read Drugs Used to Treat Diabetes, p. 182. *Adverse effects* Similar to those described under chlorpropamide. Skin rashes and intolerance to alcohol may occur and, rarely, blood disorders and jaundice. *Precautions* See chlorpropamide. Sulfonamides and phenylbutazone may increase its blood-sugar-lowering effects. *Dose* By mouth, 500 to 2000 mg. daily in divided doses.

\*TOLINASE  See tolazamide.

\*tolnaftate (TINACTIN)  An antifungal drug. It is used in creams or powders to treat ringworm and other fungal infections of the skin. Read Drugs Used to Treat Skin Disorders, p. 193, and Drugs Used to Treat Worm Infections, p. 229. It is not active against thrush or bacteria. In treatment of fungus infections of the nails or scalp it should be used along with general treatments such as griseofulvin.

tolu balsam (tolu)  Has very mild antiseptic properties and is used in cough mixtures and also as a flavoring agent. Read Drugs Used to Treat Coughs, p. 135.

\*TORECAN  See thiethylperazine.

\*TOTACILLIN  See ampicillin.

\*TRANCOPAL  See chlormezanone.

\*TRANXENE  See clorazepate.

\*tranylcypromine (PARNATE; tranylcypromine sulfate)  A monoamine oxidase inhibitor antidepressant drug. Unlike other drugs of this group, its effects persist for only about two to three days after withdrawal. Read Antidepressants, p. 56. *Adverse effects* Similar to those discussed under phenelzine. The most frequent recurring adverse effects are insomnia, dizziness, muscle weakness, dryness of the mouth, and a fall in blood pressure. In some patients the blood pressure may increase and be associated with severe headaches. *Precautions* These are important and are discussed under phenelzine. *Dose* By mouth, 20 to 60 mg. daily in divided doses, reducing to a maintenance dose of about 20 mg. daily.

\*TRASENTINE  See adiphenine.

\*TRECATOR  See ethionamide.

\*TREMIN  See trihexyphenidyl.

\*TREMONIL  See methixine.

\*TRENIMON  See triaziquone.

\*TREST  See methixine.

\*tretinoin (retinoic acid)  An irritant that causes skin-peeling. It is used in the treatment of acne. See Drugs Used to Treat Skin Disorders, p. 193.

\*triamcinolone (ARISTOCORT; KENACORT)  Has the effects, uses, and adverse effects of cortisone. It is a corticosteroid which is less likely to cause an increase of appetite than other members of the group, and it does not cause salt and water retention. It may cause dizziness, loss of appetite, muscle weakness, sleepiness, and flushing after meals. *Dose* By mouth, 4 to 48 mg. daily in divided doses. Triamcinolone acetonide (Kenalog) is also used in creams, ointments, and lotions (see Drugs Used to Treat Skin Disorders, p. 193). Read Corticosteroids, p. 160.

**TRIAMINIC** Contains pyrilamine maleate 25 mg., pheniramine maleate 25 mg., and phenylpropanolamine 50 mg. in each timed-release tablet. See pyrilamine, pheniramine, and phenylpropanolamine, and read Antihistamine Drugs, p. 127, and Drugs Used to Treat Common Colds, p. 132.

*\*triamterene* (DYRENIUM) A diuretic drug. It is weaker than the thiazide diuretics, but it causes potassium retention rather than loss. It does not trigger underlying diabetes. Read Diuretics, p. 103. *Adverse effects* May cause nausea, vomiting, and dizziness. *Precautions* Should be used with caution in patients with impaired kidney or liver function or with diabetes. *Dose* By mouth, 50 to 300 mg. daily in divided doses.

*\*TRIAVIL* Tablets contain amitriptyline hydrochloride and perphenazine in various strengths. See amitriptyline, and read Antidepressants, p. 56. See perphenazine, and read Major Tranquilizers, p. 53.

*\*triaziquone* (TRENIMON) An anticancer drug. Read Drugs Used to Treat Cancer, p. 225. *Adverse effects* Include nausea, vomiting, cystitis (with bleeding), skin rash, fever, and loss of hair. It is irritant and can produce pain and irritation at the site of injection. It depresses bone-marrow function, producing blood disorders. *Precautions* It should not be used in pregnancy. It should be given with caution to patients with impaired bone-marrow function. *Dose* Varies according to treatment program being followed.

**trichloracetic acid** A caustic and keratolytic to treat warts. Read Drugs Used to Treat Skin Disorders, p. 193. It is also used in dilute solution (1%) as an astringent to treat perspiration of the feet.

*\*trichlorethanol* A breakdown product of chloral hydrate. See chloral hydrate.

*\*trichlormethiazide* (NAQUA) A diuretic with uses and effects similar to those described under chlorothiazide. See chlorothiazide, and read Diuretics, p. 103. *Dose* By mouth, 2 to 4 mg. once daily.

*\*triclofos* (TRICLOS; triclofos sodium) Used as a sedative and sleeping drug. It has effects similar to those described under chloral hydrate. Read Sleeping Drugs and Sedatives, p. 43. *Adverse effects, precautions, and drug dependence* Similar to those described under chloral hydrate. Headache and skin rashes may occur, and triclofos may increase the effects of alcohol. *Dose* By mouth, sleeping dose, 1 to 2 G. Sedative dose, 0.5 G. twice daily.

*\*TRICLOS* See triclofos.

*\*tridihexethyl* (PATHILON; tridihexethyl chloride) Produces atropinelike effects and is used to treat patients with peptic ulcers or gut disorders. See atropine, and read Drugs Which Act on the Autonomic Nervous System, p. 145, Drugs Used to Treat Indigestion and

Peptic Ulcers, p. 74, and Drugs Used to Treat Diarrhea, p. 80. *Adverse effects* Include dry mouth, blurred vision, loss of taste, headache, nervousness, drowsiness, impotence, suppression of lactation, nausea, vomiting, constipation, urinary retention, and rashes. *Dose* By mouth, 10 to 100 mg. four times daily.

*TRIDIONE  See trimethadione.

*trifluoperazine (STELAZINE; trifluoperazine hydrochloride)  A major tranquilizer. It has effects and uses similar to those described under chlorpromazine, but it is effective in smaller doses. It may stimulate rather than sedate. Read Major Tranquilizers, p. 53, and Drugs Used to Treat Nausea, Vomiting, and Motion Sickness, p. 71. *Adverse effects* Similar to those discussed under chlorpromazine. Mild adverse effects include drowsiness, dizziness, agitation, insomnia, stuffy nose, and sweating. High doses may produce Parkinsonism symptoms and peculiar stiffness and trembling of muscles (dystonias and akathisia), particularly of the face, eyes, neck, tongue, and throat (especially in children). These symptoms are not always reversible on stopping the drug. Rarely, it causes blood disorders, jaundice, and discharge of milk from the breasts (galactorrhea). *Precautions* See chlorpromazine. *Dose* By mouth, 2 to 30 mg. daily in divided doses; to prevent nausea or vomiting, 1 to 6 mg. daily in divided doses.

*trihexyphenidyl (ARTANE; TREMIN; trihexyphenidyl hydrochloride) Diminishes salivation, increases heart rate, dilates the pupils, and reduces spasm of involuntary muscles. It is used mainly to relieve muscle rigidity and increase mobility in patients suffering from Parkinsonism. Read Drugs Used to Treat Parkinsonism, p. 149. *Adverse effects* Include dizziness, dryness of the mouth, nausea, vomiting, and blurred vision. These symptoms are dose-related, and disappear when the dose is reduced. *Precautions* Should not be used in patients suffering from closed-angle glaucoma. *Dose* By mouth, 1 to 2 mg. three times daily.

*triiodothyronine  See liothyronine.

*TRILAFON  See perphenazine.

*trimeprazine (TEMARIL; trimeprazine tartrate)  Produces antihistamine effects and also major tranquilizer effects like those described under chlorpromazine. However, its main effect and use is to prevent itching. It is slow to work, and its effects last a long time. Read Antihistamine Drugs, p. 127, and Major Tranquilizers, p. 53. *Adverse effects* Frequently produces drowsiness and occasionally dizziness, dryness of the mouth, skin rashes, blood disorders, and Parkinsonism. *Precautions* Similar to those described under chlorpromazine. It should be given with caution to patients with impaired liver function. *Dose* By mouth, to prevent itching, 10 to 40 mg. daily.

\*trimethadione (TRIDIONE) Used in the treatment of petit mal epilepsy. Read Drugs Used to Treat Epilepsy, p. 142. *Adverse effects* Most frequent is a blurring of vision in bright light (hemeralopia), which may necessitate the wearing of dark glasses. Sedation, nausea, headache, fatigue, muscle weakness, and skin rashes may occur. Rarely, allergic reactions may produce disorders of the bone marrow, skin, kidneys, and liver, which may be fatal. *Precautions* Should not be used in patients with serious kidney, liver, or eye disorders or in patients with blood disorders or drug allergy. Regular blood and urine checks should be carried out. *Dose* By mouth, 900 to 2100 mg. daily in divided doses.

\*trimethaphan (ARFONAD; trimethaphan camsylate) Used to lower blood pressure in surgery and emergencies. See manufacturer's warnings and dose recommendations. Read Drugs Used to Treat Raised Blood Pressure, p. 108.

\*trimethobenzamide (TIGAN; trimethobenzamide hydrochloride) An antinausea drug. Read Drugs Used to Treat Nausea, Vomiting, and Motion Sickness, p. 71. *Dose* By mouth, 100 to 250 mg. four times daily.

\*trimethoprim An antibacterial drug. It is active against the same range of bacteria as the sulfonamides, with which it produces a synergistic effect. It is usually given combined with sulfamethoxazole (a sulfonamide), a combination marketed as Bactrim or Septra. Read Sulfonamides, p. 220. *Adverse effects* Nausea, vomiting, and diarrhea may occasionally occur. When used over a prolonged period it may produce anemia, because it interferes with the body's use of folic acid, which is essential for the manufacture of blood. *Precautions* Should be given with caution to patients with impaired kidney function. It should not be given during pregnancy. When it is used over a prolonged period, blood tests should be carried out at appropriate intervals of time. *Dose* By mouth, 80 mg. trimethoprim in combination with 400 mg. sulfamethoxazole in each tablet, 2 or 3 tablets initially and then two tablets every 12 hours for 10 to 14 days.

\*trimethoprim-sulfamethoxazole (BACTRIM, SEPTRA) See trimethoprim and sulfamethoxazole.

\*trimipramine (SURMONTIL; trimipramine maleate) A tricyclic antidepressant drug. It has effects and uses similar to those described under imipramine, but it is more sedating. Read Antidepressants, p. 56. *Adverse effects and precautions* Similar to those described under imipramine. Drowsiness is common and so is rapid heartbeat, dryness of the mouth, and blurred vision. Trembling and stiffness of muscles (Parkinsonism) may occur, though rarely. *Dose* By mouth, 25 to 125 mg. daily in divided doses.

*trinitrin   See nitroglycerin.

*TRINSICON   Contains concentrated extract of liver and stomach 240 mg., vitamin $B_{12}$ 7.5 mcg., iron 110 mg., ascorbic acid 75 mg., and folic acid 500 mcg. Read Iron, p. 152, and Vitamins, p. 155.

*tripelennamine (PYRIBENZAMINE; tripelennamine hydrochloride) An antihistamine drug. Read Antihistamine Drugs, p. 127. *Dose* By mouth, 25 to 600 mg. daily in divided doses.

*triprolidine (ACTIDIL; triprolidine hydrochloride)   An antihistamine drug. Read Antihistamine Drugs, p. 127. *Adverse effects and precautions* Similar to those described under promethazine. *Dose* By mouth, 5 to 7.5 mg. daily.

*TROBICIN   See spectinomycin.

*TRONOTHANE   See pramoxine.

*tropicamide (MYDRIACYL)   Has effects and uses similar to those described under atropine. Read Drugs Which Act on the Autonomic Nervous System, p. 145.

*tubocurarine (tubocurarine chloride)   A muscle relaxant used along with general anesthetics in surgical operations. Read Drugs Which Act on the Autonomic Nervous System, p. 145. Its effects are increased by ether. It increases the fall in blood pressure produced by halothane, and its effects in depressing respiration may be increased by quinidine and some antibiotics. Patients with impaired liver function may be resistant to tubocurarine.

*TUINAL   Capsules contain equal quantities of secobarbital and amobarbital in 100 mg. and 200 mg. strengths. See secobarbital sodium and amobarbital sodium, and read Sleeping Drugs and Sedatives, p. 43. *Dose* By mouth, 100 or 200 mg. at bedtime.

TUMS   Each tablet contains 489 mg. calcium carbonate, 6 mg. magnesium silicate, 11 mg. magnesium carbonate, and peppermint oil. See calcium carbonate, magnesium silicate, and magnesium carbonate. Read Drugs Used to Treat Indigestion and Peptic Ulcers, p. 74.

*TUSS-ORNADE   Each spansule contains caramiphen edisylate 20 mg., chlorpheniramine 8 mg., phenylpropanolamine hydrochloride 50 mg., and isopropamide iodide 2.5 mg. Tuss-Ornade liquid contains caramiphen edisylate 5 mg., chlorpheniramine maleate 15 mg., phenylpropanolamine hydrochloride 15 mg., and isopropamide 0.75 mg. See caramiphen, chlorpheniramine, phenylpropanolamine, and isopropamide. Read Drugs Used to Treat Common Colds, p. 132, and Antihistamine Drugs, p. 127. *Dose* By mouth, 1 capsule every twelve hours, or 1 to 2 teaspoonfuls (5 to 10 ml.) three to four times daily.

*tybamate (TYBATRAN)   An antianxiety drug related to meprobamate. Read Minor Tranquilizers, p. 51. *Dose* By mouth, 750 mg. to 2 G. daily in divided doses.

*TYBATRAN   See tybamate.

**TYLENOL** See acetaminophen.

\*TYLENOL **with codeine** Tablets contain acetominophen 300 mg. and codeine phosphate 7.5 mg., 15 mg., 30 mg., or 60 mg. See acetominophen and codeine, and read Aspirin, Nonnarcotic Pain Relievers, and Drugs Used to Treat Rheumatism and Arthritis, p. 118. Also read about codeine in Morphine and Narcotic Pain Relievers, p. 115. *Dose* By mouth, Tylenol with codeine 60 mg., 1 tablet every four hours as needed. Other strengths, 1 or 2 tablets every four hours as needed.

\*TYZINE See tetrahydrozoline.

\*ULTANDREN See fluoxymesterone.

**undecenoic acid (undecylenic acid)** An antifungal drug used in skin applications. Read Drugs Used to Treat Skin Disorders, p. 193.

**undecylenic acid** See undecenoic acid.

\*UNIPEN See nafcillin.

\*unmodified insulin Read Drugs Used to Treat Diabetes, p. 182.

UNNA'S BOOT See zinc gelatin.

\*URACIL MUSTARD See uramustine.

\*uramustine (URACIL MUSTARD) An anticancer drug. Read Drugs Used to Treat Cancer, p. 225. *Adverse effects* It may produce nausea, vomiting, diarrhea, changes in mood, skin rashes, and loss of hair. It damages bone marrow, producing blood disorders. *Precautions* It should not be used in pregnancy, in patients with an infection, or in patients with severe blood disorders. It should be given with utmost caution to patients with impaired bone-marrow function. *Dose* Varies according to treatment program being followed.

\*URECHOLINE See bethanechol.

\*URITONE See methenamine mandelate.

\*VALISONE See betamethasone.

\*VALIUM See diazepam.

\*VALLESTRIL See methallenestril.

\*VALMID See ethinamate.

\*VANCERIL See beclamethasone.

\*VANCOCYN See vancomycin.

\*vancomycin (VANCOCIN; vancomycin hydrochloride) An antibiotic. It is given by intravenous injection to treat severe (staphylococci) infections caused by bacteria resistant to other antibiotics. Read Antibiotics, p. 210. *Adverse effects* Thrombophlebitis is the commonest complication caused by vancomycin; this risk may be reduced by giving the drug slowly and well diluted. Leakage into the surrounding tissues at the site of injection causes pain and tissue damage. The drug may cause nausea, fever, and skin rashes, and large doses or prolonged treatment may cause irreversible deafness, particularly in patients with impaired kidney function. *Precautions* Should not be given to patients with impaired kidney function. It should be given slowly, well diluted, and blood levels should not be allowed to go above 0.025 mg. per ml. *Dose* By slow, diluted intravenous injection, 1 to 3 G. daily.

*VANOBID See candicidin.

*VANQUIN See pyrvinium.

*VARIDASE See streptodornase.

VASELINE Contains white soft and yellow soft petroleum jelly.

*VASODILAN See isoxsuprine.

*vasopressin (PITRESSIN) Used to treat and diagnose a disorder known as diabetes insipidus, in which the patient cannot concentrate his urine and drinks and urinates excessively. It acts directly upon the kidney, producing an antidiuretic effect.

*V-CILLIN See phenoxymethylpenicillin.

*VEETIDS See phenoxymethylpenicillin.

*VELBAN See vinblastine.

*VELOSEF See cephradine.

*VENTOLIN See salbutamol.

*VERACILLIN See dicloxacillin.

*VIBRAMYCIN See doxycycline.

VICKS COUGH SYRUP 5 ml. contain 3.5 mg. dextromethorphan hydrobromide, cetylpyridinium chloride, 200 mg. sodium citrate, ammonium chloride, chloroform 0.25%, and alcohol 5%. See dextromethorphan, cetylpyridinium, sodium citrate, ammonium chloride, and read Drugs Used to Treat Coughs, p. 135.

VICKS FORMULA 44 COUGH MIXTURE 5 ml. contain 5 mg. dextromethorphan hydrobromide, 3 mg. doxylamine succinate, 250 mg. sodium citrate, 10% alcohol, and 0.5% chloroform. See dextromethorphan, doxylamine, and sodium citrate. Read Drugs Used to Treat Coughs, p. 135.

*vinblastine (VELBAN; vinblastine sulfate) Used as an anticancer drug. Read Drugs Used to Treat Cancer, p. 225. *Adverse effects* Include nausea, vomiting, diarrhea, mood changes, loss of hair, nerve damage, and convulsions. It damages bone marrow, producing blood disorders, and can affect the nerves supplying the bladder (producing retention of urine) and the gut (producing paralysis). Injections may be painful and can produce irritation and phlebitis at the site. *Precautions* Should not be used in pregnancy or in patients with an infection. It should be given with utmost caution to patients with impaired bone-marrow function. *Dose* Up to 10 mg. weekly by intravenous injection.

*vincristine (ONCOVIN; vincristine sulfate) Used as an anti-cancer drug. Read Drugs Used to Treat Cancer, p. 225. *Adverse effects* Include nausea, vomiting, constipation, mood changes, loss of hair, nerve damage, and convulsions. It damages bone marrow, leading to blood disorders, and can affect the nerves supplying the bladder (producing retention of urine) and the gut (producing paralysis). Injections may be painful and can produce irritation and phlebitis at the site. *Precautions* It should not be used in pregnancy or in patients with an infection. It should be given with utmost caution to patients with impaired bone-marrow function. It may cause severe constipation, and therefore enemas or laxatives may be needed. *Dose* Varies according to disorder being treated.

*VIOCIN See viomycin.

*VIOFORM See iodochlorhydroxyquin.

*VIOFORM WITH HYDROCORTISONE Topical applications contain iodochlorhydroxyquin and hydrocortisone. See iodochlorhydroxyquin and hydrocortisone, and read Drugs Used to Treat Skin Disorders, p. 193.

*viomycin (VIOCIN; viomycin sulfate) An antibiotic which is active against tuberculosis. Read Antibiotics, p. 210, and Drugs Used to Treat Tuberculosis, p. 224. It is used to treat tuberculosis when a safer or more effective antibiotic cannot be used because the bacteria are resistant or the patient is allergic. Viomycin treatment should be combined with other antitubercular drugs to avoid bacterial resistance. *Adverse effects* May cause skin rashes, kidney damage, disturbance of salt and water balance, abnormalities on electrical heart tracings, dizziness, and deafness. *Precautions* Should not be given along with streptomycin or kanamycin because of the risk of deafness from these drugs. Tests of urine, liver function, and blood salt levels should be carried out at frequent intervals. *Dose* By intramuscular injection, two injections of 1 G. each, twelve hours apart, not more often than twice weekly.

*VISINE See tetrahydrozoline.

*VISTARIL See hydroxyzine.

*VIVACTIL See protriptyline.

*warfarin (PANWARFIN, COUMADIN sodium; warfarin sodium) An anticoagulant drug. It is used to stop the blood from clotting and has effects and uses similar to those described under phenindione. Read Drugs Used to Prevent Blood from Clotting, p. 90. *Adverse effects* Loss of hair (alopecia) and nettle rash (urticaria) may occur. Early signs of overdosage are bleeding from the gums or elsewhere and red blood cells in the urine. *Precautions* Should be given with caution to patients with impaired liver or kidney function. It should not be used in the last few months of pregnancy. It should not be used by mothers who are breast feeding or within three days of a surgical operation or childbirth. Its effects may be increased by aspirin, other salicylates, clofibrate, dextrothyroxine, disulfiram, oxyphenbutazone, phenylbutazone, and possibly anabolic steroids, antibiotics, and quinidine. Its effects are reduced by barbiturates, glutethimide, griseofulvin, and possibly by corticosteroids. Consult your physician or pharmacist before starting or stopping any other drugs at the same time. *Dose* By mouth, 30 to 50 mg. daily initially (optional regimen), reducing to a maintenance dose of 2 to 15 mg. daily.

*warfarin sodium   See warfarin.

WHITFIELD'S OINTMENT   A benzoic acid and salicylic acid compound mixture. See benzoic acid.

*WILPO   See phentermine.

*WINSTROL   See stanozolol.

witch hazel (hamamelis water)   Used on sprains and bruises as a cooling agent.

*WYAMINE   See mephentermine.

*XYLOCAINE   See lidocaine.

xylometazoline (OTRIVIN)   Used as a nasal decongestant. Read Drugs Used to Treat Common Colds, p. 132. It may rarely cause stinging, dry nose, headache, palpitations, drowsiness, and insomnia.

yeast   A source of vitamin B. Read Tonics, p. 65, and Vitamins, p. 155. Large doses may cause diarrhea.

*YODOXIN   See diiodohydroxyquin.

*ZACTANE   See ethoheptazine.

*ZACTIRIN   Each tablet contains ethoheptazine citrate 75 mg. and aspirin 325 mg. Used as a mild pain reliever. See ethoheptazine and aspirin, and read Aspirin, Nonnarcotic Pain Relievers, and Drugs Used to Treat Rheumatism and Arthritis, p. 118. *Dose* By mouth, 1 or 2 tablets three to four times daily.

*ZARONTIN   See ethosuximide.

ZAROXOLYN   See metolazone.

ZEPHIRAN   See benzalkonium.

zinc acetate   An astringent used in eye drops.

zinc chloride   A caustic and astringent. Read Drugs Used to Treat Skin Disorders, p. 193. It is also used as a deodorant and a mouthwash.

zinc gelatin (DOME-PASTE bandage; UNNA'S BOOT)   A preparation containing zinc oxide, glycerin, and gelatin. It is used in the treatment of leg ulcers.

zinc oxide   Used in bandages and in soothing and protective skin applications. Read Drugs Used to Treat Skin Disorders, p. 193.

zinc phenolsulfonate   An astringent. Read Drugs Used to Treat Skin Disorders, p. 193.

**zinc sulfate** An astringent used in skin applications. Read Drugs Used to Treat Skin Disorders, p. 193. It is also found in mouthwashes and eye lotions.

**zinc undecylenate** An antifungal drug. Read Drugs Used to Treat Skin Disorders, p. 193.

*ZORANE Contains various amounts of norethindrone and ethinyl estradiol. See the constituent drugs, and read Oral Contraceptive Drugs, p. 173.

*ZYLOPRIM See allopurinol.

# SELECTED BIBLIOGRAPHY

*American Drug Index.* C. O. Wilson and T. E. Jones. J. B. Lippincott Co., Philadelphia, 1975.

*American Hospital Formulary Service.* American Society of Hospital Pharmacists. Washington, D.C., 1975.

*American Medical Association Drug Evaluations,* 2nd ed. AMA Department of Drugs, Publishing Sciences Group, Inc. Acton, Mass., 1973.

*Clinical Pharmacology.* K. L. Melmon and H. F. Morrelli (eds.). Macmillan Publishing Co., Inc. New York, 1972.

*Drugs of Choice.* Walter Modell (ed.). C. U. Mosby Company. St. Louis, Missouri, 1974.

*Handbook of Non-Prescription Drugs.* G. B. Griffenhagen and L. L. Hawkins, (eds.). American Pharmaceutical Association. Washington, D.C., 1973.

*Hazards of Medication.* E. W. Martin. J. B. Lippincott Co. Philadelphia, 1971.

*Iatrogenic Diseases.* P. F. D'Arcy and J. P. Griffin. Oxford University Press. New York, 1972.

*Martindale: The Extra Pharmacopoeia,* 26th ed. N. W. Blacow (ed.). The Pharmaceutical Press. London, 1972.

*The Medical Letter.* The Medical Letter, Inc., New Rochelle, N.Y.

*The Merck Index,* 8th ed. Paul G. Stecher (ed.). Merck and Co., Inc. 1968.

*The Pharmacologic Basis of Therapeutics,* 5th ed. L. S. Goodman and A. Gilman (eds.). Macmillan Publishing Co., Inc. New York, 1975.

*Pharmindex.* Skyline Publishers, Inc. Portland, Oregan.

*Physicians' Desk Reference,* 29th ed. Medical Economics Co. Oradell, N.J., 1975.

Side Effects of Drugs, 7th ed. L. Meyler and A. Herxheimer (eds.). Excerpta Medica, Amsterdam, 1972.

# INDEX

diphenadione, 92, 282
diphenhydramine, 72, 150, 196, 204, 282
diphenoxylate, 81, 82, 283
diphenylhydantoin, *see* phenytoin
dipyridamole, 102, 283
disinfectants and antiseptics, 201–2, 209
disulfiram, 93, 283–4
dithranol (anthralin), 207, 210, 284
diuretics, 103–8; action of, on kidneys, 104, 107; with cardiac glycosides, 88; and the elderly, 16; fast-acting, 106; for glaucoma, 103, 106; to lower blood pressure, 104; osmotic, 106–7; and potassium conservation, 107–8; and potassium loss, 88, 104, 105, 106; for pulmonary edema, 103–4; for reducing, 69; thiazides and related drugs, 104–5, 186; xanthines, 108
dizziness, *see* vertigo
domiphen, 136, 201, 284
dopamine, 150, 151, 152
dosage, and intervals between, 10–12
doxepin, 60, 284
doxorubicin, 227, 285
doxycycline, 217, 218, 285
doxylamine, 50, 285
drivers: drinking by, 19, 20, 26; vulnerability of, to drugs, 19–20
dromostanolone, 165, 285
dropsy, *see* edema
drug(s): absorption of, 5–6, 11–12; administration of, 4–5, *see also* injections; adverse effects of, 13–23; bioavailability of, 5–6; biotransformation of, 7; dependence on, 23–36; distribution of, in body, 6–7; dosage of, 8, 10–12; effect of excipients on, 12–13; endorsements for, 10; excretion of, 6, 7; over-the-counter drugs, 36–9; regimens, 10–13; shelf life of, 12–13; testing, 8–10;

therapeutic index of, 8, 11; in variety of forms, 12; warnings about use of, 22–3
drug automatism, 46
dydrogesterone, 172, 285–6
dysentery, amoebic, 230
dyspepsia, 75

ear(s): drops, 38; drugs for infections, 199; softening wax in, 85
eczema, treatment of, 207, 209
edema: causes of, 86; pulmonary, 103–4; *see also* heart failure
edrophonium, 90, 286
elderly, the, vulnerability of, 15–16
embolism, 91
embryos, vulnerability of, 16–18, 29, 31; *see also* pregnancy
emetine, 230, 286
emollients, 194–5
emphysema, 139
ephedrine, 66, 139, 140, 141, 287
epilepsy, 142–5; drugs for, *see* anticonvulsants
epinephrine (adrenaline), 21, 59, 160, 182, 191, 287–8; for asthma, treatment of, 139, 140, 141; with local anesthetic, 62, 191; sympathetic nervous system, effect on, 148–9, 150; shock in allergic reactions, treatment of, 287
ergonovine, 288
ergotamine, 127, 288–9
erythrityl, 103, 289
erythromycin, 216, 224, 289; for acne, 208
estradiol, 170, 181, 289
estrogens, 100, 169–71; adverse effects, 171; conjugated, 170, 269; esterified, 170; in oral contraceptives, 173–4; precautions with, 171; replacement therapy, 171; synthetic, 170–1; uses of, 170
estrone, 170, 289
ethacridine, 202

## A Note About the Type

The text of this book was set in a film version of Palatino, a type face designed by the noted German typographer Hermann Zapf. Named after Geovanbattista Palatino, a writing master of Renaissance Italy, Palatino was the first of Zapf's type faces to be introduced to America. The first designs for the face were made in 1948, and the fonts for the complete face were issued between 1950 and 1952. Like all Zapf-designed type faces, Palatino is beautifully balanced and exceedingly readable.

The book was composed by The Haddon Craftsmen, Inc., ComCom Division, Allentown, Pennsylvania; printed and bound by R.R. Donnelley, Crawfordsville, Indiana. The typography and binding design are by Camilla Filancia.